DENTAL
MATERIALS

Properties and Manipulation

DENTAL MATERIALS

Properties and Manipulation

ROBERT G. CRAIG, Ph.D.

Marcus Ward Professor of Dentistry
Director, Biomaterials Program
Department of Biologic and Materials Sciences

WILLIAM J. O'BRIEN, Ph.D.

Professor of Biomaterials
Department of Biologic and Materials Sciences
The University of Michigan School of Dentistry
Ann Arbor, Michigan

JOHN M. POWERS, Ph.D.

Professor and Chairman
Department of Oral Biomaterials
The University of Texas Health Science Center at Houston
Dental Branch
Houston, Texas

FIFTH EDITION

With 193 illustrations

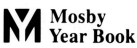
Mosby
Year Book

St. Louis   Baltimore   Boston   Chicago   London   Philadelphia   Sydney   Toronto

Mosby
Year Book

Dedicated to Publishing Excellence

Editor   Robert W. Reinhardt
Assistant Editor   Melba Steube
Project Manager   Patricia Tannian
Manuscript Editor   Bess Wilfong
Designer   David Zielinski

Fifth edition

Copyright © 1992 by Mosby–Year Book, Inc.

A Mosby imprint of Mosby–Year Book, Inc.

Previous editions copyrighted 1975, 1979, 1983, 1987

Printed in the United States of America

Mosby–Year Book, Inc.
11830 Westline Industrial Drive
St. Louis, Missouri 63146

Library of Congress Cataloging in Publication Data

Craig, Robert G. (Robert George), 1923-
    Dental materials : properties and manipulation / Robert G. Craig,
    William J. O'Brien, John M. Powers. — 5th ed.
        p.   cm.
    Includes bibliographical references and index.
    ISBN 0-8016-1075-3 : $29.95
    1. Dental materials.   I. O'Brien, William J. (William Joseph),
    1935-   . II. Powers, John M., 1946-   III. Title.
    [DNLM: 1. Dental Materials.   WU 190 C886d]
    RK652.5.C7   1991
    617.6'95—dc20
    DNLM/DLC
    for Library of Congress   91-4831
                                                                   CIP

ISBN 0-8016-1075-3

CL/PH/DC   9 8 7 6 5 4 3 2 1

preface

The fifth edition of *Dental Materials: Properties and Manipulation* presents new and revised information about materials used in the dental office and laboratory, with emphasis on their manipulation and its effect on properties. The level of instruction is at the macroscopic rather than the atomic level, and although chemical formulas and equations are used, word descriptions are included.

Major changes have been made in sections discussing preventive and esthetic restorative materials: cements, adhesives, impression materials, alloys, and ceramics; however, each section includes the most recent changes and developments.

A second color has been used for the production of this book to highlight chapter titles, tables, key terms, and summaries. The format has been altered to provide improved study guides. Definitions of words are placed prominently in the text where they are introduced. Particularly important statements in the text are identified in bold type, and concise summaries are presented at the end of major sections. The final study aids are the objective self-tests at the end of each chapter, which have been updated.

Robert G. Craig
William J. O'Brien
John M. Powers

c o n t e n t s

chapter one

Introduction to Dental Materials

The main aim of restorative dentistry is to replace diseased or lost tooth structure with materials that restore function and appearance.

Rather than one universal material, many are used for different types of restorations. Each of these materials has qualities that make it more suitable for certain restorations. Selection of the restorative material must be made before the tooth is prepared for restoration. Therefore understanding the properties that distinguish one material from another is important.

A brief survey of the types of restorations, along with a description of restorative materials, illustrates the factors involved in the selection process.

First, the loss of tooth structure in restoration of a portion of an anterior tooth may have been caused by either injury (Fig. 1-1, *A*) or caries. Resin composite materials are usually chosen for this restorative task. These materials, discussed later, are shaded to match the teeth in appearance. Their strength is a secondary factor, since the anterior teeth are usually not subject to high biting forces. Although resin composite materials are weaker than metals, their excellent appearance, along with acceptable durability, is the main reason for their choice (Fig. 1-1, *B*).

A metallic restoration may be preferable to a resin composite material for the restoration of the portion of a posterior tooth subject to considerably greater biting forces because of strength considerations. Since a posterior restoration is not so noticeable, the appearance factor is not so important. Dental silver amalgam restorations and gold inlays are most often used for this type of restoration. An amalgam paste is placed directly into the prepared tooth cavity and carved to the

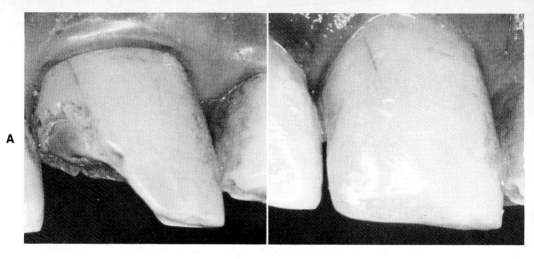

Fig. 1-1. A, Fracture of a central incisor from injury. **B,** Restoration of incisor with composite resin. (Courtesy Dr. JB Dennison, University of Michigan School of Dentistry, Ann Arbor, Mich.)

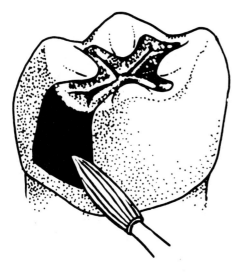

Fig. 1-2. Two-surface amalgam restoration being finished with bur. (From Chapman CE, editor: *Manual of dental operative techniques,* Edinburgh, 1969, E & S Livingstone.)

Fig. 1-3. Posterior inlay restoration.

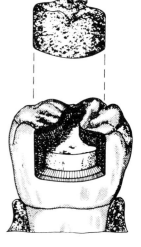

correct anatomy (Fig. 1-2). An **inlay** is a restoration prepared outside the mouth and cemented to the prepared tooth (Fig. 1-3).

If a deep posterior restoration is required, a cement base is placed below the metallic restoration (Fig. 1-4). Such a base serves to insulate the pulp of the tooth from the irritation of thermal sensations transmitted through metallic restorations. A number of cements are available for this application and are discussed in a later chapter.

A **crown** is a restoration of part or all of the coronal portion of a tooth. A full cast gold crown is illustrated in Fig. 1-5. This type of restoration is suitable for the posterior portion of the mouth, where high strength is needed and appearance is secondary.

Inlay: a restoration that is made to fit into a tapered cavity preparation.

A crown is a restoration that restores the anatomy and function of part or all of the coronal portion of the tooth.

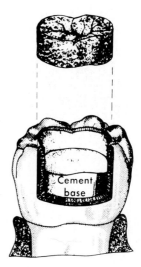

Fig. 1-4. Use of a cement base beneath a metallic restoration.

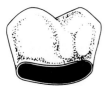

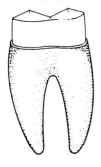

Fig. 1-5. Full gold crown. (Modified from Morrey LW, Nelsen RJ: *Dental science handbook,* Washington, DC, 1970, U.S. Government Printing Office.)

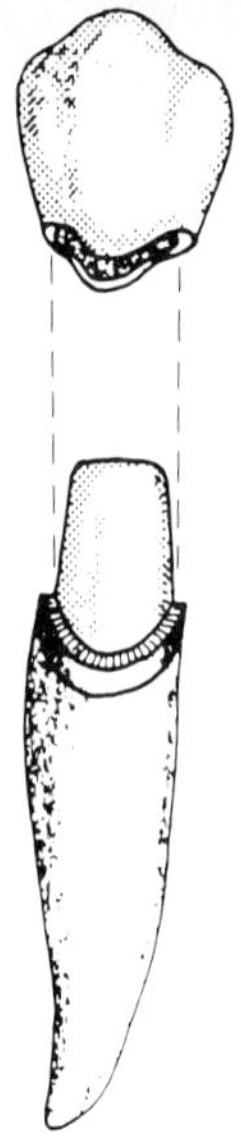

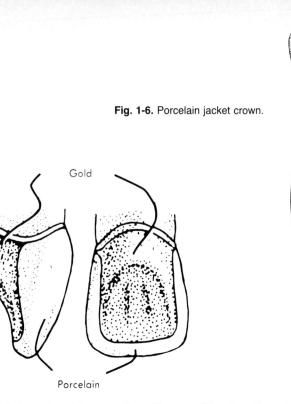

Fig. 1-6. Porcelain jacket crown.

Gold

Porcelain

Fig. 1-7. Porcelain-fused-to-metal crown. (From Chapman CE, editor: *Manual of dental operative techniques,* Edinburgh, 1969, E & S Livingstone.)

Frequently, the entire crown portion of an anterior tooth requires restoration. A crown made from porcelain could be used (Fig. 1-6), since this material combines strength with excellent esthetic properties. Different types of porcelains are discussed in a later chapter. A **porcelain-fused-to-metal crown** may be used that combines the esthetics of a porcelain veneer and the strength and fit of a cast crown (Fig. 1-7).

The dental **bridge** is used to replace a missing tooth or teeth (Fig. 1-8). The two teeth adjacent to the space must be prepared with abutment (anchor) restorations to support the artificial tooth. Gold or nickel-chromium alloys are used for dental bridgework because of their strength, tarnish resistance, and ease of casting (fabrication). A dental bridge may be made with a facing of acrylic resin or veneered with porcelain (Fig. 1-9). Cements are used for retention to hold the bridge permanently in place on the abutment teeth. Again, different cement products are available and are discussed in detail.

A jacket crown is an all-porcelain crown.

A porcelain-fused-to-metal crown consists of a metal crown with a veneer of porcelain.

A bridge is a fixed partial denture that is cemented on anchoring teeth.

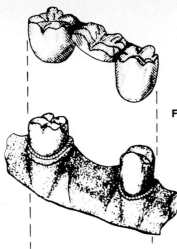

Fig. 1-8. Three-unit dental bridge.

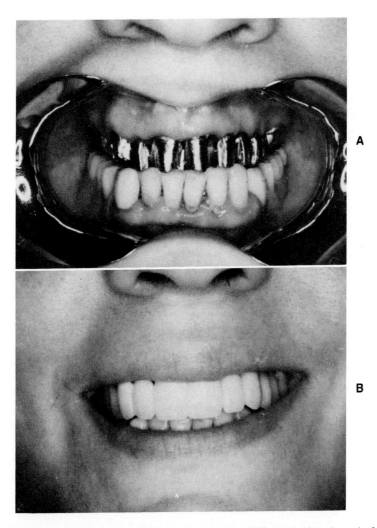

A

B

Fig. 1-9. A, Large dental bridge before finishing with porcelain. **B,** Dental bridge shown in **A** finished with porcelain. (Courtesy Dr. James Yee, Jr., New York City.)

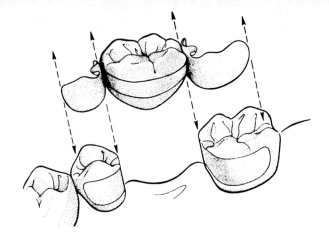

Fig. 1-10. Resin bonded or "Maryland bridge" is bonded to etched enamel of abutment teeth by means of polymer adhesives. (Courtesy G Mora, CDT, Ann Arbor, Mich.)

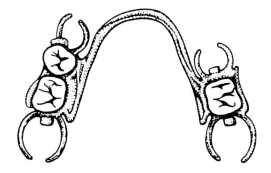

Fig. 1-11. Partial denture made with a cobalt-chromium-nickel alloy and acrylic resin.

A similar type of bridge known as a resin-bonded or "Maryland bridge" has been used for several years. As shown in Fig. 1-10, the pontic is attached to the two abutment teeth by concave metal extensions that clasp the lingual and interproximal surfaces. These abutments are bonded to the enamel of the abutment teeth with adhesive cements. The enamel and metal surfaces should be etched so that the resin adhesive cements form a micromechanical attachment.

If a number of teeth are missing, a more complex prosthetic appliance known as a removable partial denture may be used. As illustrated in Figs. 1-11 and 1-12, artificial teeth are mounted on a metal framework. **Clasps** are used to attach the partial denture to the remaining abutment teeth. Silver-colored metals mainly composed of cobalt, chromium, and nickel are strong and highly resis-

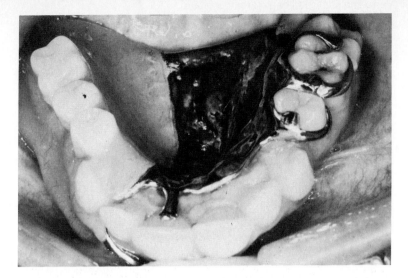

Fig. 1-12. Partial denture in the mouth. (Courtesy Dr. LW Seluk, Plymouth, Mich.)

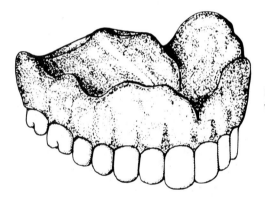

Fig. 1-13. Complete upper denture made with acrylic resin.

tant to corrosion. Since partial dentures are removable, the clasps must be capable of springlike action without being distorted or broken. Acrylic resin materials possessing excellent esthetic qualities are used to fabricate artificial teeth on the partial denture. Here, as in other situations, materials are combined in a restoration or appliance to use the best properties of each.

A clasp is a clawlike metal attachment of a partial denture that grasps the natural teeth.

Finally, if all the natural teeth in an arch are lost, a full, or complete, **denture** is required. As shown in Figs. 1-13 and 1-14, the denture consists of a base with artificial teeth. Most denture bases are made from acrylic resins that are pigmented to match the pink shades of the oral tissues. The teeth used in con-

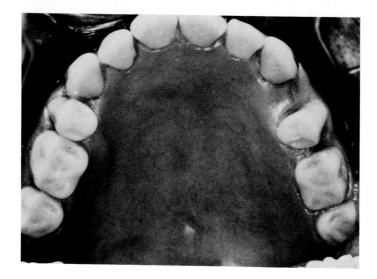

Fig. 1-14. Full denture in the mouth. (Courtesy Dr. LW Seluk, Plymouth, Mich.)

structing a denture may be made with acrylic resin or porcelain. The porcelain teeth are more resistant to wear but more brittle than acrylic resins.

Resins, alloys, and ceramics, as can be seen from this brief survey of dental restorations, are all used in dentistry, in addition to the many other materials that are used in the fabrication of these restorations. Studying dental materials enables members of the dental health team to understand the properties of these materials and how best to use them. The correct selection and manipulation of dental materials largely determine the service a restoration will give to the patient.

A denture is a removable prosthesis that replaces all the teeth of the lower or upper arch.

Self-test questions

In the following multiple choice questions, one or more of the responses may be correct.
1 A small portion of an anterior tooth would most likely be restored with:
   a. Amalgam
   b. Composite resin
   c. Gold alloy
   d. Porcelain
2 The restorative material used to restore a small portion of an anterior tooth should have which of the following properties?

a. Esthetics
b. High strength
c. Durability
d. Ease of casting

3 A portion of a posterior tooth subject to high biting forces might be restored with:
a. Amalgam
b. Composite resin
c. Gold inlay
d. Acrylic resin

4 A direct restorative material used frequently to restore a portion of a posterior tooth subject to large biting forces has the following properties:
a. Esthetics
b. High strength
c. Ease of casting
d. Thermal insulation

5 A full crown on a maxillary anterior tooth may be restored with which of the following restorative materials?
a. Porcelain
b. Gold alloy
c. Composite resin
d. Porcelain fused to metal

6 An anterior bridge could have facings constructed of which of the following materials?
a. Composite resin
b. Acrylic resin
c. Porcelain
d. Gold alloy

7 Which of the following sentences describe the construction of partial dentures?
a. They are attached to natural teeth with cements.
b. They are removable and attached to teeth with clasps.
c. Cobalt, chromium, and nickel alloys are used for the framework.
d. Artificial acrylic teeth are attached.

8 Full denture bases are usually made from the following material:
a. Composite restorative resins
b. Gold alloys
c. Acrylic resins
d. Porcelain

9 The following metals are currently used in dental alloys:
a. Gold
b. Mercury
c. Cobalt and chromium
d. Nickel

10 Acrylic resins are used in the following:
a. Posterior inlays
b. Denture bases
c. Artificial teeth
d. Porcelain-fused-to-metal crowns

chapter
two

Properties of Materials

An understanding of the physical, electrical, and mechanical properties of materials used in dentistry is of tremendous importance. First, materials used to replace missing portions of teeth are exposed to attack by the oral environment and subjected to biting forces. In addition, the restorative materials are cleansed and polished by various prophylactic procedures. Second, their properties are the basis for the selection of materials to be used in particular dental procedures and restorations. Clinical experience and research have related clinical success to certain properties of materials, which have been used as guides in the improvement of dental materials. Third, the establishment of critical physical properties for various types of dental materials has led to the development of minimum standards, or specifications. The American National Standards Institute and the American Dental Association, in conjunction with federal and international standards organizations, have established more than 48 standards, or specifications, for dental materials and periodically publish lists of materials that satisfy the minimum standards of quality. These lists are helpful in the selection of materials for dental practice and ensure quality control of certified materials.

This chapter emphasizes the dimensional change, electrical properties, solubility and sorption, and mechanical properties of dental materials. It is also important in the selection of materials to have knowledge of their effect on the oral tissues and of possible toxic effects if they are ingested. The color and optical qualities of materials likewise are important in the selection of restorative materials.

DIMENSIONAL CHANGE

Maintaining dimensions during dental procedures, such as taking impressions and pouring models, is highly important in the accuracy of dental res-

torations. Dimensional changes may occur during setting as a result of a chemical reaction, such as with rubber impression materials or composite tooth restorative materials. To compare materials easily, the **dimensional change** is usually expressed as a percentage of an original length or volume. A typical example is the linear dimensional change of a polysulfide impression material from a time just after setting until 24 hours after setting. An impression is taken of two marks on a metal plate approximately 51 mm apart; then the distance between the two marks transferred to the impression is measured with a measuring microscope just after the impression sets, l_0, and, again, 24 hours later, l_1. The percentage is calculated as indicated by the following formula:

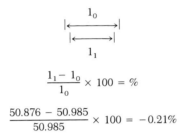

$$\frac{l_1 - l_0}{l_0} \times 100 = \%$$

$$\frac{50.876 - 50.985}{50.985} \times 100 = -0.21\%$$

The result of -0.21% indicates that a linear shrinkage took place within 24 hours after setting. Values for other elastic impression materials can be used to compare their accuracy.

Volumetric dimensional change is more difficult to measure and is not described here. Usually the volumetric dimensional change is assumed to be three times the linear dimensional change for a specific material.

> **Dimensional change is the percent shrinkage or expansion of a material.**

Thermal dimensional change

Restorative dental materials are subjected to temperature changes in the mouth. These changes result in dimensional changes in the materials, as well as in the neighboring tooth structure. Since the thermal expansion of the restorative material usually does not match that of the tooth structure, a differential expansion occurs that **results in leakage of oral fluids between the restoration and the tooth.**

The linear thermal expansion of materials can be measured by determining the difference in length of a specimen at two temperatures. To make comparison between materials easier, the linear thermal expan-

> **The linear thermal expansion coefficient of a material is a measure of how much it expands per unit length if heated one degree higher.**

Table 2-1. Linear Thermal Coefficient of Expansion of Dental Materials in the Temperature Range of 20° to 50° C

Material	Coefficient ($\times 10^{-6}/°$ C)
Human teeth	10-15
Dental amalgam	22-28
Composite plastics	25-50
Gold alloys	12-15
Unfilled plastics and sealants	70-100
Porcelain	8
Porcelain enamel	13.5
Inlay wax	300-1000

sion is expressed as a **coefficient of thermal expansion,** which is calculated according to the following formula:

$$\left(\frac{1_{t_2} - 1_{t_1}}{1_{t_1}}\right) \div (t_2 - t_1) = \text{Linear coefficient of thermal expansion}$$

The first term converts the change to unit length and the second to unit temperature. The value represents the change in length per unit length for each degree of temperature change. Following is a typical calculation for an unfilled dental plastic:

$$\frac{50.500 - 50.409}{50.409} \div (40 - 20) = 90.3 \times 10^{-6}/° \text{ C}$$

The dimensions are per degree because the first term in the equation is dimensionless, since it is a length per unit length. Typical values for selected restorative dental materials and human teeth are listed in Table 2-1.

The thermal coefficient of expansion is not uniform throughout the entire temperature range and is usually higher for liquids than for solids. The thermal coefficient of expansion for a solid, such as a dental wax, generally increases at some point as the temperature is increased. The linear rather than the volumetric coefficient of thermal expansion is usually reported.

The relationship between the coefficients of thermal expansion of human teeth and restorative materials is important, and Table 2-1 shows that the values for amalgam and composite plastics are about two to three times those of human teeth. The values for unfilled plastics, however, are five to seven times those of teeth, with porcelain being one half to one third and gold alloys being approximately the same as for human teeth. If a tooth containing an unfilled plastic restoration is cooled by the drinking of a cold liquid, the restoration contracts substantially more than the tooth, and a small space results at the junction between the two materials. Oral fluids can penetrate this space. When the

Table 2-2. Thermal Conductivity of Dental Materials

Material	Thermal conductivity (cal/sec/cm²[°C/cm])
Human enamel	0.0022
Human dentin	0.0015
Dental amalgam	0.055
Composite plastics	0.0025
Gold alloys	0.710
Unfilled acrylic plastics	0.0005
Porcelain	0.0025
Zinc phosphate cement	0.0028
Zinc oxide–eugenol cement	0.0011

temperature returns to normal, this fluid is forced out of the space. This phenomenon is called percolation and occurs to a greater or lesser extent with all restorative materials, depending on the relationship of the thermal coefficient of expansion of the material and human teeth. **Percolation is thought to be undesirable because of possible irritation to the dental pulp and recurrent decay.** Dental amalgam is unusual in that percolation decreases with time after insertion, presumably as a result of the space being filled with corrosion products from the amalgam.

THERMAL CONDUCTIVITY

Qualitatively, materials have different rates of conducting heat, with metals having higher values than plastics and ceramics. When a portion of a tooth is replaced by a metal restoration such as amalgam or gold alloy, the tooth may be temporarily sensitive to temperature changes in the mouth. Individuals wearing orthodontic appliances or complete acrylic dentures also notice temperature effects different from those experienced without these appliances.

Thermal conductivity has been used as a measure of the heat transferred and is defined as the number of calories per second flowing through an area of 1 cm² in which the temperature drop along the length of the specimen is 1° C/cm. This is a rather complicated quantitative term, but

Materials with high thermal conductivity values are good conductors of heat and cold.

qualitatively it is simply related to the rate of heat flow. The thermal conductivity of a variety of materials is reported in Table 2-2.

Human enamel and dentin are poor thermal conductors compared with gold alloys and dental amalgam, although amalgam is substantially lower than gold. Zinc oxide–eugenol and zinc phosphate cements approximately replace lost tooth structure with respect to thermal conductivity. The reason for using ce-

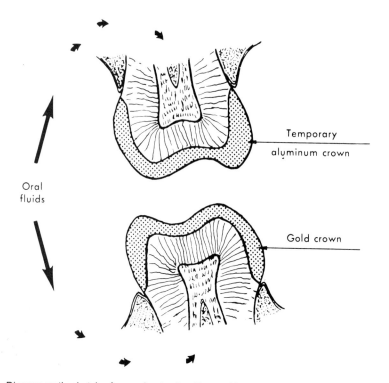

Oral
fluids

Temporary
aluminum crown

Gold crown

Fig. 2-1. Diagrammatic sketch of opposing teeth with a gold crown and a temporary aluminum crown indicating how galvanism can occur.

ments as thermal insulating bases in deep cavity preparations is because although dentin is a poor thermal conductor, a thin layer of it does not provide enough thermal insulation for the pulp unless a cement base is used under the metal restoration. Composite restorations have thermal conductivities comparable to tooth structure and do not present a problem with this property. Cavity varnishes have low thermal conductivities, as do unfilled acrylics, but are used in layers so thin that they are ineffective as thermal insulators.

ELECTRICAL PROPERTIES

Two electrical properties of interest are galvanism and corrosion. **Galvanism** results from the presence of dissimilar metals in the mouth. Metals placed in an electrolyte (a liquid containing ions) have various tendencies to go into solution. Aluminum, which is sometimes used as a temporary crown, has a strong tendency to go into solution and has an electrode potential of $+1.33$ volts. Gold, on the other hand, has little tendency to go into solution, as indicated by an electrode potential of -1.36 volts. A schematic sketch of two opposing teeth, one with a temporary aluminum crown and the other with a gold crown, is shown in Fig. 2-1. The oral fluids function as the electrolyte, and the system is similar to that of an electrical cell. When the two restorations touch, current flows because the potential difference is 2.69 volts, and the patient experiences pain and frequently complains of a metallic taste. The same effect can be experienced if a piece of aluminum foil from a baked potato becomes wedged between two teeth and contacts a gold restoration. Temporary plastic crowns are used to prevent this problem, since they are poor electrical conductors.

Galvanism is the generation of electrical currents that the patient can feel.

Corrosion can also result from this same condition when adjacent restorations are of dissimilar metals. **As a result of the galvanic action, material goes into solution, and roughness and pitting occur.** This effect may also occur if a gold alloy is contaminated with a metal such as iron during handling in the dental laboratory or because of variations in concentration of elements from one part of the restoration to another. Corrosion may also result from chemical attack of metals by components in food or saliva. Dental amalgam, for example, reacts with sulfides and chlorides in the mouth, as shown by polished amalgams becoming dull and discolored with time. This effect is sometimes referred to as **tarnish.**

Corrosion is the dissolution of metals in the mouth.

Tarnish is a surface reaction of metals in the mouth from components in saliva or foods.

SOLUBILITY AND SORPTION

The solubility of materials in the mouth and the sorption (adsorption plus absorption) of oral fluids by the material are important criteria in their selection. Frequently, laboratory studies have evaluated materials in distilled water, at times giving results that were inconsistent with clinical observations, since materials in the mouth are covered with plaque and therefore are exposed to various acids and organic materials. An example of the inconsistency is that zinc phosphate cements are considerably more soluble in the mouth than laboratory tests in water indicate. Also, the loss of zinc phosphate cement retaining a gold crown is a result of dissolution followed and accompanied by disintegration. Nevertheless, laboratory tests usually rank materials correctly, so only the actual numbers should be taken with a grain of salt.

Solubility and sorption are reported in two ways: (1) in weight percent of soluble or sorbed material, and (2) as the weight of dissolved or sorbed material per unit of surface area (e.g., milligrams per square centimeter).

Absorption refers to the uptake of liquid by the bulk solid; for example, the equilibrium absorption of water by acrylic plastics is in the range of 2%. Adsorp-

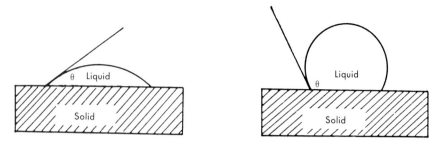

Fig. 2-2. Good wetting of a solid by a liquid with a low contact angle *(left)*; poor wetting by a liquid on a solid forming a high contact angle *(right)*. (From O'Brien WJ, Ryge G: *J Prosthet Dent* 15:304, 1965.)

tion indicates concentration of molecules at the surface of a solid or liquid, an example being the adsorption of components of saliva at the surface of tooth structure.

WETTABILITY

The **wettability** of solids by liquids is quite important in dentistry, with some examples being the wetting of denture base plastics by saliva, the wetting of tooth enamel by pit and fissure sealants, and the wetting of wax patterns by dental investments.

Wettability is a measure of the affinity of a liquid for a solid as indicated by spreading of a drop.

The wettability of a solid by a liquid can be observed by the shape of a drop of the liquid on the solid surface. Profiles of drops of liquids on solids are shown in Fig. 2-2 above. The shape of the drops is identified by the contact angle θ, by the angles through the drops bounded by the solid surface, and by a line through the periphery of the drop and tangent to the surface of the liquid.

If a low contact angle occurs, as in the left of Fig. 2-2, the solid is readily wetted by the liquid (hydrophilic if the liquid is water). If a contact angle is greater than 90 degrees, as in the right of Fig. 2-2, poor wetting occurs (hydrophobic if the liquid is water).

The degree of wetting depends on the relative surface energies of the solids and the liquids and on their intermolecular attraction. High-energy solids and low-energy liquids encourage good wetting; thus liquids generally wet higher-energy solids well (e.g., water on metals and oxides). On the other hand, liquids bead up on lower-energy solids such as wax, Teflon, and many polymers. The high contact angle of water on these solids can be decreased by the addition of a wetting agent such as a detergent to the water.

MECHANICAL PROPERTIES

A knowledge of the magnitude of biting forces is essential in understanding the importance of the mechanical properties of dental materials. Maximum biting forces decrease from the molar to the incisor region, and the average biting forces on the first and second molars are about 130 pounds force, whereas the average forces on bicuspids, cuspids, and incisors are about 70, 50, and 40 pounds force. In metric units these values are 578, 311, 222, and 178 newtons (N), respectively. To convert pounds to newtons, pounds are multiplied by 4.44.

Patients exert lower biting forces on bridges and dentures than on their normal dentition. For example, when a first molar is replaced by a fixed bridge, the biting force on the restored side is approximately 50 pounds compared with 130 pounds when the patient has natural dentition. The average biting force on partial and complete dentures has been measured to be about 25 pounds (111 N); therefore **patients with dentures can apply only approximately 19% of the force of those with normal dentition.**

Stress. When a force is applied to a material, there is a resistance in the material to the external force. The force is distributed over an area, and the ratio of the force to the area is called the **stress:**

$$\text{Stress} = \frac{\text{Force}}{\text{Area}}$$

Thus, for a given force, the smaller the area over which it is applied, the larger the value of the stress. This effect can be visualized by examining Fig. 2-3. A distributed force has been applied in Fig. 2-3, *A,* and the same force

Stress is the force per unit area.

has been applied in a concentrated manner in Fig. 2-3, *B.* The number of lines in the plastic model of a tooth is directly proportional to the stress, and the stress is shown to be inversely proportional to the area of application. This effect can be demonstrated as follows: place an unsharpened pencil against the palm of your hand, apply a force by placing a book on the end with the eraser, and note any pain. Then sharpen the pencil, repeat the procedure, and note the increase in pain as a result of the increase in stress.

The relationship of force, area, and stress is also shown in Table 2-3. It can be seen that a force of 25 pounds (111 N), which can readily be applied in the mouth, can produce a large stress, such as 25,000 psi (172 meganewtons per square meter, or MN/m^2), when the area of application of the force is small. Such conditions readily exist in the mouth, where contact areas of 0.001 in^2 (0.645 mm^2) frequently occur.

Several types of stress may result when a force is applied to a material. These are referred to as **compressive, tensile,** and **shear stress** and are shown diagrammatically in Fig. 2-4. A material is subjected to compressive stress when

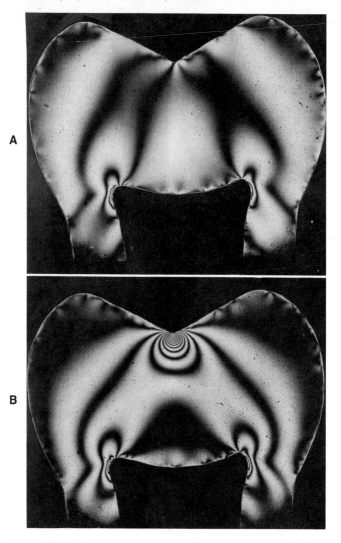

Fig. 2-3. Cross-sectional model of a tooth under distributed force, **A,** and concentrated force, **B.** Higher stress in **B** is indicated by the number of lines of stress.

Table 2-3. Relationship of Force, Area, and Stress

Force		Area		Stress	
lb	N	in²	mm²	psi	MN/m²
25	111	1	645	25	0.1724
25	111	0.1	64.5	250	1.724
25	111	0.01	6.45	2500	17.24
25	111	0.001	0.645	25,000	172.4
25	111	0.0001	0.0645	250,000	1724.0

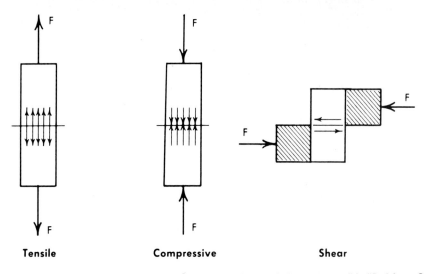

Tensile   Compressive   Shear

Fig. 2-4. Schematic representation of tensile, compressive, and shear stress. (Modified from Craig RG, editor: *Restorative dental materials,* ed 8, St. Louis, 1989, Mosby–Year Book.)

the material is squeezed together, or compressed, and to tensile stress when pulled apart. Shear stress occurs when one portion (plane) of the material is forced to slide by another portion. These types of stresses are considered to evaluate the properties of various materials.

Strain. The change in length, or deformation per unit length, when a material is subjected to a force is defined as **strain:**

$$\text{Strain} = \frac{\text{Deformation}}{\text{Length}}$$

Strain is easier to visualize than stress, since it can be observed directly. For example, if a rubber band 1 inch (2.54 cm) long is stretched ½ inch (1.27 cm), the strain is $\frac{0.5 \text{ inch}}{1 \text{ inch}}\left(\frac{1.27 \text{ cm}}{2.54 \text{ cm}}\right)$, or 0.5. Note that the units of strain are dimensionless, and the value is the same regardless of whether English or metric units are used. Some dental substances, such as rubber impression materials, exhibit considerable strain when a stress is applied; others, such as gold alloys or human enamel, show low strain under stress.

> **Strain is the change in length per unit length of a material produced by stress.**

Stress-strain curves. A convenient means of comparing the mechanical properties of materials is to apply various forces to a material and to determine the corresponding values of stress and strain. A plot of the corresponding values of stress and strain is referred to as a stress-strain curve. Such a curve may be obtained in compression, tension, or shear. An example of a stress-strain curve in

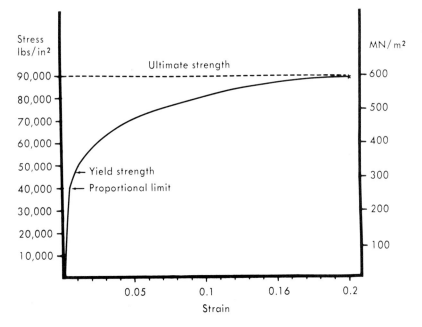

Fig. 2-5. Stress-strain curve in tension for dental gold alloy.

tension for a dental gold alloy is shown in Fig. 2-5. The shape and magnitude of the stress-strain curve are important in the selection of dental materials. Fig. 2-5 clearly shows that the curve is a straight line, or linear, up to a stress of about 40,000 psi (276 MN/m²), after which it is concave toward the strain axis. The curve ends at a stress of 90,000 psi (621 MN/m²) and a strain of 0.2 because the sample ruptured.

Elastic modulus. The following is the elastic modulus for the gold alloy in Fig. 2-5:

$$\text{Elastic modulus} = \frac{\text{Stress}}{\text{Strain}} = \frac{40{,}000 \text{ psi}}{0.0029} \text{ or } \frac{275.9 \text{ MN/m}^2}{0.0029} = 13{,}790{,}000 \text{ psi or } 95{,}100 \text{ MN/m}^2$$

The elastic modulus is a measure of the stiffness of a material, and high numbers are not unusual for this property. Values for selected materials are listed in Table 2-4, which shows that gold alloys have approximately the same stiffness as human enamel and that composite plastics and zinc phosphate cement are in the same range as human dentin. Unfilled acrylic plastics and zinc oxide–eugenol cements are much more flexible, with polysulfide

The elastic modulus is equal to the ratio of the stress to the strain in the linear or elastic portion of the stress-strain curve.

Table 2-4. Elastic Moduli of Selected Dental Materials

Material	Elastic modulus	
	psi	MN/m²
Human dentin	2,700,000	18,600
Human enamel	12,000,000	83,000
Dental amalgam	4,000,000	27,600
Gold alloy	14,000,000	96,600
Composite restorative materials	2,410,000	16,600
Unfilled acrylic plastic	400,000	2760
Zinc phosphate cement	3,300,000	22,800
Zinc oxide−eugenol cement	300,000	2070
Zinc polyacrylate cement	718,000	4950
Glass ionomer cement	1,400,000	9800
Polysulfide rubber	100-400	0.7-2.8

rubber being the most flexible. Stiffness is important in the selection of restorative materials, since large deflections under stress are not desired.

Proportional limit and yield strength. Proportional limit and yield strength indicate the stress at which the material no longer functions as an elastic solid. The strain recovers below these values if the stress is removed, and permanent deformation of the material occurs above these values. The **proportional limit** is the stress on the stress-strain curve when it ceases to be linear or when the ratio of the stress to the strain is no longer proportional. The **yield strength** is the stress at some arbitrarily selected value of permanent strain, such as 0.001, and thus is always slightly higher than the proportional limit. For example, the proportional limit for the gold alloy in Fig. 2-5 is 40,000 psi (276 MN/m²), and the yield strength is 47,000 psi (324 MN/m²). These values indicate that stresses in excess of 40,000 to 47,000 psi (276 to 324 MN/m²) in the gold alloy will result in permanent deformation after the applied force has been removed.

Proportional limit and yield strength are measures of the stress allowed before permanent deformation.

These two properties are particularly important, since a restoration can be classified as a clinical failure when a significant amount of permanent deformation takes place even though the material does not fracture. Materials are said to be elastic in their function below the proportional limit or yield strength and to function in a plastic manner above these stresses.

Typical yield strength values for a variety of materials are listed in Table 2-5, which shows that unfilled acrylic plastics deform permanently at a considerably lower stress than composite plastics but that both have much lower values than human enamel. It might seem that none of these materials would deform permanently with such high numbers for the yield strength except that, as has been shown in the section on stress, biting forces can readily produce stresses that could exceed the yield strength.

Ultimate strength. If higher and higher forces are applied to a material, a stress will eventually be reached at which the material will fracture, or rupture. This point on the stress-strain curve in Fig. 2-5 is denoted with a star. If the fracture occurs from tensile stress, the property is called the **tensile strength,** and, if in compression, the **compressive strength.** As can be seen in Fig. 2-5, the tensile strength of the gold alloy was 90,000 psi (621 MN/m^2).

> The stress at which fracture occurs is called the ultimate strength.

The tensile and compressive strength of a material may be significantly different, as illustrated in Table 2-6. Brittle materials such as human enamel, amalgam, and composite plastics have large differences and are stronger in compression than in tension.

Table 2-5. Yield Strength of Selected Dental Materials

Material	Yield strength	
	psi	MN/m^2
Human dentin	24,000*	165
Human enamel	50,000*	344
Gold alloys	30,000-90,000†	207-620
Composite plastics	20,000-25,000*	138-172
Unfilled acrylic plastics	7000-8000*	43-55
Nickel-chromium alloy	52,000†	359
Cobalt-chromium alloy	103,000†	710

*, Yield strength in compression.
†, Yield strength in tension.

Table 2-6. Ultimate Strength of Some Dental Materials

Material	Tensile strength		Compressive strength	
	psi	MN/m^2	psi	MN/m^2
Human dentin	7000	48	43,000	297
Human enamel	1500	10	58,000	400
Dental amalgam	7000-10,000	48-69	45,000-70,000	310-483
Gold alloys	60,000-120,000	414-828	—	—
Composite plastics	6000-10,000	41-69	25,000-43,000	170-300
Unfilled acrylic plastics	4000	28	14,000	97
Porcelain (feldspathic)	5000	40	22,000	150
Nickel-chromium alloy	61,000	421	—	—

Limited data are available on the shear strength of dental materials. The shear strength of composite plastics is about 8000 to 10,000 psi (55 to 69 MN/m^2) and is about 6000 psi (41 MN/m^2) for unfilled acrylic plastics; these values are only slightly higher than and are comparable to the corresponding tensile strengths.

The bond between two materials is usually measured in tension or shear and is expressed as the stress necessary to cause rupture of the bond. Depending on the system, the bond may be chemical, mechanical, or a combination of the two types. The bond between acrylic denture teeth and acrylic denture bases is essentially chemical and is frequently greater than 5000 psi (34 MN/m^2) measured in tension. On the other hand, the bond between composite plastics and acid-etched tooth enamel is essentially mechanical and has a value of 2500 to 4500 psi (17 to 31 MN/m^2) in tension.

Elongation and compression. The percent of elongation at rupture of the gold alloy shown in Fig. 2-5 can be readily determined from the strain at rupture simply by multiplying the strain (deformation per unit length) by 100 to convert it to percent of elongation. In the example the percent of elongation is 20%. In practical tests the plastic strain (the strain between the proportional limit and the ultimate tensile strength) is used in the calculations, and thus, for the example in Fig. 2-5, the percent of elongation is (0.20 to 0.01) × 100 = 19%. Similar calculations can be made for materials in compression and would represent the percent of plastic strain at rupture.

The amount of deformation that a material can withstand before rupture is reported as the percent of elongation when the material is under tensile stress or the percent of compression when it is under compressive stress.

The **percent of elongation and compression** are important properties in that they **are measures of ductility and malleability,** respectively. These two properties are indications of the amount of plastic strain, or deformation, that can occur before the material fractures and, as such, indicate the brittleness of the material. For example, the gold alloy with a percent of elongation of 19 can be deformed considerably before fracture, and it would be classed as a ductile alloy. Considerable burnishing and adaptation of the margins of castings from this alloy could be done without fear of fracturing the margin. In general, gold alloys with elongations of less than 5% are considered brittle, and those with values higher than 5% are classed as ductile materials.

Composite plastics are considered brittle materials, since the percent of compression at failure is in the range of 2% to 3%. Clinical observation has been that these materials under excessive stress fail as a result of brittle fracture.

Resilience and toughness. Up to this point, properties related only to stress or strain have been discussed. Two properties involve the area under the stress-strain curve and thus involve the energy required to reach specified points on the curve.

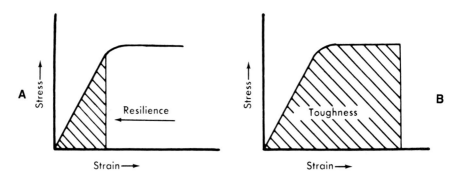

Fig. 2-6. Stress-strain curves illustrating the areas that give a measure of the resilience, **A,** and toughness, **B.**

The energy required to deform a material permanently is a criterion of its resilience, whereas the energy necessary to fracture a material is a measure of its toughness. These areas are shown as shaded portions of the stress-strain curves in Fig. 2-6.

These two properties are more complex than strength or deformation, since their magnitude is a product of stress and strain. Two materials may have the same resilience, with one having a high yield strength and low corresponding strain and the other having a lower yield strength and a higher corresponding strain. Two such materials are composite plastics and unfilled acrylic plastics, both of which have a resilience of approximately 100 in-lb/in³ (7 cm-kg/cm³) despite considerable differences in yield strength. Toughness also is not a simple quantity; for example, although composite plastics have considerably higher yield strengths than unfilled acrylic plastics, the latter may be deformed so much more before rupture that they are tougher than composite plastics (Fig. 2-7).

Hardness. A material is considered hard if it strongly resists indentation by a hard material such as diamond. One might expect that hardness would be related to yield strength; however, the property is complex, and, in general, no direct relationship exists between the two properties. The only exception is in the comparison of materials of the same type, such as a series of similar gold alloys.

The hardness of dental materials generally is reported in Knoop hardness numbers. Rockwell hardness numbers, however, may be used for composite

> Resilience and toughness indicate the energy absorbed up to the proportional limit and the ultimate strength, respectively, and relate to the resistance to deformation and fracture under impact.

> Hardness is the resistance of a material to indentation.

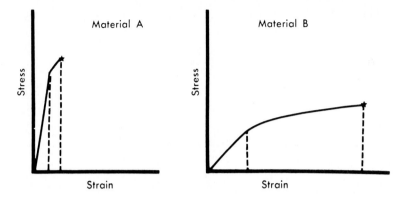

Fig. 2-7. Stress-strain curves for composite (material A) and unfilled acrylic plastic (material B). The two materials have approximately the same resilience, but material B is considerably tougher.

plastics. The Knoop hardness number is obtained by measuring the length of the long diagonal of an indentation from a diamond indenter and calculating the number of kilograms required to give an indentation of 1 mm^2. Thus the larger the indentation, the smaller the number. An example of indentations in dentin and cementum is seen in Fig. 2-8, with the larger indentations being in cementum and the smaller being in dentin. Examples of Knoop hardness numbers of various materials are listed in Table 2-7. Enamel and porcelain are two of the hardest, and unfilled acrylic plastic is the softest of the materials listed.

Rockwell numbers are usually found by making an indentation using a steel ball and measuring the depth of the indentation. The ball used with the Rockwell test on composite plastics is ½ inch in diameter and is intentionally large so that it will be supported by both phases of the composite.

Strain-time curves. For materials in which the strain is independent of the length of time that a load is applied, stress-strain curves are important. However, for materials in which the strain is dependent on the time the load is maintained, strain-time curves are more useful than stress-strain curves in explaining their properties. Examples of materials that have strain-time-dependent behavior are alginate and rubber impression materials, dental amalgam, and human dentin.

A strain-time curve for a rubber impression material is shown in Fig. 2-9. A compressive load was applied at t_0, and an initial rapid increase in strain occurred from O to A. The load was maintained until t_1, with the strain gradually increasing from A to B; this increase resulted from a combination of viscoelastic strain (time dependent but recoverable) and viscous flow (time dependent and not recoverable). The load was removed at t_1, which resulted in a rapid decrease in strain from B to C. This recovery took place because of the release of elastic

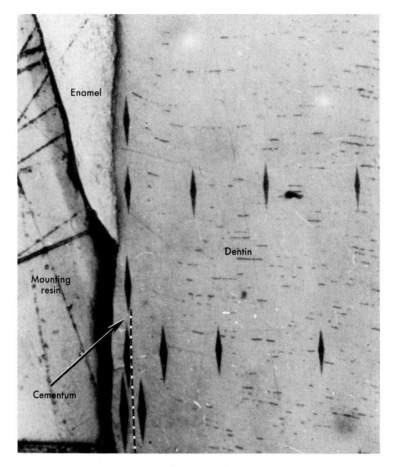

Fig. 2-8. Knoop hardness indentations in dentin and cementum. Longer indentations are in cementum, indicating lower hardness than for dentin.

Table 2-7. Knoop Hardness of Selected Dental Materials

Material	Knoop hardness number (kg/mm^2)
Human enamel	343
Human dentin	68
Human cementum	43
Dental amalgam	110
22-k gold alloy	85
Unfilled acrylic plastic	20
Porcelain	460
Zinc phosphate cement	40
Nickel-chromium alloy	330

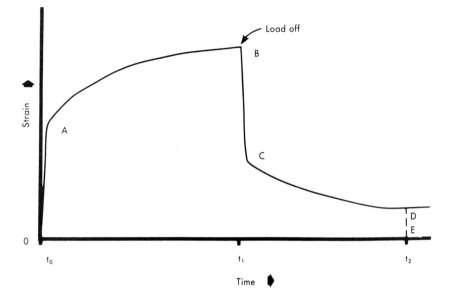

Fig. 2-9. Strain-time curve for elastic impression material.

strain. A continued gradual decrease in strain occurred from *C* to *D* as a result of the recovery of the viscoelastic strain. At t_2 no further decrease in strain took place, and a permanent strain remained, the magnitude being represented by *DE*.

If the load had been applied for a longer time than t_1 or the magnitude of the load had been greater, the amount of permanent strain would have been more. Clinically this means the shorter the time and the less force applied to the impression material, the lower the permanent strain and the more accurate the impression.

The strengths of such materials are also dependent on the rate of application of the load, with higher tensile strengths resulting at more rapid rates of applying the load. As a result, **it is recommended that alginate impressions be removed rapidly with what is described as a "snap" removal.**

Dental amalgam is stronger the more rapidly the force is increased; however, in this instance the values for the compressive strength obtained at low rates of speed have been shown to correlate better with rankings of clinical service. As a result, the testing of amalgam is conducted at low rates of application of force.

Dynamic properties. The properties described so far are classified as static properties because of the relatively slow rate of application of the load. The properties at extremely high rates of loading, such as from an impact, are also important in dentistry. They are classified as dynamic properties and are of importance in the evaluation of materials such as athletic mouth protectors.

Properties of particular importance are the dynamic modulus and dynamic resilience. The dynamic modulus is a measure of the stiffness of the material at a high rate of strain and is important for mouth protector materials for which the mechanical properties are strain-rate dependent. The dynamic resilience measures the energy absorbed at high rates of strain such as from a blow to an athletic mouth protector.

The properties of materials are major criteria for the performance of dental materials in service. Dimensional stability is an important property requirement of impression and restorative materials. Thermal conductivity is important as a measure of how much heat and cold are transmitted to pulpal and soft tissues under restorations. Electrical properties are important in terms of galvanic currents generated by dissimilar metals and the discomfort they cause patients. Solubility is especially important in regard to cements that hold restorations in place. Wetting of dental materials by liquids is important in the processing of dental materials and in their relation to saliva in the mouth. Mechanical properties, including hardness, strength, and stiffness, determine how much stress materials can withstand in the mouth. Toughness is especially important for materials such as denture resins to withstand the shocks of being accidentally dropped without breaking.

Self-test questions

In the following multiple choice questions, one or more of the responses may be correct.
1 Which of the following statements describe the purpose of the American National Standards Institute and the American Dental Association specifications?
   a. The specifications measure clinical properties of materials to establish minimum standards.
   b. The specifications measure critical physical and mechanical properties of materials to establish minimum standards.
   c. Lists of certified materials ensure clinical success.
   d. Lists of certified materials ensure quality control and are helpful in the selection of materials for dental practice.
2 An impression of the vertical dimension of a cavity preparation 8 mm in length shows a linear contraction of 0.5%. Compute the actual dimensional change in micrometers (μm).
   a. −4 μm
   b. −40 μm
   c. +40 μm
   d. −0.04 μm

3 A pattern 8 mm in length made from a wax with a linear coefficient of thermal expansion of $380 \times 10^{-6}/°$ C cools from $37°$ to $22°$ C. Compute the actual dimensional change in micrometers (μm).
   a. $-45.6\ \mu$m
   b. $-0.0456\ \mu$m
   c. $-4.56\ \mu$m
   d. $+4.56\ \mu$m

4 Rank the following dental materials in order of increasing values of their coefficient of thermal expansion: dental amalgam, human teeth, porcelain, and unfilled acrylic plastics.
   a. Human teeth, porcelain, dental amalgam, and unfilled acrylic plastics
   b. Porcelain, human teeth, unfilled acrylic plastics, and dental amalgam
   c. Porcelain, human teeth, dental amalgam, and unfilled acrylic plastics
   d. Human teeth, porcelain, unfilled acrylic plastics, and dental amalgam

5 Which of the following statements describe percolation?
   a. Percolation usually decreases with time after insertion of dental amalgam.
   b. Percolation is caused by differences in the coefficient of thermal expansion between the tooth and the restorative material when heated or cooled.
   c. Percolation is thought to be undesirable because of possible irritation to the dental pulp and recurrent decay.
   d. Percolation is not likely to occur with unfilled acrylic restorations.

6 Which of the following restorative materials have values of thermal conductivity similar to human enamel and dentin?
   a. Dental amalgam
   b. Composite plastics
   c. Zinc phosphate cements
   d. Gold alloys

7 Which of the following are examples of galvanism in restorative dentistry?
   a. A piece of aluminum foil from a baked potato becomes wedged between two teeth and contacts a gold restoration.
   b. A temporary plastic crown contacts a gold restoration.
   c. A temporary aluminum crown contacts a gold restoration.
   d. A metallic taste is a frequent complaint of patients.

8 Which of the following conditions could lead to corrosion in restorative dentistry?
   a. A gold alloy contaminated with iron during handling in the dental laboratory
   b. A chemical attack of a metal by components in food or saliva
   c. Polished amalgams that have become dull and discolored with time
   d. Adjacent restorations constructed of dissimilar metals

9 The contact angle of water on a dental wax is 105 degrees. Which of the following terms describe the wettability of the wax?
   a. Hydrophobic
   b. Hydrophilic
   c. Hydroscopic
   d. Hygroscopic

10 Which of the following factors increase the wetting of a solid by a liquid?
  a. High surface energy of the solid
  b. Low surface energy of the liquid
11 Which of the following statements are true?
  a. The average biting force on an incisor is about 40 pounds.
  b. The average biting force on a first molar is about 250 pounds.
  c. The average biting force on complete dentures is about 25 pounds.
  d. When a first molar is replaced by a fixed bridge, the biting force on the restored side is about 50 pounds.
12 An amalgam has a compressive strength of 60,000 psi. A restoration made of this amalgam is loaded by an occlusal force over an area of 0.004 in². What is the probable force the restoration can withstand?
  a. 15 pounds
  b. 60,000 pounds
  c. 240 pounds
  d. 60,000 psi
13 An alginate impression can withstand a strain of 10% without permanent deformation. If the impression must be deformed 0.5 mm to pass over an undercut, how thick should the material be between the tray and the tooth?
  a. 10 mm
  b. 5 mm
  c. 0.5 mm
  d. 0.05 mm
14 Which of the following dental materials have an elastic modulus value that is similar to human enamel?
  a. Zinc phosphate cement
  b. Human dentin
  c. Dental amalgam
  d. Gold alloy
15 Which of the following statements are true?
  a. The yield strength is always slightly higher than the proportional limit.
  b. Above the stress associated with the yield strength, a material no longer functions as an elastic solid.
  c. Above the stress associated with the yield strength, a material will be permanently deformed, even after the applied force is removed.
  d. Most restorations are not classified as clinical failures until fracture has occurred.
16 Rank the following dental materials in order of increasing tensile strength: dental amalgam, gold alloy, human dentin, and human enamel.
  a. Dental amalgam, human dentin, human enamel, and gold alloy
  b. Human enamel, human dentin, dental amalgam, and gold alloy
  c. Human dentin, human enamel, dental amalgam, and gold alloy
  d. Human dentin, human enamel, gold alloy, and dental amalgam

17 Rank the following dental materials in order of increasing compressive strength: unfilled acrylic plastics, dental amalgam, human dentin, and human enamel.
   a. Human enamel, human dentin, dental amalgam, and unfilled acrylic plastics
   b. Unfilled acrylic plastics, human enamel, human dentin, and dental amalgam
   c. Unfilled acrylic plastics, human dentin, human enamel, and dental amalgam
   d. Dental amalgam, unfilled acrylic plastics, human dentin, and human enamel
18 Which of the following are tests for measuring hardness?
   a. Knoop
   b. Toughness
   c. Rockwell
   d. Resilience
19 Which of the following dental materials have mechanical properties that are time dependent?
   a. Human dentin
   b. Gold alloy
   c. Dental amalgam
   d. Alginate hydrocolloid
   e. Rubber impression materials
20 If a load is applied to a rubber impression for a long rather than a short time:
   a. The permanent strain will be greater.
   b. The permanent strain will be less.
   c. The elastic strain will be greater.
   d. The viscoelastic strain will be less.

chapter three

Preventive Dental Materials

Preventive dental materials are designed to prevent disease or injury to the teeth and supporting tissues. Three materials that may be classified as preventive are fluoride gels, pit and fissure sealants, and mouth protectors. Fluoride gels are applied in a tray to the teeth after a dental prophylaxis or at home to prevent smooth-surface caries. Fluoride rinses are also available. Pit and fissure sealants are **polymers** applied to the occlusal surfaces of posterior teeth for the purpose of preventing pit and fissure caries. Mouth protectors are made from polymers that are formed by heat to fit over the teeth of the maxillary arch to protect the mouth from sudden blows that could fracture or dislodge the teeth. Mouth protectors may also be used as trays, or carriers, to provide topical fluoride or bleaching applications or as shields to prevent damage from bruxism.

Polymers are organic molecules of high molecular weight made up of many repeating units.

FLUORIDE GELS AND RINSES

Numerous clinical studies have established the effectiveness of the fluoride ion in lowering the incidence of dental caries. Two methods to accomplish topical application of fluoride are by the use of acidulated phosphate-fluoride (APF) gels in trays and with rinses.

Composition

Typical commercial APF gels contain 2% sodium fluoride, 0.34% hydrogen fluoride, and 0.98% orthophosphoric acid with thickening, flavoring, and coloring agents in an aqueous gel. Some commercial gels, however, contain more sodium fluoride (2.6%) but less hydrogen fluoride (0.16%). The fluoride ion con-

Table 3-1. Examples of FDA–ADA-Accepted Office and Prescription Fluoride Application Systems

Fluoride delivery system	Type	Concentration	Product	Manufacturer
Acidulated phosphate-fluoride	Office Use	1.23% F	Checkmake Gel Fluorident Liquid Karidium Thixotropic Gel	Oral-B Premier Dental Lorvic
	Daily-use rinse	0.05% NaF	Phos-Flur Supplement	Colgate-Hoyt
	Daily-use gel	1.1% NaF	Thera-Flur Gel-Drops	Colgate-Hoyt
Sodium fluoride	Office use	2% NaF	Sodium Fluoride Solution	Young Dental
	Daily-use gel	1.1% NaF	Karigel-N Neutral Gel	Lorvic
	Weekly-use rinse	0.2% NaF	Iradicav Neutral	Johnson & Johnson
Stannous fluoride	Daily-use gel	0.4% SnF_2	Gel-Kam Gel Perfect Choice Gel	Scherer Challenge Products

Modified from Farah JW, Powers JM, editors: Fluorides, *Dental Advis* 4(3):1, 1987.

centration of most gels ranges from 1.22% to 1.32%. Sodium fluoride gels and rinses and stannous fluoride gels are also available. Examples of office and prescription fluoride application systems accepted by the Food and Drug Administration and the American Dental Association are listed in Table 3-1.

Recently, a neutral gel-like topical sodium fluoride agent, Nupro (Johnson & Johnson), has been developed. The product is **thixotropic**, and it contains sodium fluoride and is thickened by polyacrylic acid and a gum. The pH is adjusted to between 6 and 8. Values of pH in this range should minimize acid etching of restorative materials such as composites, glass ionomers, and ceramics compared with APF gels.

A thixotropic material has low flow under no load but flows readily when placed under load.

Properties

The clinical effectiveness of acidulated phosphate-fluoride gels has varied, apparently depending in part on the method and frequency of application. Reductions in dental caries of 37% and 41% were observed in two studies of 2 years' duration in which the gel was applied annually. A reduction of 26% was observed at the end of 3 years in another study. A reduction of 80% after 2 years

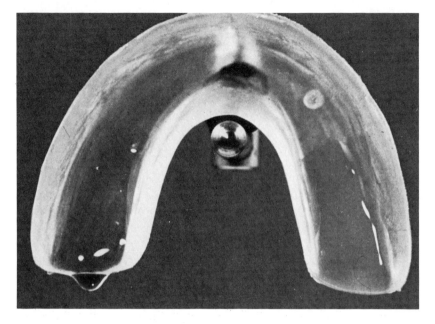

Fig. 3-1. Tray with thixotropic fluoride gel. (From Beal JF, Rock WP: *Br Dent J* 140:307, 1976.)

was observed in a study in which a gel with a lower fluoride content (0.5% vs 1.23%) and a higher pH (pH 4.5 vs pH 3) than that used in the aforementioned studies was self-applied each school day. One clinical study showed no significant reduction in the incidence of dental caries after 2 years.

A gel should be viscous enough to provide for ease of handling during loading of the tray and insertion, yet fluid enough to allow efficient contact of the gel with the enamel surfaces of the teeth. Presumably, more viscous gels would have less tendency to flow from the tray and into the throat, thereby causing nausea. A thixotropic gel could be advantageous clinically because the gel would be highly viscous during rest (Fig. 3-1) but would become more fluid when sheared (forced to flow) during insertion in the mouth. The viscosity of a gel should decrease with increasing temperature.

Manipulation

Acidulated phosphate-fluoride gels are usually applied in soft, spongy trays after a dental prophylaxis. The teeth should be as free from saliva as possible before application of the tray. A ribbon of gel is placed in the troughs of the maxillary and mandibular trays, the trays are placed in position, pressure is applied by squeezing the buccal and lingual surfaces to mold the tray tightly around the teeth so that the gel penetrates between the teeth, and the patient is instructed

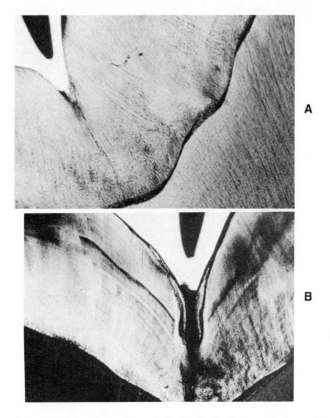

Fig. 3-2. Anatomy of the occlusal surface of a posterior tooth. **A,** Groove. **B,** Fissure in which debris has collected. Dental caries has initiated in enamel.

to bite lightly for 4 minutes. After application of a gel, the patient should not eat for 30 minutes.

PIT AND FISSURE SEALANTS

The reduction of smooth-surface caries has been accomplished by the use of established preventive measures such as fluoridation of communal water supplies, topical application of fluoride during enamel development, and individual plaque-control programs. These measures, however, have not been completely effective in reducing the incidence of dental caries in pits and fissures, which are sites susceptible to dental caries because of their anatomic construction.

The uniqueness of pit and fissure caries is a result of the special anatomy of the occlusal surfaces of posterior teeth. A smooth-based depression on the occlusal surface of a tooth is termed a groove, an example of which is shown in a histologic section in Fig. 3-2, *A*. The tip of an explorer in the upper left corner of

Table 3-2. Examples of Commercial Dimethacrylate Pit and Fissure Sealants

Product	Color	Manufacturer
Visible light-activated		
Delton (light cured)*	Clear, opaque	Johnson & Johnson
Fluro-Shield	Tooth-colored, white	Dentsply/Caulk
Helioseal*	White	Vivadent (USA)
Prisma-Shield*	Tooth-colored, white	Dentsply/Caulk
Sealite†	Clear, white	Sybron/Kerr
Visio-Seal*	Pink	ESPE-Premier
Amine-accelerated		
Concise*	White	3M
Delton*	Clear, opaque, red	Johnson & Johnson
Oralin*	Red	Mission White

*Acceptable product of ADA Acceptance Program.
†Provisionally acceptable product of ADA Acceptance Program.

this figure indicates the relative size of such a groove. A groove is readily cleansed by the excursion of food or of a toothbrush bristle. The pit and fissure, however, is an enamel fault that is the result of noncoalescence of enamel during tooth formation. This lack of enamel coalescence may extend to the dento-enamel junction, or it may be incomplete, with the fissure extending some lesser depth into the enamel. The debris and microbial masses that collect in a fissure are readily apparent in Fig. 3-2, *B*. Under appropriate conditions, pit and fissure caries is initiated. The unusual anatomy of the pit and fissure causes such sites to exhibit a high incidence of dental caries. In fact, **84% of dental caries in children ages 5 to 17 involve pits.**

One approach to the prevention of pit and fissure caries has been a restorative procedure whereby occlusal fissures are cut away and filled with dental amalgam. A newer approach is the use of pit and fissure sealants. **The purpose of a pit and fissure sealant is to penetrate all cracks, pits, and fissures on the occlusal surfaces of both deciduous and permanent teeth** in an attempt to seal off these susceptible areas and provide effective protection against caries.

Composition and reaction

Most commercial pit and fissure sealants, examples of which are listed in Table 3-2, are bisphenol A-glycidyl methacrylate (BIS-GMA) or urethane dimethacrylate materials in which polymerization is accelerated by light or an organic amine. The chemistry of sealants is similar to that of the composite restorative materials that are discussed in Chapter 4. The principal difference in the sealants is that they must be much more fluid to penetrate the pits and fissures as well as the etched areas produced on the enamel, which provide for retention of the sealant.

Sealants polymerized by visible light (420 to 450 nm wave length) are one-component systems that require no mixing. The resin is a dimethacrylate mono-mer, the polymerization of which is initiated by an activa-tor such as a diketone in the presence of an organic amine. Several sealants contain up to 50% inorganic filler to improve durability, and many contain a white pigment to improve the contrast between the sealants and enamel. The sealants polymerize in the mouth when exposed to a curing light to become a cross-linked polymer, as indi-cated in the following simplified reaction.

> A monomer is a single organic molecule used to prepare a high–mo-lecular weight polymer.

$$\text{Dimethacrylate} + \text{Diluent} + \text{Activator} \rightarrow \text{Sealant}$$

The sealants polymerized by an organic amine accelerator are supplied as two-component systems. One component contains a monomer and a benzoyl peroxide initiator, and the second component contains a diluted monomer with 5% organic amine accelerator. The two components are mixed thoroughly be-fore being applied to the prepared teeth.

In addition to the dimethacrylate sealants, some glass ionomer cements are being evaluated as pit and fissure sealants (see Chapter 4).

Properties

Physical and mechanical properties of commercial pit and fissure sealants of the BIS-GMA type are listed in Table 3-3. Additional properties of clinical impor-tance include retention and efficacy.

Retention of a sealant in a fissure is the result of mechanical bonding caused by penetration of the sealant into the fissure and the etched areas of enamel to form tags. Filling the fissure completely is difficult because air fre-quently is trapped in the bottom of the fissure (Fig. 3-3, A), or the accumulation of debris at the base of the fissure prevents it from being completely sealed (Fig.

Table 3-3. Properties of BIS-GMA Pit and Fissure Sealants

Property	Amine-accelerated sealant
Setting time (seconds)	60
Compressive strength (psi [MN/m²])	13,000-22,000 (92-150)
Tensile strength (psi [MN/m²])	2900-4500 (20-31)
Elastic modulus ($\times 10^6$ psi [GN/m²])*	0.30-0.75 (2.1-5.2)
Knoop hardness (kg/mm²)	20-25
Water sorption, 7 days (mg/cm²)	1.3-2.0
Water solubility 7 days (mg/cm²)	0.2
Penetration coefficient, 22° C (cm/sec)	4.5-8.8
Wear ($\times 10^{-4}$ mm³/mm)	22-23

*1 GN/m^2 = 1000 MN/m^2.

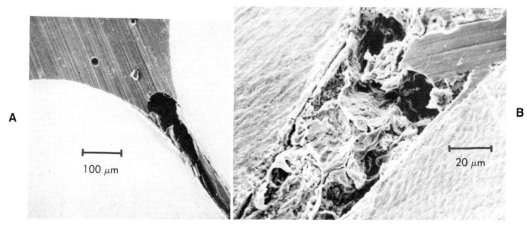

Fig. 3-3. Section showing a fissure incompletely filled with sealant as a result of air, **A,** and debris, **B.** (From Gwinnett AJ: *J Am Soc Prev Dent* 3:21, 1973.)

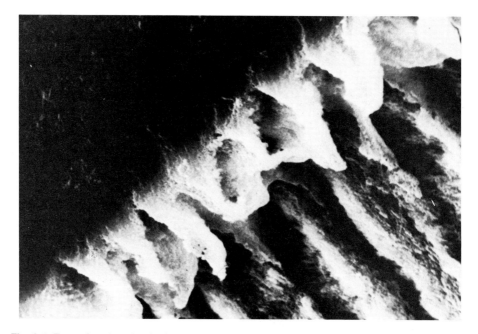

Fig. 3-4. Tags of sealant that had penetrated the etched enamel. (From Dennison, JB: Restorative materials for direct application. In Craig RG, editor: *Dental materials: a problem-oriented approach,* St. Louis, 1978, Mosby–Year Book.)

3-3, *B*). Acid etching of the enamel surface improves the retention of the sealant by cleaning the area to be sealed, improving the wettability of the enamel, increasing the surface area, and forming spaces into which the sealant can penetrate to form tags (Fig. 3-4).

Penetration of a sealant into the fissure must occur before the sealant has polymerized. The rate of penetration is determined by the geometry (length [1] and radius [r]) of the pit or fissure and by the penetration coefficient (PC) of the sealant:

$$\text{Rate} = \frac{(r)(PC)}{2(1)}$$

The penetration coefficient is related to the surface tension (γ) and viscosity (η) of the sealant and the contact angle (θ) of the sealant on the enamel:

$$PC = \frac{\gamma \cos \theta}{2(\eta)}$$

The containers in which the sealant components are supplied must be kept closed tightly during storage to minimize the evaporation of volatile monomers that would cause the sealant to become more viscous.

Many clinical studies have been reported, but caution should be used in comparing some of these studies because materials, technics, teeth studied, and clinical criteria for judging success or failure have varied from study to study. Three parameters that are important in the evaluation of a clinical study of a sealant are (1) a statistical test of the significance, (2) the net gain as a result of treatment, and (3) the percent of effectiveness. When pairs of teeth are studied, the net gain is the number of pairs in which the treated tooth is sound and the untreated tooth is decayed minus the number of pairs in which the treated tooth is decayed and the untreated tooth is sound. The percent effectiveness is the net gain divided by the total number of carious controls expressed in percent. A summary of a 5-year clinical study on schoolchildren is listed in Table 3-4. The effectiveness of a single application of a sealant clearly decreases with time. In another clinical study, the teeth of schoolchildren were maintained free of caries for 2 years by reapplication of sealant as indicated by clinical reexamination at 6-month intervals. The highest retreatment rate (18%) occurred 6 months after initial treatment but was as low as 4% at subsequent 6-month recalls. The pit and fissure sealants are effective in preventing caries in sealed tooth surfaces when the sealant is retained. Periodic clinical observation is recommended to determine the success or potential failure of the sealant treatment.

One concern is what happens to dental caries that are purposely or inadvertently left beneath sealed pits and fissures. Several studies have reported that the number of cultivable microorganisms from carious dentin left in situ in sealed

Table 3-4. Summary of a Clinical Study After Single Application of a Pit and Fissure Sealant (Sybron/Kerr)

Type of teeth and patients	Duration of study (years)	Total retention (%)	Net gain (number of teeth)	Effectiveness (%)
First permanent molars in	1	79.2	77	82.8
children ages 5-9 years	2	71.0	96	74.4
	3	60.1	91	63.6
	4	52.4	78	53.8
	5	31.0	58	39.7
Second primary molars in	1	72.5	—	—
children ages 5-9 years	2	59.5	2	28.6
	3	44.6	7	53.8

Modified from Charbeneau GT, Dennison JB: *J Am Dent Assoc* 98:559, 1979.

pits and fissures for up to 5 years was considerably less than before sealant was applied. Sealing a suspected carious pit and fissure appears to be a reasonable clinical service if appropriate clinical observation is maintained.

The use of sealants requires clinical judgment and continued observation. Modes of failure that have been observed include direct loss of sealant, absence of bonding of an area within an otherwise intact sealant, and wear that uncovers the terminal ends of the fissures. Current evidence indicates that **sealants should not be used on the teeth of a patient who does not cooperate in maintaining good oral hygiene, on occlusal surfaces where pits and fissures do not exist, on teeth that have been free of caries for a number of years, or on teeth with many proximal lesions.**

Manipulation of sealants

The technic for handling the pit and fissure sealants involves six basic steps that must be followed sequentially, including cleansing and etching the occlusal surfaces, washing these areas, drying them, applying the sealant to the pit and fissure, polymerizing, and finishing.

Visible light-activated sealants. The advantages of acid etching the enamel before the application of a sealant have been discussed earlier. The cleansing or etching solutions, which are known as preconditioning solutions, are generally 37% or 50% solutions of orthophosphoric acid in water. Some solutions are buffered by the addition of 7% zinc oxide, and some etching agents are phosphoric acid gels. Typically the enamel surface is cleansed with pumice before etching.

The preconditioner is applied liberally to the central fissure area of the occlusal surface with a small cotton pellet held by tweezers or with a fine brush. The solution should be left on the tooth for 60 seconds before the surface is washed with a liberal amount of water for at least 15 seconds. **Rinsing is important be-**

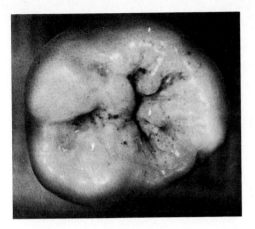

Fig. 3-5. Dark areas of a preconditioned occlusal surface indicate location of pits and fissures.

cause residual phosphoric acid would interfere with the bonding of the sealant. Care should be taken not to apply the preconditioning solution to other surfaces of the tooth or to allow the acid to overetch the enamel. **If a preconditioned tooth should become contaminated by saliva, etching and rinsing must be repeated.**

The washed surface of the tooth should then be dried for 15 seconds with an air syringe. **This step is critical to the success of the sealant because moisture interferes with the retention of the sealant by the fissure.** At this point the occlusal surface will have an appearance similar to that shown in Fig. 3-5. During application of the sealant, the isolation of the area from moisture should be maintained by use of cotton rolls and high-volume evacuation.

Applying the pit and fissure sealant to the occlusal surface on the tooth should be done carefully with a small tube (cannula), as shown in Fig. 3-6, *A*, or ball applicator, *B*. The application of an excessive amount of sealant is wasteful. In particular, **application of the sealant to unetched areas of enamel should be avoided.**

Once the sealant has been applied to the etched enamel, polymerization is activated by the use of a visible light source, such as shown in Fig. 3-7. The protective plastic tip of the light source is positioned on the occlusal surface (Fig. 3-8) and held there for at least 20 seconds.

Once the sealant has set, finishing can be accomplished with the use of a small cotton pellet held by tweezers. The pellet is used on the surface to remove sealant that has failed to polymerize because of exposure to air. When successfully polymerized, the sealant should offer considerable resistance to attempts to penetrate it with the tip of an explorer. **The coating should be inspected for areas of incomplete coverage and voids.** Defects can be corrected by repeating the entire procedure and reapplying sealant to the defective areas. A completed

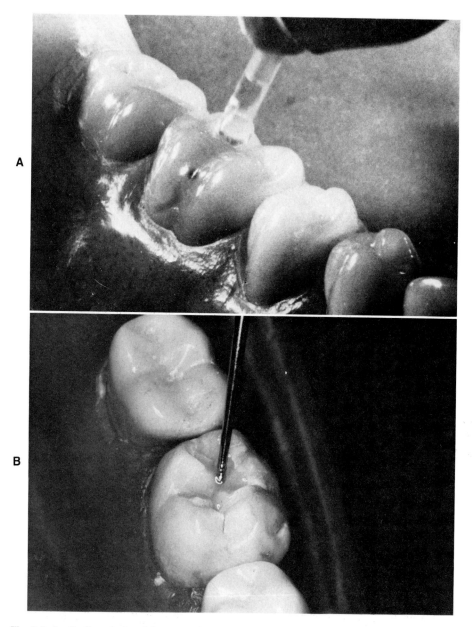

Fig. 3-6. Application of pit and fissure sealant with a small tube (cannula), **A,** and a ball applicator, **B.** (Courtesy Dr. JB Dennison, University of Michigan School of Dentistry, Ann Arbor, Mich.)

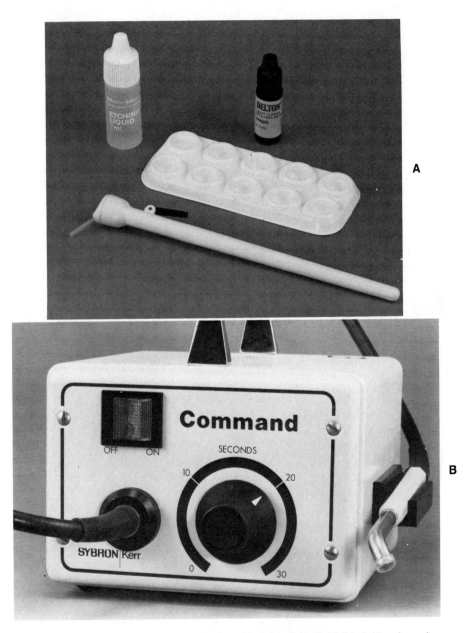

Fig. 3-7. A, Sealant polymerized by activation with visible light. **B,** Visible light-curing unit.

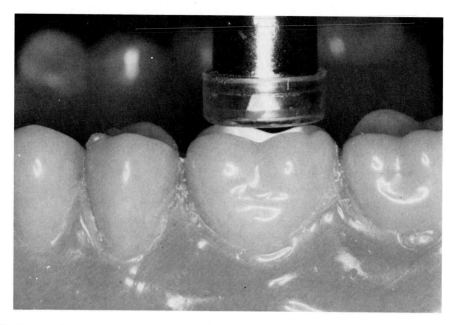

Fig. 3-8. Tip of a visible light source positioned on the occlusal surface of a molar containing sealant.

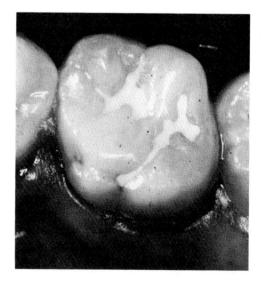

Fig. 3-9. Tooth with completed sealant treatment. (Courtesy Dr. JB Dennison, University of Michigan School of Dentistry, Ann Arbor, Mich.)

sealant treatment is shown in Fig. 3-9. If a fluoride treatment is used in conjunction with the pit and fissure sealant, the treatment should be applied after the sealant has polymerized.

Amine-accelerated sealants. The procedure for manipulation of these sealants is similar to that just described for sealants polymerized by visible light. These sealants require mixing of the base and initiator components. They should be mixed thoroughly to ensure that polymerization will be homogeneous, but gently to minimize incorporation of air. Typically the mixing time is 10 to 15 seconds. The sealant should be applied promptly because its ability to penetrate the fissure and etched enamel decreases rapidly as it begins to polymerize.

With most products, setting will occur within several minutes after application of the liquid sealant. Once polymerized, the sealant can be finished as already described.

MOUTH PROTECTORS

The incidence of oral injuries in contact sports such as football, hockey, lacrosse, soccer, basketball, boxing, and wrestling has been shown to be at least 50% of the total injuries sustained. Although most surveys have concentrated on sports played by men, evidence shows that many injuries to the mouth and teeth are occurring in women's field hockey. Furthermore, a direct relationship exists between inexperience and injury. Therefore a youngster participating in contact sports, even before becoming a member of an organized team, is in need of protection. Players wearing orthodontic appliances have an additional need for protection.

Surveys have shown conclusively that extraoral protectors such as face guards prevent only about 50% of the oral injuries of athletes playing football. The most prevalent causes of dental injury in football (in the presence of a face guard) are (1) blows under the chin resulting from forearm blocking; (2) blows that slip past the face bar, including blows by the bars of a face guard worn by another player; (3) gritting the teeth or snapping the jaws shut, especially as a result of unexpected body blocks and tackles; and (4) blows on top of the head that cause the jaws to snap shut. The injuries most frequently observed are chipped, broken, or dislodged teeth and concussions resulting from blows to the chin. **For maximum protection, intraoral devices such as mouth protectors are needed in addition to extraoral protection.**

The mouth protector program has been particularly effective in the area of preventive dentistry. The original mandate by the National Football Alliance Rules Committee that all high school athletes be equipped with internal mouth protectors has influenced other athletic programs. Most junior colleges and many amateur hockey and football leagues have now adopted this rule, and The National Collegiate Athletic Association adopted a mouth protector rule in 1973.

Furthermore, professional hockey and football players who have worn mouth protectors in college or elsewhere usually continue to wear them in professional sports. It is estimated that at least 1.5 million athletes have been equipped with mouth protectors and that this number increases by 70,000 each year. In fact, 25,000 to 50,000 injuries are estimated to be prevented each year by the use of the intraoral mouth protector.

Types and composition

The three types of mouth protectors, all of which offer some protection to the athlete, are stock, mouth-formed (Fig. 3-10), and custom-made. The results of studies that have evaluated the effectiveness of the various types of mouth protectors can be broadly summarized by the statement that any of the mouth protectors will reduce oral injuries. The results of these studies, however, are not in complete agreement with respect to the superiority of one or the other type. **Players prefer the custom-made protectors because of cleanliness, lack of taste or odor, durability, low speech impairment, and comfort.**

A thermoplastic material becomes softer on heating and harder on cooling with the process being reversible.

The custom-made mouth protectors are generally formed from thermoplastic polymers that are supplied in the form of clear or colored sheets approximately 5½ inches square (Fig. 3-11). The thickness of these sheets varies from ¹⁄₁₆ to ⅛ inch, depending on the product. The most common material used in custom-made protectors is a polyvinylacetate-polyethylene polymer. Other products have used polyurethane, rubber latex, and a vinyl plastisol.

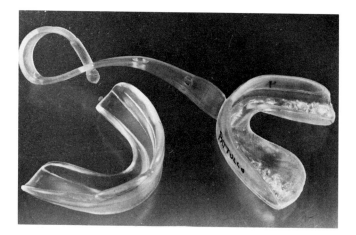

Fig. 3-10. Stock and mouth-formed mouth protectors.

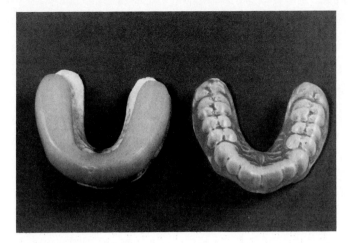

Fig. 3-11. Custom-made mouth protectors made from colored *(left)* and clear *(right)* thermoplastics.

Table 3-5. Properties of Polyvinylacetate-Polyethylene Mouth Protector After Processing and After Being Worn

Property	Processed	Worn
Tensile strength (psi [MN/m^2])	454 (3.13)	310 (2.14)
Tear strength (lb/in [N/cm])	140 (240)	146 (250)
Elongation (%)	975	—
Hardness (Shore A Durometer)	71	66
Water sorption, 24 hours (mg/cm^2)	0.05	—
Water solubility, 24 hours (mg/cm^2)	0.001	—
Dynamic modulus, 37° C (psi [MN/m^2])	1360 (9.4)	1050 (7.2)
Dynamic resilience, 37° C (%)	23.4	20.2

Properties

Laboratory studies have compared the physical and mechanical properties of a number of materials used for custom-made mouth protectors. These properties include tensile strength, percent of elongation, tear strength, hardness, water sorption, solubility, dynamic modulus, and dynamic resilience. The properties of a polyvinylacetate-polyethylene mouth protector after processing and after being worn are compared in Table 3-5. After exposure to the oral environment, the mouth protector becomes more flexible and better able to absorb an impact (energy) but has less strength in tension.

Compared to the polyvinylacetate-polyethylene material, the polyurethanes possess higher strength, hardness, and energy absorption but also have higher values of water sorption and require higher processing temperatures. The vinyl plastisols and latexes possess only slightly lower values of strength, hardness, and energy absorption than the polyvinylacetate-polyethylene materials, but their greatest disadvantage is the difficulty of processing. In general, polyvinyl-acetate-polyethylene materials are the easiest to fabricate.

Clinical studies of custom-made mouth protectors made of polyvinylacetate-polyethylene have been concerned with the following clinical variables: gagging, taste, irritation, impairment of speech, feel, durability, staining, deformation, and changes in the mouth.

Gagging, taste, irritation, and impairment of speech are problems not common to properly fabricated custom-made protectors. The elimination of these four variables as potential excuses for an athlete not to wear the protector is one reason that custom-made protectors are more desirable than the stock variety. Staining is a problem that can be expected regardless of the protector material.

There appears to be an optimum hardness at which an athlete will accept the protector. Complaints may be received from athletes who dislike the "feel" of the harder materials. If this dislike is sufficient motivation for an athlete not to wear the protector, a softer material should be selected.

The breakdown of a mouth protector usually results from one of three causes: "bite-through," tearing, or a general deterioration that results from chewing the protector. Both bite-through and chewing problems are compounded by the emotional involvement of the athlete. If the mouth protector is used to counteract high emotional stress during periods such as player assignments or the "big game," breakdown of the mouth protector can be expected regardless of the material of construction. In addition, some athletes may react to the harder mouth protector materials by chewing them, in which case a softer material should be selected. Examples of deteriorated mouth protectors are shown in Fig. 3-12.

Tearing of a protector generally is caused by an excessive force applied to the protector. If this force is the result of a blow to the jaw, for example, tearing of the protector would be a dissipation of part of the energy of the blow. The energy absorbed by the mouth protector is not available to do damage to the mouth, and thus, from this point of view, tearing of a mouth protector from a blow is probably desirable.

As a result of the aforementioned three causes of breakdown of a mouth protector, its durability is highly dependent on both the athlete's acceptance of the protector and his or her reaction to emotional stress. A protector may last 1 week in a highly emotional high school athlete or a whole season (4 months) in a more experienced college player. As a general rule, mouth protectors should be evaluated for breakdown on a game-to-game basis and should be replaced when necessary.

Observations have shown that mouth protectors permanently deform. A pri-

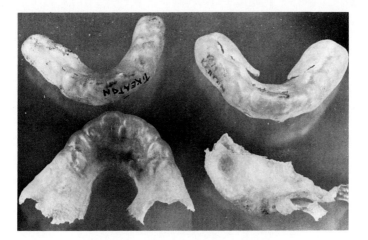

Fig. 3-12. Deteriorated mouth protectors.

mary cause is the mode of storage. Permanent deformation can occur as the result of pressure (such as that occurring when the mouth protector is squeezed together in a locker) or heat (such as that resulting when the mouth protector is stored in a helmet left in the hot sunlight). **When not in use between games or practice, the mouth protector should be stored in a rigid plastic container or on the model on which it was fabricated.**

An attempt to provide additional protection has resulted in the development of a laminated protector that contains a hard insert bonded to the softer polyvinyl-acetate-polyethylene material. The insert is located immediately palatal to the incisal edges of the central maxillary teeth after fabrication. Examination has shown that, once a tear occurs in proximity to the insert, the presence of saliva accelerates further tearing of the vinyl surrounding the insert, and loosening of the insert occurs. Since the insert is small and could be aspirated into the trachea, this type of protector must be evaluated for deterioration continually and discarded when the insert is no longer firmly bonded to the vinyl.

The use of extraoral instead of intraoral mouth protection on young athletes has been advocated because of the continued eruption of teeth. However, in view of the fact that many injuries result from a blow that drives the mandible into the maxillary arch, the protection afforded by the extraoral protector is not considered adequate. It is therefore best to start the athlete with the intraoral protector.

Fabrication of mouth protectors

The fabrication of a custom-made mouth protector from a thermoplastic material such as polyvinylacetate-polyethylene requires four basic steps: taking an

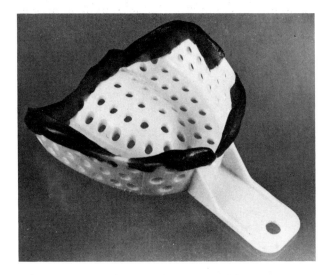

Fig. 3-13. Disposable impression tray modified with utility wax.

impression of the arch, pouring a model, forming the thermoplastic material over the model, and finishing the mouth protector.

An alginate impression is made of the maxillary arch. If a number of protectors are being made in a short time, such as in a clinic, it is convenient to use disposable impression trays, modified as necessary with utility wax (Fig. 3-13), to provide adequate extension of the labial portion of the tray and to prevent gagging of the patient. Further information on manipulation of alginate and impression taking can be found in Chapter 8.

Athletes should not wear any removable appliances when participating in contact sports. Thus impressions for mouth protectors should be made with such appliances removed. Orthodontic appliances that are fixed to the teeth need not be removed, since an impression can be made with them in place. The areas occupied by the appliances can then be blocked out on the model with dental stone or wax (Fig. 3-14), so that the mouth protector will fit over them.

After disinfection, the impression should be poured immediately in stone. Since the model may be reused to form a number of mouth protectors, the high-strength stone provides the most durable model. It is not necessary to pour the palate in the model (Fig. 3-14), since only areas to be included in the mouth protector are poured. The model should be identified with the athlete's name written in pencil. Further information on the manipulation of gypsum products can be found in Chapter 9.

Forming the mouth protector can be accomplished by a vacuum method or by hand. Regardless of the technic used, remember that the goal is to attain an op-

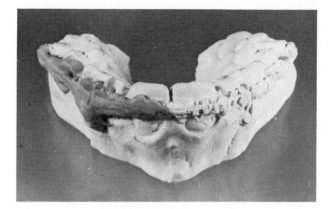

Fig. 3-14. Orthodontic appliance blocked out on model with dental stone. Note that the model has no palate.

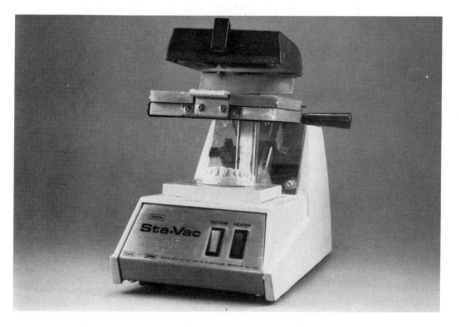

Fig. 3-15. Equipment for vacuum forming a custom-made mouth protector.

timum fit so that the mouth protector will distribute a blow over the entire dental arch. In addition, **the protector should provide as little distortion of normal occlusion as is necessary for maximum protection.**

The vacuum method of forming the protector is desirable, since it reproduces the occlusal anatomy more accurately than does forming by hand. Vacuum forming equipment, as shown in Fig. 3-15, is available. A simple and inexpen-

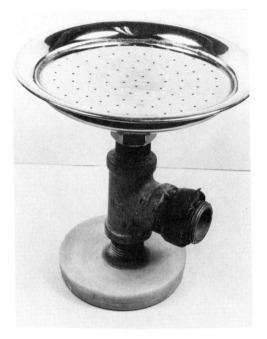

Fig. 3-16. Shower head adapted for vacuum forming a mouth protector.

sive device for vacuum forming can be constructed from an old style shower head (Fig. 3-16) attached to a vacuum cleaner.

To form the protector, the model should be centered on the shower head. By eliminating the palatal area of the model, a higher vacuum can be attained more readily; thus the adaptation of the protector will be better.

The thermoplastic material can be warmed by heating in boiling water for approximately 20 seconds. Since the material has a tendency to lose its shape, it should be heated by holding first one corner and then another. The fingers can be protected from the sticky material by wetting them with water or by using tongs.

Once the material is heated, the vacuum can be turned on and the softened material centered on the model. As the material is pulled over the model by the vacuum (Fig. 3-17), the edges of the material can be sealed to the shower head with finger pressure. Care should be taken to avoid applying heavy pressure to the occlusal surface, since heavy pressure may cause a thinning of the material in this area. After the vacuum is allowed to run for 2 minutes, it may be shut off and the material allowed to cool for 1 additional minute. The model and material may then be removed from the shower head and chilled thoroughly in cold wa-

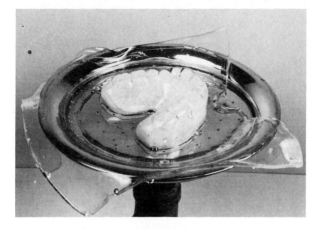

Fig. 3-17. Softened material pulled over the model by a vacuum.

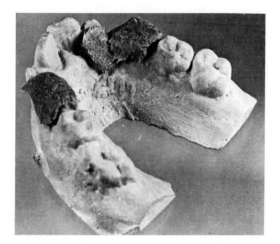

Fig. 3-18. Space left to accommodate rapidly emerging deciduous teeth by placing a portion of a damp towel over these teeth on the model.

ter or allowed to air-cool before handling. Examples of commercial sheets for the fabrication of custom-made mouth protectors are Proform (Dental Resources), Sta-Guard (Buffalo Dental), and Mira-Guard (World Wide Dental).

If the athlete has rapidly emerging deciduous teeth, space to accommodate this growth can be allowed in the mouth protector by placing portions of a damp towel over these teeth on the model as shown in Fig. 3-18. The damp towel serves as a spacer during fabrication but can be easily removed once the material has cooled.

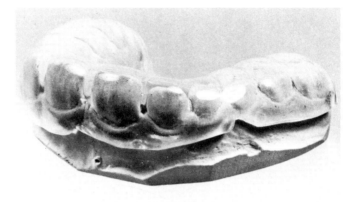

Fig. 3-19. Mouth protector, on a model, trimmed and notched in the area of the labial frenum.

The mouth protector can be removed from the model and trimmed ⅛ inch short of the labial fold (Fig. 3-19) with a curved pair of surgical scissors. **Care should be taken to provide clearance for the buccal and particularly the labial frenum by notching the mouth protector in these areas.** The mouth protector may have to be replaced on the model and have its edges flamed with an alcohol torch. These edges can then be easily smoothed with moist fingers.

Only a small percentage of mouth protectors need adjustment to equalize the occlusion. Should equalization be necessary, it can be accomplished by the following procedure. The contacting surfaces of the mouth protector are gently heated with an alcohol torch. Only enough heat should be used to barely soften the material. The appliance is dipped in warm water and is placed in the athlete's mouth; he or she should close gently until all the teeth contact the mouth protector. The athlete should open his or her jaws, and the mouth protector should be removed to cool. The protector is replaced in the mouth to examine the occlusion. All the teeth must contact the appliance. If it is desirable to open the athlete's vertical dimension, a layer of the thermoplastic material is heated and adapted to the occlusal surface of the stone model. A second layer is vacuum processed over the entire model, enclosing the first layer. The increased occlusal thickness of the appliance allows the vertical dimension and the occlusion to be adjusted.

In forming a mouth protector by hand, the heated material is adapted to the model by using finger pressure. Once the protector has been cooled, any areas not adapted can be reheated with a suitable torch and readapted. The mouth protector is trimmed in the same manner described in the vacuum technic.

A strap can be attached to a custom-made mouth protector as shown in Fig.

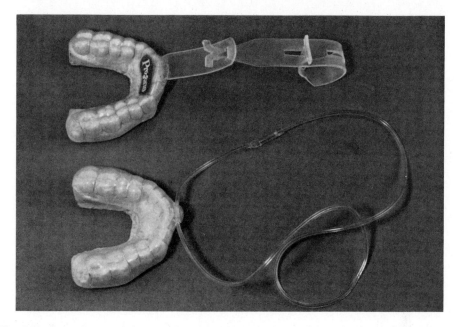

Fig. 3-20. Straps heat-sealed to custom-made mouth protectors. *Top,* Proform with strap provided; *bottom,* Sta-Guard with custom-made tubular strap.

3-20. The wide strap is heat-sealed into a slit made in the mouth protector at the incisal edge of the maxillary central incisors. The tubular strap is fabricated from three sizes of Tygon tubing. Both straps "break away" at low forces of 5 to 25 newtons (1 to 6 lb).

Two mistakes that are common to the fabrication of mouth protectors are (1) using a sooty flame during smoothing and (2) reproducing flaws in the model that do not exist in the arch. A sooty flame should not be used during smoothing operations, since this type of flame blackens the mouth protector. When handling and trimming a model, one should take care not to change the anatomy, since the protector will reproduce any changes in the model and thus not fit properly or comfortably on the arch.

The athlete should be instructed in the proper hygiene of a mouth protector. It may be convenient to enclose the following instructions in the plastic storage case given to the athlete:

After each use:

1. Rinse your mouth protector under cold tap water.
2. Occasionally clean your mouth protector in a solution of soap and cool water.
3. Do not scrub your mouth protector with an abrasive dentifrice.

4. Do not use alcohol solutions or denture cleansers to clean your mouth protector.

5. Store your mouth protector in the container provided.

If necessary, identification can be placed on the buccal flange of the mouth protector with a laundry-marking pencil.

Fluoride gels and rinses, pit and fissure sealants, and mouth protectors are dental materials designed to prevent disease or injury to the teeth and supporting tissues. Fluoride gels and rinses are effective in lowering the incidence of dental caries depending on the method and frequency of application. Pits and fissures are responsible for the majority of dental caries in children. Sealants are effective in preventing caries when they are properly applied and completely retained. Intraoral mouth protectors prevent numerous athletic injuries each year. Players prefer custom-made protectors. Mouth protectors should be evaluated for breakdown frequently and replaced when necessary.

Self-test questions

In the following multiple choice questions, one or more of the responses may be correct.
1 Which of the following statements best describes the clinical effectiveness of fluoride gels?
   a. The clinical effectiveness of fluoride gels varies, depending in part on the method and frequency of application.
   b. There is no significant reduction in the incidence of dental caries.
   c. Reductions in dental caries vary between 37% and 41% when a gel is applied annually.
   d. A reduction in dental caries of 80% occurs when a gel is self-applied daily.
2 Which of the following statements are true?
   a. The reduction of pit and fissure caries has been accomplished by fluoridation of communal water supplies, topical application of fluoride during the development of enamel, and individual plaque-control programs.
   b. A smooth-based depression on the occlusal surface of a posterior tooth is termed a fissure.
   c. The uniqueness of pit and fissure caries is the result of the special anatomy of the occlusal surfaces of posterior teeth.
   d. The anatomy of the pit and fissure causes difficulty in diagnosing the early stages of dental caries.
3 An amine-accelerated sealant contains:
   a. Bisphenol A-glycidyl methacrylate monomer diluted with methyl methacrylate to lower the viscosity
   b. An organic amine

  c. An organic peroxide initiator
  d. An absorber of visible light, such as a diketone
4 Which of the following statements are true?
  a. The compressive strength of pit and fissure sealants is less than that of enamel but more than that of dentin.
  b. The hardness of pit and fissure sealants is less than that of enamel and dentin.
  c. Retention of sealants is the result of chemical bonding to enamel.
  d. The penetrativeness of a sealant could be reduced if evaporation of the diluent caused the viscosity of the sealant to increase.
5 Which of the following statements are true?
  a. The evaluation of any clinical study on sealants requires a statistical test of significance, the net gain as a result of treatment, and the percent of effectiveness.
  b. A patient with sealant treatment should be recalled at 6-month intervals and have sealant reapplied after 2 years.
  c. After 2 years, values of retention and effectiveness of sealants are both about 70%.
  d. Sealants appear to be retained better on permanent than on primary teeth.
6 The preconditioning solution:
  a. Is usually a 37% or 50% solution of phosphoric acid
  a. Is usually a 37% or 50% solution of phosphoric acid
  b. Is allowed to overetch the immediate vicinity of the fissure
  c. Is applied liberally to the central fissure area but not allowed to contact other surfaces of the tooth
  d. Is left on the tooth for 60 seconds and then rinsed away with water for 15 seconds
7 Application of the sealant:
  a. Can be done with a small tube (cannula)
  b. Should be done carefully to avoid overextending the sealant to unetched areas of enamel
  c. Should be done with isolation to prevent contamination of the etched surface with saliva
  d. Should be preceded by re-etching, rinsing, and drying if contamination of the enamel occurs
8 Which of the following statements are true?
  a. The setting time of an amine-accelerated sealant is about 60 seconds.
  b. A visible light-activated sealant will polymerize within 15 to 20 seconds after the light source is applied.
  c. A cotton pellet is used to remove sealant that fails to polymerize because of exposure to air.
  d. When successfully polymerized, the sealant should offer considerable resistance to attempts to penetrate it with the tip of an explorer.
  e. The occlusal surfaces of the teeth should be etched and sealed after a fluoride treatment has been applied.
9 Which of the following are used as athletic mouth protectors?
  a. Stock protector
  b. Mouth-formed protector
  c. Custom-made poly(methyl methacrylate) protector
  d. Custom-made polyvinylacetate-polyethylene protector

10 Which of the following statements concerning the properties of a mouth protector are true?

a. A harder material should be selected if the athlete complains about the "feel" of the protector and will not wear it.

b. Pressure and heat can cause a mouth protector to deform permanently.

c. Staining is generally not a problem with a mouth protector.

d. Tearing of a mouth protector may be desirable if the tearing dissipates the energy of a blow.

11 When not in use, a mouth protector should be stored:

a. In distilled water

b. In an immersion denture cleanser

c. In a rigid plastic container

d. On the model on which it was fabricated

12 The fabrication of a custom-made mouth protector requires:

a. A rubber base impression of the mandibular arch

b. An alginate impression of the maxillary arch

c. An alginate impression of the mandibular arch

d. Alginate impressions of both arches

e. Removable appliances to remain in the mouth when the impression is made

13 Which of the following statements concerning the fabrication of a mouth protector are true?

a. Improved stone provides the most durable model.

b. The model should be poured within 24 hours.

c. It is not necessary to pour the palate in the model.

d. Orthodontic appliances should be blocked out in the model with dental stone or wax.

14 Steps involved in finishing a mouth protector include:

a. Trimming ⅛ inch short of the labial fold

b. Notching the protector in the areas of the buccal and labial frenum

c. Flaming the edges of the protector to smooth them

d. Polishing the labial surfaces with extra-fine pumice

15 To form the protector from a polyvinylacetate-polyethylene material:

a. The model should be centered on a shower head.

b. The thermoplastic material can be warmed in boiling water for about 20 seconds.

c. Heavy pressure should be applied to the occlusal surface of the model to reproduce the occlusal anatomy.

d. The material should cool for 1 minute before being chilled thoroughly in cold water.

Suggested supplementary readings

Fluoride gels

Council on Dental Materials, Instruments and Equipment, and Council on Dental Therapeutics: Accepted dental products, *J Am Dent Assoc* 116:249, 1988.

Farah JW, Powers JM, editors: Fluorides, *Dent Advis* 4(3):1, 1987.

Pit and fissure sealants

Charbeneau GT, Dennison JB: Clinical success and potential failure after single application of a pit and fissure sealant: a four-year report, *J Am Dent Assoc* 98:559, 1979.

Council on Dental Health and Health Planning and Council on Dental Materials, Instruments, and Equipment: Pit and fissure sealants, *J Am Dent Assoc* 114:671, 1987.

Dennison JB, Straffon LH, Corpron RE, Charbeneau CT: A clinical comparison of sealant and amalgam in the treatment of pits and fissures. Part I: Clinical performance after 18 months, *Pediatr Dent* 2:167, 1980.

Dennison JB, Straffon LH, Corpron RE, Charbeneau CT: A clinical comparison of sealant and amalgam in the treatment of pits and fissures. Part II: Clinical application and maintenance during an 18 month period, *Pediatr Dent* 2:176, 1980.

Farah JW, Powers JM, editors: Radiography and sealants, *Dent Advis* 3(1):6, 1986.

Mertz-Fairhurst EJ, Fairhurst CW, Della-Giustina VE, Brooks JD: A comparative clinical study of two pit and fissure sealants: six year results in Augusta, Ga., *J Am Dent Assoc* 105:237, 1982.

Mertz-Fairhurst EJ: Arresting caries by sealants: results of a clinical study, *J Am Dent Assoc* 112:194, 1986.

Ripa LW: Occlusal sealing: rationale of the technique and historical review, *Am Soc Prev Dent J* 3:32, 1973.

Mouth protectors

Bureau of Health Education and Audiovisual Services and Council on Dental Materials, Instruments and Equipment: Mouth protectors and sports team dentists, *J Am Dent Assoc* 109:84, 1984.

Godwin WC, Craig RG, Koran A, Lang BR, Powers JM: Mouth protection in junior football players, *Phys Sportsmed* 10:41, 1982.

Wilkinson EE, Powers JM: Properties of stock and mouth-formed mouth protectors, *J Mich Dent Assoc* 68:83, 1986.

Wilkinson EE, Powers JM: Properties of custom-made mouth protector materials, *Phys Sportsmed* 14:77, 1986.

chapter four

Direct Esthetic Restorative Materials

The need for restorative materials that have the appearance of natural tooth tissue and that can be placed directly into a cavity preparation in a plastic condition is obvious. The patient desires esthetic restorations, particularly in the anterior portion of the mouth, and a direct filling material is advantageous in terms of the time required and the cost of the restoration.

Four types of materials have been used as direct esthetic dental restorations: (1) silicates, (2) acrylic polymers (unfilled), (3) dimethacrylate polymers containing inorganic reinforcing agents (composites), and (4) ionomer restoratives. Silicate restorative materials were introduced in the late 1800s and were used extensively until about 1970. The silicates had high solubility and did not resist disintegration in the oral environment; as a result they were a short-term restorative system. The silicates also discolored and increased in opacity as staining and dehydration occurred; thus their esthetic qualities degraded with time. Unfilled acrylic polymers were introduced about 1945 and were improved so that they were in moderate usage in the 1960s. The unfilled acrylic materials possessed improved resistance to solubility and had no problems with dehydration, although staining was a problem. The undesirable qualities of unfilled acrylics were large dimensional change on setting and with temperature, resulting in percolation of saliva at margins; low mechanical strength and stiffness; low resistance to wear; and problems with recurrent decay.

The composite dimethacrylates were introduced about 1960 and have been used increasingly until they now dominate the materials used for direct esthetic restorations. Ionomers were introduced in 1972 and have been used primarily for restoration of cervically eroded areas. Therefore only composites and ionomer restorative materials are discussed.

COMPOSITE RESTORATIVES

The composite restoratives represent a major improvement in direct esthetic restorations. They are generally recommended for Classes III to V and for Class I when occlusal stress is not a problem and appearance is crucial. Although less durable than amalgam, composites designed for Class II posterior applications are available.

Composition and reaction

Composite restorations consist mainly of two phases: a polymer matrix and dispersed filler particles. Inorganic fillers are surface treated with chemicals (coupling agents) to produce a good bond between the matrix and the filler.

Filler size. Dental composites may be classified on the basis of the particle size and distribution of the inorganic filler. Commercial composites may contain (1) fine irregularly shaped filler particles from 0.5 to 5 μm in diameter (Fig. 4-1, *A*), (2) microfine particles having a diameter of 0.04 to 0.2 μm (Fig. 4-1, *B*), or (3) blends (hybrids) of these two particle sizes. Fine particle-filled composites con-

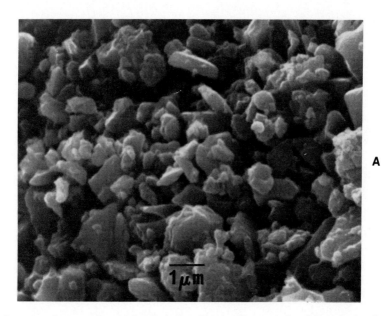

A

Fig. 4-1. Scanning electron micrographs of, **A,** fine, **B,** microfine, and, **C,** reinforced microfine fillers for composites. (From Craig RG, editor: *Restorative dental materials,* ed 8, St. Louis, 1989, Mosby–Year Book.)   *Continued.*

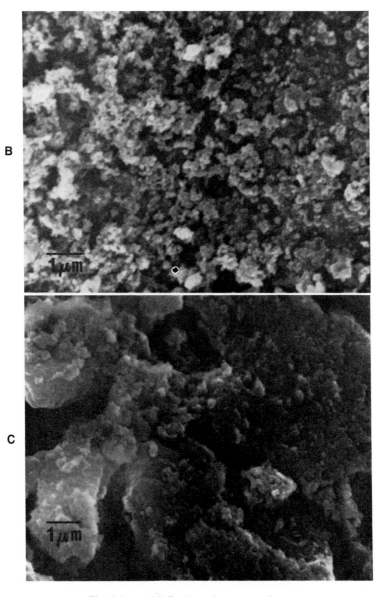

Fig. 4-1, cont'd. For legend see preceding page.

tain 60% to 70% of filler by volume, which is equivalent to 77% to 88% of filler by weight. The volume percentage is lower than the weight percentage because the filler is more dense than the polymer matrix. The microfine particles in microfilled composites have high surface areas of about 100 to 300 m^2/g and greatly increase the viscosity of the mixture when mixed with the organic component **(oligomer).** As a result low–molecular weight organic diluents are added to reduce the viscosity, but even then only about 25% of the filler by volume or 38% of the filler by weight can be added and still result in a paste with workable viscosity. Further increases in microfiller concentrations have been accomplished by polymerizing the filler-resin mixture and then grinding this into particles of 10 to 20 μm and using these reinforced particles as filler in a composite (Fig. 4-1, *C*); this method can increase the microfiller concentration to 32% by volume or about 50% by weight.

An oligomer is a moderate molecular weight organic made from two or more organic molecules.

Composites containing blends of fine and microfine filler particles have higher filler concentrations than the fine or microfilled composites alone, since the microfine particles can fit into the spaces between the fine particles. These hybrid composites can have filler concentrations of about 70% by volume when the microfiller concentration is about 15% by volume. Most current composites can be classified as hybrids, since they are fine-particle composites plus some microfiller.

Filler composition. Quartz, lithium aluminum silicate, and barium, strontium, or zinc glasses have been used as fillers. In some instances the glass particles have been etched. Microfine fillers are colloidal silicas, sometimes referred to as pyrolytic silica, since they are prepared by burning **silanes.** The reinforced fillers consist of colloidal silica surrounded by bisphenol A-glycidyl methacrylate (BIS-GMA) or another dimethacrylate polymer, which is described later in the chapter.

Silanes are metal-organic compounds containing silicon.

Quartz, lithium aluminum silicate, and colloidal silica are not opaque to radiographs and sizable amounts of barium, strontium, or zinc glasses must be used if a radiopaque composite is to be made. Manufacturers specify on the product if it is radiopaque or not.

Coupling agents. To provide a good bond between the inorganic fillers and the polymer matrix, the surface of the filler must be treated. The most common treatment by the manufacturer is the use of an organic silicon compound (a silane), which has groups that react with the inorganic filler and other groups that react with the organic matrix; thus the filler and matrix are coupled.

Organic matrix. The most common organic matrices are based on dimethacrylate identified as BIS-GMA or urethane dimethacrylate (UDMA). A highly simplified formula follows in which R represents any of a large number of organic groups (e.g., phenyl-, methyl-, carboxyl-, hydroxyl-, and amide-).

$$CH_2 = C—R—C = CH_2$$
$$\qquad \; | \qquad \quad |$$
$$\qquad CH_3 \quad\; CH_3$$

BIS-GMA or UDMA

BIS-GMA and UDMA oligomers are viscous liquids, and low–molecular weight monomers (dimethacrylates) are added to control the consistency of the materials. Both oligomers and the low–molecular weight monomers are characterized by carbon double bonds that react to convert them to a polymer.

Initiators and accelerators. Two principal systems used to achieve polymerization are the **chemically activated** system and the **visible light-activated** system, the latter being more common. In the former, polymerization (setting) is accomplished with an organic peroxide initiator and an organic amine accelerator. The initiator and accelerator must be kept separated and not mixed until just before the restoration is placed. Therefore the chemically activated systems usually are supplied as two pastes, with the initiator in one and the accelerator in the other (Fig. 4-2).

In the visible light-activated system, the composite is exposed to an intense blue light. The light is absorbed by a diketone, which, in the presence of an or-

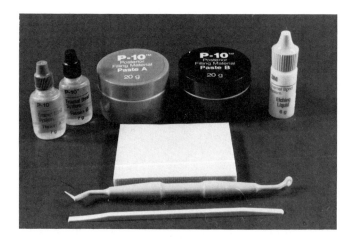

Fig. 4-2. Chemically initiated two-paste composite.

ganic amine, starts the polymerization reaction. Exposure times of 20 to 60 seconds are needed for polymerization. Since blue light is necessary to start the reaction, the diketone and amine can be in the same paste and no reaction occurs until it is exposed to blue light. Thus the material is supplied as a single paste in a light-tight syringe (Fig. 4-3).

Regardless of the system used, the following general reaction takes place.

Dimethacrylate +   Initiator   + Accelerator + Treated inorganic or → Dental composite

(peroxide or   **(amine)**   reinforced filler
diketone plus
blue light)

Pigments. Inorganic pigments are added in small amounts so that the color of the composite matches tooth structure. Typically, four or more shades are supplied, covering the normal range of human teeth (yellow to gray). Highly pigmented tints are available that can be mixed with the standard shades to match the color of teeth outside the normal range.

Composite systems

Composites most commonly are packaged as a single-paste system in a syringe or in compules and less commonly as a two-paste system supplied in two jars.

Two-paste system. An example of a product supplied as two pastes is shown in Fig. 4-2. Although each jar contains a paste consisting of the dimethacrylates and filler, one paste contains the peroxide initiator (sometimes called catalyst) and the other paste includes the amine accelerator. The materials are usually

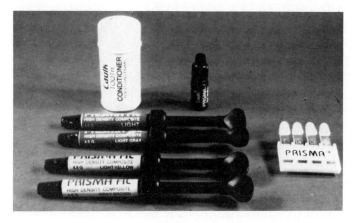

Fig. 4-3. Single-paste visible light-initiated composite.

pigmented to a universal shade that matches the majority of teeth. Additional shades are available, as well as tints that can be mixed with the universal shade, and these provide the dentist with composites to match teeth of other shades. The manufacturers usually supply an acid etchant for enamel, plus an enamel and dentinal bonding agent. Although dentinal bonding agents are usually sold separately, a few manufacturers include them in the composite system. These bonding agents are described later.

Single-paste system. All of the components are contained in a single-paste system and are combined by the manufacturer. The mixture is supplied in various shades in disposable syringes, examples of which are shown in Fig. 4-3. The syringes are made of opaque plastic to protect the material from exposure to light and thus provide adequate shelf life. After the desired amount of composite is dispensed, it is packed into the cavity preparation or is placed in a syringe, such as the one shown in the section on manipulation, and syringed into the preparation (see Fig. 4-8).

Single-paste composites are also supplied in compules as shown in Fig. 4-4. A colored protective tip identifies the various shades. The compule is placed on the end of the syringe, and the paste is extruded after removal of the protective tip.

Properties

Important physical and mechanical properties of composites are polymerization shrinkage, thermal conductivity, linear coefficient of thermal expansion, water sorption, radiopacity, compressive strength, tensile strength, elastic modulus, hardness, abrasive wear, and bond strength to etched enamel and dentin. Values of various composites are presented in Table 4-1. Values are given for fine particle and microfilled composites and not for blends, which will have properties depending on the ratio of the fine to microsized particles.

Polymerization shrinkage. Fine particle composites shrink less during polymerization (setting) than microfilled types, since the shrinkage is a direct function of the amount of organic matrix. It has been shown that, even with the acid etching of enamel and the use of bonding agents, stresses from polymerization shrinkage exceed the bond strength of the composites to tooth structure and, as a result, marginal leakage is not prevented.

Two technics have been proposed to overcome or minimize the effect of polymerization shrinkage. One method has been to **insert and polymerize the composite in layers,** thus reducing the effective shrinkage. The second method has been to **prepare a composite inlay** in the mouth or on a die, then to cement the inlay to the tooth with a thin layer of composite cement. The composite inlays are usually heated outside the mouth, after curing, which increases the polymerization and the wear resistance.

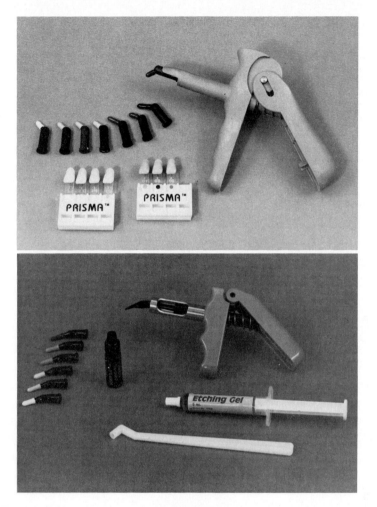

Fig. 4-4. Single-paste composites supplied in compules and the injection syringe.

Thermal conductivity. The thermal conductivity values (Table 4-1) are lower for microfilled than for fine particle composites, since the organic matrix is a good thermal insulator. The values for either type of composite are much lower than those for metallic restorations (see Table 2-2) and closely match those of enamel and dentin. Therefore composites provide good thermal insulation for the dental pulp.

Thermal expansion. Typical values for the two types of composites are shown in Table 4-1. The higher the amount of organic matrix, the higher the linear coefficient of thermal expansion, since the polymer has a higher value than the filler. As a result, the **microfilled composites have the higher values for ther-**

Table 4-1. Properties of Fine Particle and Microfilled Composites

Property	Fine particle composite	Microfilled composite
Polymerization shrinkage (% by volume)	1.0-1.7	2-3
Thermal conductivity (10^{-4} cal/sec/cm^2 [° C/cm])	25-30	12-15
Linear coefficient of thermal expansion ($\times 10^{-6}$/° C)	25-38	55-68
Water sorption (mg/cm^2)	0.3-0.6	1.2-2.2
Radiopacity (mm Al)*	2.7-5.7	—
Compressive strength lb/in^2 [M Pa]	35,000-57,000 or 241-393	25,000-32,000 or 172-221
Diametral tensile strength lb/in^2 [M Pa]	5000-9000 or 34-62	3800-4800 or 26-33
Elastic modulus lb/in^2 [M Pa]	1.3-2.3 $\times$ 10^6 or 9000-10,000	0.4-0.6 $\times$ 10^6 or 2800-4100
Knoop hardness (kg/mm^2)	55-80	22-36
Abrasive wear (mm^3/mm travel $\times$ 10^{-4})	7-10	12-15
Bond strength to etched enamel (lb/in^2 [kg/cm^2])	2400-2900 or 170-205	1400 or 100
Bond strength to dentin (lb/in^2 [kg/cm^2])	500-2400 or 71-170	500-2400

*If advertised as radiopaque, enamel is 4.0 and dentin is 2.5 mm.

mal expansion; therefore restorations from these composites will have a greater change in dimensions with changes in oral temperatures and probably will have more marginal leakage than fine particle types.

Water sorption. Values for various types of composites are given in Table 4-1. The higher values of the microfilled composites are apparent. These results occur because the organic matrix is mainly responsible for the absorption of water. Thus the **microfilled composites have a greater potential for being discolored by water-soluble stains.** Water sorption is accompanied by swelling of the composite, but this has not been an effective way to counteract polymerization shrinkage.

Radiopacity. For a composite to be radiopaque, it must contain an element with a high atomic number, such as barium, strontium, bromine, zinc, zirconium, or iodine, since carbon, hydrogen, oxygen, and silicon are not sufficiently high to attenuate x-rays. Microfilled composites are filled with silica, and some fine particle composites are filled with quartz (SiO_2); thus these products are not radiopaque. Fine particle or hybrid composites containing sufficient amounts of heavy metal glasses are radiopaque and are identified as such by the manufacturer. Argument exists whether radiopacity is an advantage in diagnosis; nevertheless, one should be aware that not all composites appear radiopaque on dental radiographs.

Compressive and tensile strength. The compressive strengths of the fine particle composites are higher than those of the microfilled composites. At the same volume fraction of inorganic filler, decreasing the particle size increases the strength. However, the fine particles of the microfilled composites increase the viscosity of the materials so that only low-volume fractions of filler are possible and thus their compressive strengths are lower than those for the fine particle composites. Since these restorations probably fail in tension, their values are of special interest (see Table 4-1).

Elastic modulus. The elastic modulus, or stiffness, of the composites is dominated by the amount of filler as shown in Table 4-1. The lower filler content of the microfilled or reinforced macrofilled composites results in elastic moduli of one quarter to one half of the more highly filled fine particle composites. This stiffness is important in applications where high biting forces are involved and wear resistance is essential.

Hardness, penetration resistance, and wear. Knoop hardness of composites (see Table 4-1) is directly related to filler content and is less related to the hardness of the filler. The higher filler content of fine particle composites is important in providing higher resistance to nonrecoverable penetration (Knoop hardness) and abrasive wear. Abrasive wear is, however, only one aspect of the wear process and is described in the section on clinical qualities.

Bond strength. The maximum bond strengths of composites to acid-etched enamel are about twice as high as the bond strengths to dentin (see Table 4-1). Dentinal bonding agents are as effective as enamel bonding agents and thus separate enamel bonding agents need not be purchased.

Dentinal bonding agents are designed to bond to the hydroxyapatite of enamel and dentin or the collagen of the dentin, or both. They all contain molecules with two types of reactive groups: one bonds to hydroxyapatite or collagen and the other reacts with the organic components in the composite during setting.

Etching of the enamel is recommended, and most bonding procedures recommend removal of the smear layer of collagen on the dentin, resulting from cavity preparation before application of the bonding agent. Some bonding agents require polymerization before placement of the composite, and some polymerize at the same time as the composite. Both chemically and light-initiated systems are available. Considerable controversy exists in this area, since the polymerization stresses are of the same magnitude as the bond strengths to dentin, and thus marginal leakage is not entirely prevented. Therefore dentinal bonding of direct composites is still inadequate and should be used in conjunction with acid etching of enamel, bonding to enamel, and mechanical retention in the cavity preparation.

Clinical qualities

The finishing of composites has been a major clinical concern, since a smooth surface is desired to prevent retention of plaque and is needed to maintain good oral hygiene. The surfaces of composites are generally contoured with a plastic

Table 4-2. Surface Roughness (μm) of Composites Finished with Various Disks and Polishing Pastes

Surface treatment	Fine particle composite	Hybrid composite	Microfilled composite
Mylar strip	0.13	0.12	0.09
Disks	1.96	2.00	1.87
Coarse disk			
Medium disk	0.61	0.59	0.71
Fine disk	0.33	0.26	0.25
xx Fine disk	0.17	0.14	0.16
Superfine disk	0.12	0.06	0.10
Polishing paste			
Sof-Lex fine	0.33	0.26	0.25
Moore xx-fine	0.17	0.15	0.16
Command Lustre Paste	0.14	0.09	0.13
Sof-Lex superfine	0.12	0.06	0.10
Prisma Gloss	0.11	0.03	0.09

Modified from Herrgott AML, Ziemiecki TL, Dennison JB: *J Am Dent Assoc* 119:729, 1989.

matrix, but some finishing is usually required to obtain proper contour. Producing a smooth surface on early composites was a problem because of the large particle size (~20 μm) of the hard filler. Polishing procedures preferentially removed the polymer leaving filler particles protruding from the surface. Current fine particle and microfilled composites can be polished, and the surface roughness is independent of the size of their filler particles (Table 4-2); the small differences in roughness of the three types of composites do not represent significant differences.

Even with the use of a plastic matrix strip, gross reduction with finishing diamonds and burs is often necessary. The roughness of surfaces of composites with various instrumentation is listed in Table 4-3. After the use of these instruments, final finishing and polishing are done using finishing disks and polishing pastes.

Table 4-3. Surface Roughness (μm) of Composites After Using Finishing Diamonds and Burs

Instrumentation	Surface roughness (μm)
12-Fluted bur	2.0
Diamond SF-1	1.4
30-Fluted bur	0.85
Diamond SF-2	0.80
Diamond SF-3	0.60
No. 57 fissure bur	0.60

Modified from Herrgott AML, Ziemiecki TL, Dennison JB: *J Am Dent Assoc* 119:729, 1989.

Microfilled

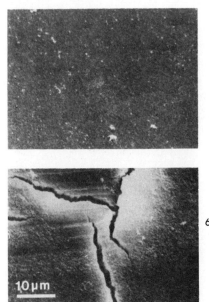

0 hours

Fig. 4-5. Photomicrographs of a microfilled composite processed against a Mylar matrix (0 hours) and after erosion with water spray and exposure to ultraviolet light (600 hours). (Modified from Fan PL, Powers JM: *Wear* 68:241, 1981.)

600 hours

10 µm

Although the fine particle and microfilled composites yield surfaces of the same smoothness, laboratory abrasive wear tests show that the microfilled composites wear more rapidly. Another cause of the loss of surface contour of composites is erosive wear in the oral environment. This type of wear has been simulated in the laboratory by exposing surfaces to ultraviolet light and water spray. Photomicrographs of surfaces processed against a Mylar matrix with 0 and 600 hours of laboratory erosion are shown in Fig. 4-5. Degradation of the surface of a microfilled composite is visible, appearing dull and rough even with the unaided eye. Thus loss of surface contour of composite restorations in the mouth results from a combination of abrasive wear from chewing, toothbrushing, and erosive wear from degradation of the composite in the oral environment.

Early wear studies of composites resulted in recommendations that their use be restricted to anterior low-stress-bearing areas; however improvements have resulted in their use in posterior applications. An example of wear of composites used in posterior teeth from an early study is shown in Fig. 4-6, *A*. A magnified view of an area of the margin of one of the restorations is shown in Fig. 4-6, *B*. The wear of the composite resulted in a rather uniform loss of material over the entire surface of the composite rather than just in the areas in contact with the opposing occlusion. This type of wear would be expected when the wear process involves a combination of erosion and abrasion.

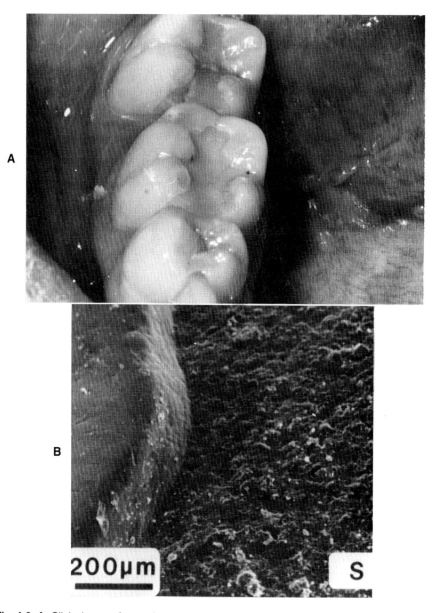

Fig. 4-6. A, Clinical wear of posterior composites. **B,** Magnified view of a margin with enamel on the left and composite on the right. (Courtesy Dr. JB Dennison, University of Michigan School of Dentistry, Ann Arbor, Mich.)

The use of composites for posterior restorations has resulted from several factors. The volume fraction of filler in the composites has been increased by use of graded sizes of filler particles. In these composites small size filler particles fit into the spaces between larger filler particles; the higher percentage of filler increases the wear resistance. Also, the restoration may be built up in increments and polymerized stepwise, which reduces the effective shrinkage during setting.

It also was found that significant numbers of unreacted groups from the monomers and oligomers existed after setting of the composite. Near the surface of the restoration the concentration of unreacted groups was about 75%, whereas in the bulk of the restoration it was about 25%. Furthermore, it was established that heating (after curing) the set composite to 120° C for 7 minutes decreased the number of unreacted groups and increased the wear resistance. Since this temperature could not be used in the mouth, a partially indirect technic was developed so that the set composite could be heated in an oven outside the mouth. To accomplish this, a cavity preparation without undercuts, such as that used for the preparation of gold inlays, was used. This allowed the composite restoration to be removed after setting and then heated to increase the extent of polymerization. The composite restoration was then cemented to the teeth using a lower viscosity composite as a cement.

A second totally indirect technic has been developed in which an impression of the nonretentive cavity preparation is taken and then a die made using a stiff rubber impression material or a fast-setting epoxy. The composite restoration is made on the die and heated after setting. The postcured restoration is then cemented using a composite cement. These indirect methods also allow development of better proximal contacts than the direct procedures.

Manipulation

To provide a bond between the composite and the tooth structure, the enamel portion of the cavity preparation is acid etched for 1 minute with an etchant supplied by the manufacturer, frequently a 36% phosphoric acid solution or an acid gel. The acid is flushed away with water, and the surface is dried with a stream of air. The etched area will appear dull; a magnified view of an etched surface is shown in Fig. 4-7. The composite or the bonding agent of the composite system penetrates the etched surface when the composite is placed and provides mechanical retention of the restoration. If a dentinal bonding agent is used, it may be applied to both the dentin and the enamel surface, following the manufacturer's recommendations.

The manipulation of the two-paste and single-paste systems is described here in general. Manufacturers have special recommendations that should be followed.

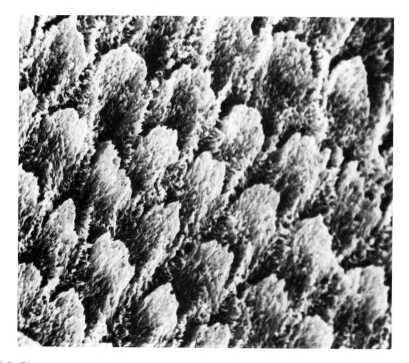

Fig. 4-7. Photomicrograph of enamel surface etched with phosphoric acid solution for 1 minute. (Courtesy Dr. JB Dennison, University of Michigan School of Dentistry, Ann Arbor, Mich.)

Two-paste system. It may be advisable to stir the contents of the two pastes when a new package is opened, since settling of the inorganic particles may have occurred. Disposable plastic or wooden mixing sticks or spatulas are supplied; one end of the stick should be used to stir the universal paste or another shade paste and the other end to stir the catalyst paste. If the same end is used, the cross-contamination will cause hardening in the jars. Some manufacturers claim no settling of the contents, and thus no mixing is required.

One end of an unused disposable mixing spatula is used to place an amount of universal paste equal to about half the size of the restoration on the mixing pad, and the other end is used to place about an equal amount of catalyst paste nearby on the pad. When the dentist needs the material, the two portions of paste are thoroughly mixed, requiring 20 to 30 seconds. The pastes are stiff, and care should be taken during mixing to avoid incorporation of air. A plastic, wooden, or even agate spatula can be used, but metal spatulas are not recommended, especially with fine particle composites, since the inorganic particles are abrasive and small amounts of the metal can be abraded and discolor the composite.

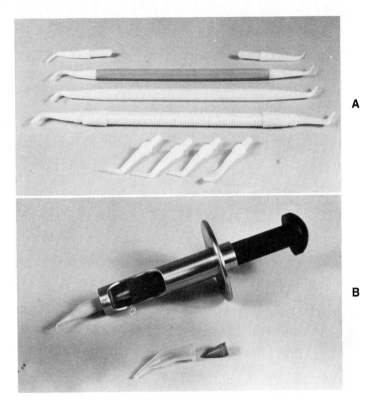

Fig. 4-8. A, Instruments for placement of composites. **B,** Syringe for injecting composites.

If the universal shade is to be altered, a small amount of the correct tint or other shade should be mixed with the universal paste *before* mixing it with the catalyst paste. The universal paste plus the tint will not set; thus time and care can be taken in arriving at the correct shade. Remember that an equal amount of catalyst paste will be added later and that it will dilute the color. Also note that the addition of the tint will increase the opacity of the set composite.

When the mixing of the universal and catalyst paste has been completed, the mix has a working (or insertion) time of 1 to 1½ minutes. The mix will begin to harden, and the material should not be disturbed from this time until the setting time of about 4 to 5 minutes from the start of the mix.

The mixed material may be inserted into the cavity preparation by several methods. It may be placed with plastic instruments, such as those shown in Fig. 4-8, *A,* which do not stick to the composite during insertion, and they avoid discoloration of the composite by metal instruments. The mixed material may also be placed in the plastic tip of a syringe, such as shown in Fig. 4-8, *B,* and then injected into the cavity preparation. The syringe allows the use of small mixes, reduces the problem of incorporating voids in the composite during insertion, and facilitates placement of the material in the areas of retention.

Various matrix materials have been used, such as polyester or polyethylene plastic strips, as well as foil-lined compound or wax pattern matrices. They should be placed immediately after insertion of the composite and held firmly in position for about 2 minutes. At this time, 3½ to 4 minutes from the start of the mix, the matrix may be removed, and initial contouring can be done readily with a sharp knife. At least 2 additional minutes should be allowed for the composite to become hard enough that final finishing can be started.

Gross reduction can be accomplished with diamonds, carbide finishing burs, finishing disks, or strips of zirconium silicate or alumina. Final finishing of either fine particle or microfilled composites is accomplished with abrasive-impregnated rubber rotary instruments or with a rubber cup and various polishing pastes. Finishing should be done in a wet field with a water-soluble lubricant. The final finishing can generally be started about 6 minutes after the start of the mixing.

Since the best final surface finish is the matrix finish, as little finishing as possible should be carried out. It is essentially impossible to obtain the proper contour without providing some excess, so it is especially important to use proper finishing methods. It may be necessary to refinish the composite restoration if staining occurs during service. If refinishing is required, the recommendations for final finishing should be followed.

Composites placed in Class III or V preparations, or in Class IV restorations with pins, generally are used in combination with enamel-bonding agents, which consist of unfilled dimethacrylate liquids that are polymerized by chemical activation. Bevels are placed on the peripheral enamel for a space of approximately 1 mm, and the enamel is etched with an acid solution, usually for 1 minute. The acid is flushed off, the preparation dried, and the bonding agent painted on the etched bevel. The restoration is then completed with the composite as described previously in this section.

Single-paste system. Composites activated with visible light are supplied as single pastes. The paste, available in many shades, is held in a syringe that contains all of the necessary ingredients, and the proper amount is dispensed and placed into the cavity preparation with an injection syringe or with instruments mentioned earlier. An example of a visible light used to activate polymerization of composites is shown in Fig. 4-9. The light source is usually a quartz-halogen bulb. Light is transmitted to the hose tip by a fiber-optic bundle or a fluid hose. Although the light is filtered to provide only blue light, one should not look directly at the tip or the reflected light from the enamel because of the high intensity. In addition, some lamps produce considerable heat, which can produce pulpal irritation. Too much heat is being generated if one cannot hold a finger 2 to 3 mm from the tip for 20 seconds.

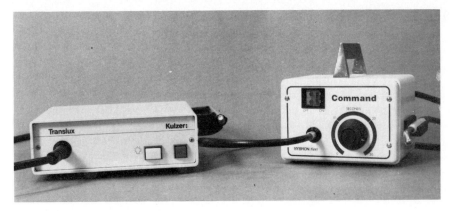

Fig. 4-9. Example of lamp for activating visible-light polymerizing composite.

Exposure times for polymerization vary depending on the type of lamp, the depth of the composite, and the type of the composite. Times may vary from 20 to 60 seconds for a restoration 3 mm thick. **Microfilled composites require longer exposure than fine particle composites because the small filler particles scatter the light more.** In deep restorations the composite may be added and polymerized in layers, with one layer bonding to another without any loss of strength.

Before the composite is inserted, exposed dentin may be protected with a cavity liner $[Ca(OH)_2]$ or a dentin bonding system may be used. The enamel is etched with an acid solution, and a bonding agent is applied and is polymerized by exposure to light. The proper amount of paste is placed in the cavity preparation, where the peripheral surfaces of enamel have been etched with a phosphoric acid solution. The instruments for placement and contouring should be nonmetallic. The material is exposed to visible light for the appropriate time. If the cavity preparation is large, the material should be placed in increments and each layer exposed to visible light. As soon as the exposure to light is completed, finishing may be started by methods described for the two-paste system.

The products described have been used to restore Class I, II, III, IV, and V restorations. Composites have been used for a variety of other applications, which are listed in Table 4-4.

Enamel-bonding agents. In the absence of an adequate chemical agent for permanently bonding composites to enamel, mechanical retention to acid-etched enamel is essential. The composites are highly viscous, and getting the composite to penetrate sufficiently into the etched areas to produce a good bond is often a problem. Enamel-bonding agents usually consist of a BIS-GMA system that has been diluted with dimethacrylates of lower molecular weight to decrease the viscosity. Also, the bonding agents contain little or no fillers, further reducing

Table 4-4. Other Applications of Composites and Associated Materials

Application	Type of material	Quality of viscosity	System
Enamel-bonding agents	Dimethacrylates with no filler Chemically activated or visible light-activated	Low	Liquid-liquid or single liquid
Restoration of incisal or cervical area	Dimethacrylate + filler Chemically activated or light-activated	Variable	Powder-liquid
Core buildups	Dimethacrylates + filler + colorant Chemically activated	High	Paste-paste
Temporary bridge construction	Dimethacrylates + filler Chemically activated	High	Paste-paste
Repair of porcelain or composite	Silanating agent followed by a variety of composites	Low	Liquid

the viscosity. If the bonding agents are chemically activated, they are supplied as two liquids, one containing the initiator and the other the accelerator. The material is mixed with equal amounts of the two liquids. Bonding agents are also available as a single liquid for light activation. Bonding agents for dentin function effectively as enamel-bonding agents.

After the area is acid etched, flushed with water, and dried, the bonding agent is applied in a thin layer to the etched area. After polymerization, the exposed surface is tacky because air inhibits the reaction. This tacky layer is an advantage and should not be removed.

The composite is applied on top of the bonding agent, and polymerization occurs between the composite and the bonding agent through the tacky layer.

Restoration of incisal or cervical area. Materials for applications to incisal or cervical areas are supplied as a powder and a liquid that can be mixed to a variety of consistencies. The powder is an inorganic filler, and the liquid is a diluted dimethacrylate. Greater translucency in the set material is obtained by using less powder. Materials are available that are chemically activated or visible light-activated.

Core buildups. In instances in which so much tooth structure has been lost that the crown of the tooth must be built up to receive a gold crown, composites have found application. The materials are typical two-paste composites that have been tinted gray, pink, or another color to provide a contrasting color with the tooth structure.

Temporary bridge construction. Temporary fixed bridges have been constructed by attaching a pontic to the adjacent teeth by using composites. A variety of technics are used, but they all involve acid etching of the enamel of the adjacent teeth and using a composite to bond the pontic to the teeth.

Repair of porcelain or composite. One of the main concerns in these repairs is the amount of bond strength between the remaining porcelain or composite and the added composite. To achieve the maximum bond strength, the remaining porcelain is cleaned and surface-treated with a silane supplied in a liquid form. The silane is an organic silicon compound that reacts with the porcelain and the newly placed composite. The silanating agent is supplied separately, and a composite of choice is used with it.

The repair of composites is accomplished in a similar manner. The remaining composite is freshened by abrading its surface, then keeping it well isolated from saliva and moisture. The surface of the composite is treated with silane, and the new composite is added, which may be either chemically activated or light-activated.

Clinical studies have shown that composites are superior materials for anterior restorations in which esthetics are essential and occlusal forces are low. Color changes are minimal, marginal adaptation good, and recurrent decay low. One problem with composites is the loss of surface contour as a result of abrasive and erosive wear. Disagreement between studies exists concerning whether microfilled composites wear faster than macrofilled composites. One difficulty in evaluating many of the clinical studies dealing with this subject is that, at the time the studies were started, anterior composites were used in posterior teeth because products especially designed for posterior applications did not exist. Clinical studies using posterior composites have shown mixed results.

Currently accepted composites for posterior applications require clinical studies that demonstrate over a 5-year period a loss of surface contour less than 250 μm or an average of 50 μm per year of clinical service. In general, the fine particle composites have better wear resistance than the microfilled composites.

Current composites can be classified as (1) fine particle, (2) microfilled, and (3) hybrid based on the particle size and distribution of the filler. The trend has been toward the hybrid composites that contain mostly fine filler particles plus some microfiller particles. These composites permit high concentrations of filler that can be polished to a smooth surface. Both BIS-GMA and UDMA oligomers are used, with a trend toward the latter, which has lower water sorption. Currently, most composites are polymerized using blue light to initiate the reaction and thus are single-paste systems supplied in syringes or compules; two-paste systems are still available and are used mainly for core buildups. Although composites were initially introduced as anterior restorative materials, they have been modified for use as posterior restorations. Graded sized fillers have allowed the volume fraction of filler to be increased, as well as the wear resistance. Postcuring of the composites, using an indirect procedure, has also increased the wear resistance and improved the quality of proximal contacts. Dentin bonding agents function well as enamel-bonding agents and thus are used for both. However, chemical bonding of composites to tooth structure still is inadequate, and acid etching of enamel and retentive cavity preparations are required.

IONOMER RESTORATIVES

Ionomers are supplied as powders of various shades and a liquid. Two commercial products are shown in Fig. 4-10, one in which the powder and the liquid are in bottles and the other in which the powder and the liquid are in predispensed capsules. The powder is an aluminosilicate glass, and the liquid is a water solution of polymers and copolymers of acrylic acid.

The powder and liquid are dispensed in proper amounts on the paper pad, and half the powder is incorporated to produce a homogeneous milky consistency. The remainder of the powder is added, and a total mixing time of 30 to 40 seconds is used with a typical setting time of 4 minutes. **After placing the restorative and carving the correct contour, the surface should be protected from saliva by an application of varnish.** Trimming and finishing is done after 24 hours.

The liquid in the predispensed capsule is forced into the powder by using the press (Fig. 4-10, *B*) and is mixed by using a mechanical amalgamator (see Chapter 5). The mixture is injected through the use of the special syringe (Fig. 4-10, *B*).

The material sets as a result of the metallic salt bridges between the Al^{+3} and Ca^{+2} ions and the acid groups on the polymers. The reaction goes to completion slowly and is protected from saliva with a varnish.

The properties of ionomer restoratives are listed in Table 4-5. Properties especially noteworthy are a modulus that is similar to dentin, a bond strength to dentin of 300 to 400 lb/in^2, an expansion coefficient comparable to tooth structure, low solubility, and fairly high opacity. The opacity varies for different products from values of 88%, which are similar to composites, to nearly complete opaqueness at 99%.

Clinical studies have shown that the retention of ionomers in areas of cervical erosion are considerably better than for composites. Examples of cervical erosion and ionomer restorations are shown in Fig. 4-11, *A* and *B*. When the dentin is etched with a citric acid solution, the ionomer may be used without a cavity preparation. If a rim of enamel is available, acid etching of it is recommended to provide additional retention of the ionomer restorative. Four-year clinical data showed a retention rate for ionomer cervical restorations of 75%. The surfaces of the restorations seen in the studies were noticeably rough, and some shade

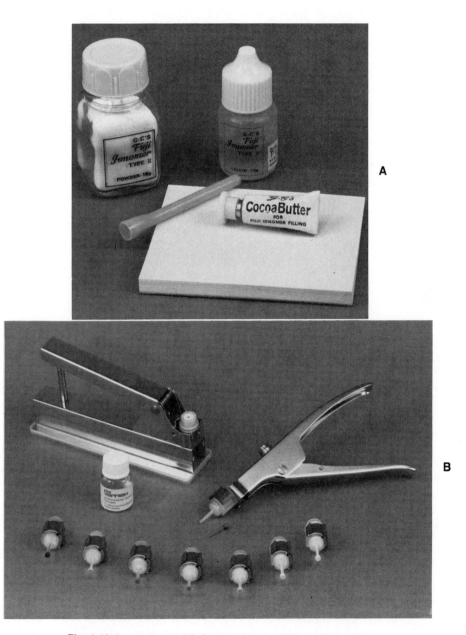

Fig. 4-10. Ionomer materials for restoring cervically eroded teeth.

Table 4-5. Properties of Ionomers for Restoration of Cervically Eroded Areas

Property	Ionomer
Inorganic content (% by weight)	63-66
Compressive strength (psi [MN/m²])	16,000-22,000 (110-150)
Tensile strength (psi [MN/m²])	1450-2200 (10-15)
Modulus of elasticity (psi [MN/m²])	2,900,000 (20,000)
Indentation resistance of ½ -inch steel ball under 30-kg load (inches [μm])	0.0022 (53-57)
Recovery from indentation (%)	69-74
Bond strength to dentin (psi [MN/m²])	300-400 (2-3)
Abrasive wear (mm³/mm × 10⁻⁴)	15
Linear coefficient of expansion (/° C × 10⁻⁶)	10-11
Solubility (% in 24 hours)	0.3-0.5
Opacity (%)	88-99

Modified from Powers JM, Fan PL, Hostetler RW: *J Mich State Dent Assoc* 63:275, 1981.

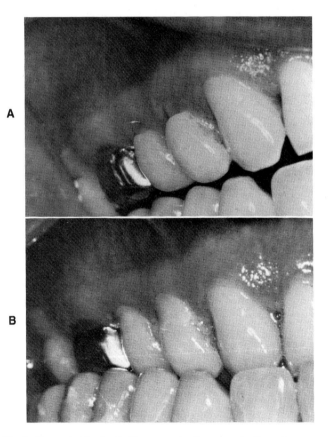

Fig. 4-11. A, Cervically eroded teeth. **B,** The same teeth restored with an ionomer restorative material. (Courtesy Dr. LW Seluk, Plymouth, Mich.)

mismatches were present. Pulp reaction to ionomers was mild and comparable to that of zinc polyacrylate cement; however, the cervical restorations did not contribute to inflammation of gingival tissues.

Clinical technic for ionomers must be adhered to rigidly, with maintenance of isolation, adequate etching procedures, protection of the restoration from saliva after placement, and delay of final finishing for 1 day or longer.

Glass ionomers have also been used in limited applications as pit and fissure sealants, although the viscosity of the mixes is adjusted so they will flow into the fine crevices.

Self-test questions

In the following multiple choice questions, one or more of the responses may be correct.

1 Which of these statements apply to the particle size of fillers in composites?
  a. Fine particle fillers range from 8 to 25 µm.
  b. Microfillers range from 0.4 to 2 µm.
  c. Reinforced microfillers range from 100 to 200 µm.
  d. Fine particle fillers range from 0.5 to 5 µm.

2 Which statements are true for the amount of inorganic filler in composites?
  a. Fine particle composites contain about 77 weight percent.
  b. Microfilled composites contain about 25 volume percent.
  c. Fine particle composites contain about 60 volume percent.
  d. Microfilled composites contain about 38 weight percent.

3 Which of the composites with the following fillers may be radiopaque?
  a. Quartz
  b. Lithium aluminum silicate
  c. Colloidal silica
  d. Barium glass

4 Which of the following polymer systems are used for the organic matrix in composites?
  a. Bisphenol A-glycidyl methacrylate (BIS-GMA)
  b. Polymethyl methacrylate
  c. Urethane dimethacrylate (UDMA)
  d. Polystyrene

5 Which of the following initiator-accelerator systems is needed for a light-activated composite?
  a. Peroxide-amine
  b. Diketone-amine
  c. Organic acid-peroxide
  d. Organic acid-metal ion

6 Which of the following properties are higher for fine particle composites than for microfilled composites?
  a. Polymerization shrinkage
  b. Thermal expansion

    c. Water sorption

    d. Modulus

    e. Abrasive wear

7 With respect to the finishing of composites, which of the following statements are true?

    a. The matrix finish produced against a Mylar strip is smoother than the final finish produced with a fine particle composite.

    b. The final finish produced with a microfilled composite is equally smooth as a Mylar matrix finish.

    c. The smoothest final finish possible with a fine particle composite is with Sof-Lex fine polishing paste.

8 With respect to the wear of composites, which of the following statements are correct?

    a. Wear of composites in the mouth is only related to loss of contour from abrasive conditions.

    b. Fine particle and microfilled composites are equally resistant to abrasive wear.

    c. Erosive wear is only a problem with fine particle composites and not with the microfilled type.

    d. Wear resistance of composites is sufficiently low that they cannot be recommended for posterior applications.

9 Which of the following statements about acid-etched composite restorations are true?

    a. Bonding is achieved by application of an acid etchant to enamel, usually followed by application of a bonding agent and then the composite resin.

    b. The bonding agent bonds chemically to the enamel and composite resin.

    c. The bonding agent forms a mechanical bond with enamel but a chemical bond with composite resin.

10 Which of the following statements about the mixing of a two-paste composite are true?

    a. Plastic, wooden, or metal spatulas should be used.

    b. Care must be taken to dispense the base paste first, followed by the catalyst paste with the spatula.

    c. Equal amounts of the two pastes are mixed thoroughly in about 20 to 30 seconds.

    d. Any tinting should be added after mixing of the two pastes is completed.

11 Which of the following statements are true for visible light-activated composites?

    a. The working time is about 2 to 3 minutes after correct mixing is completed.

    b. Yellow light is essential to initiate polymerization.

    c. No mixing is required for these composites.

    d. Larger exposure times to light are required for polymerization of microfilled composites compared with fine particle composites.

12 Which of these statements apply to the indirect technic for preparing composites?

    a. Postcuring increases the extent of polymerization.

    b. Postcuring increases the wear resistance.

    c. A nonretentive cavity preparation is required.

    d. It allows better development of proximal contacts.

13 Which of the following statements apply to ionomer restorations?
 a. The powder is an aluminosilicate glass, and the liquid is a low-viscosity BIS-GMA polymer.
 b. The material is not water soluble, and thus isolation from saliva is not critical.
 c. They have higher bond strength to dentin than composites.
 d. They have higher elastic modulus values than composites.
 e. Finishing may be satisfactorily done at the first appointment.

Suggested supplementary readings

Craig RG: Chemistry, composition, and properties of composite resins, *Dent Clin North Am* 25:219, 1981.

Farah JW, Powers JM, editors: Composites, *Dent Advis* 1(2): 1, 1984.

Herrgott AML, Ziemiecki TL, Dennison JB: An evaluation of different composite resin systems finished with various abrasives, *J Am Dent Assoc* 119:729, 1989.

Horn HR, editor: *The dental clinics of North America symposium on composite resins in dentistry,* Philadelphia, 1981, WB Saunders.

Jones DW: Composite restorative materials, *J Canad Dent Assoc* 56:851, 1990.

Letzel H: Survival rates and reasons for failure of posterior composite restorations in multicentre clinical trial, *J Dent* 17:S10, 1989.

Powers JM, Fan PL, Hostetler RW: Properties of Class V restorative materials, *J Mich State Dent Assoc* 63:275, 1981.

chapter
five

Dental Amalgam

Dental amalgam is an alloy that results when mercury is combined with an alloy containing silver, tin, copper, and sometimes zinc. This reaction is indicated as follows:

$$Mercury + Silver\ alloy \rightarrow Dental\ amalgam$$

The silver alloy powder is commercially produced as small spherical or comminuted (irregular) particles. It is reacted with mercury in the dental office to produce dental amalgam.

Amalgams are alloys of mercury with other metals.

The freshly mixed mass of amalgam has a plasticity that permits it to be conveniently packed or condensed into a cavity prepared in a tooth. Amalgam restorations usually are limited to the replacement of tooth tissue in posterior teeth and are recognized by their silvery gray metallic appearance. Amalgam accounts for a significant portion of all dental restorations. Amalgam will continue to be used until more esthetic restoratives that can function in stress-bearing areas are developed.

MERCURY

Mercury is a dense liquid metal that is highly toxic. Mercury of high purity possesses a shiny surface. The formation of a thick scum indicates that contamination has occurred and is reason to replace the mercury.

If mercury is improperly handled in the dental office, a health hazard may result from (1) systemic absorption of liquid mercury through the skin, (2) inhalation of mercury vapor, and (3) inhalation of airborne particles. Simple precautions, however, can permit the safe use of mercury. It should not be handled in the palm or with the fingers. Because small droplets of mercury have a high vapor pressure that increases with the temperature, spills should be cleaned up,* particularly in offices with baseboard heating. The possible inhalation of airborne droplets of mercury can be greatly reduced if the capsules in which the amalgam is mixed are replaced when old or damaged. Care should be exercised in handling mercury so that it does not come in contact with articles made of precious metals, such as rings and other jewelry.

Studies of the ambient mercury levels in dental offices have revealed that in most of the offices the levels of mercury vapor are below the maximum safe environmental concentration of mercury vapor in air of 0.05 mg Hg/m^3 of air in the breathing zone for a 40-hour week. In a recent survey of 1555 dentists, 99% displayed blood mercury values of less than 30 ng Hg/ml of blood. These blood mercury values were well below those of 100 ng Hg/ml for which typical symptoms of inorganic mercury poisoning have been seen. Gross spillage of mercury has been identified as the most significant factor causing high levels of mercury vapor in air.

Studies reporting the level of mercury vapor in the breath of patients with amalgam restorations after chewing gum have caused concern. The levels reported were sometimes greater than 0.05 mg Hg/m^3. However, these values are *not* time weighted, and recent studies have shown that patients with numerous amalgams injest about 0.001 mg of Hg/day, which is well below the safe environmental level. The injestion of Hg from dental amalgam is less than that from food, water, and the atmosphere of about 0.005, 0.001 and 0.0005 mg/day, respectively.

The American Dental Association (ADA) has recommended certain procedures for the handling of mercury. **Single-use capsules containing a measured amount of mercury and alloy are recommended.** These capsules eliminate mercury dispensers and possible spillage. Mercury and amalgam scrap should be stored in capped, unbreakable jars that hold water containing finely divided sulfur. Mercury has a high vapor pressure and should be stored in a cool place. Baseboard heaters should be avoided, since spills collect at the edges of rooms and the higher temperature at the baseboard will raise the mercury vapor level above the safe limit. Carpeting of operatories is not recommended to avoid absorption of any spilled mercury. A no-touch technic of handling mercury should be used. Water spray and high-volume evacuation should be used when removing old amalgam restorations or finishing new ones, since heating releases some mercury vapor. A face mask should be used to avoid breathing amalgam dust (or any other metal dust). Ultrasonic condensers should not be used to avoid

---

*A convenient way to reduce the health hazard of spilled mercury is to swab the floor of the office with a chemical marketed as Mercury Hg Absorb (Science Related Materials, Inc., Thomas Scientific).

mercury vapor release. The ADA also recommends regular monitoring of the mercury vapor levels in operatories and offices and provides a urine analysis service to its members. **A small but possible risk to the patient from mercury is an allergic reaction, which usually manifests as a skin reaction that appears after placement of the amalgam restoration.** Prevention involves including questions regarding allergic reactions to metals in the medical history.

Mercury is generally supplied in 1-pound unbreakable plastic containers. Because of its high density (13.6 gm/cm^3), mercury in a bottle is deceptively heavy; therefore mercury dispensers should be handled with care. Mercury should be chosen from products certified by the ADA to meet or exceed properties listed in the American National Standards Institute (ANSI) and the ADA Specification No. 6 for dental mercury.

SILVER ALLOYS FOR DENTAL AMALGAMS

Low-copper alloys are available as **comminuted particles (lathe-cut and pulverized) and spherical particles,** and high-copper alloys (now the most common type) are supplied as **spherical, comminuted, or combinations (admixed) of particles.** The general compositions of low-copper and high-copper alloys are listed in Table 5-1. Among the comminuted alloys, both zinc and zinc-free alloys are available. The lathe-cut particles are shown in Fig. 5-1, *A,* and spherical particles are shown in Fig. 5-1, *B.* The comminuted particles are available in various sizes such as fine-cut and microcut. The admixed alloys are mixtures of spherical and comminuted particles, as shown in Fig. 5-1, *C.* The original admixed alloys were known as "dispersed phase alloys" (e.g., Dispersalloy) and consisted of a mixture of a comminuted traditional silver alloy and spherical particles of the silver-copper **eutectic** alloy.

A eutectic alloy is made up of elements that when solid are insoluble and form a layered structure.

Table 5-1. Composition of Silver Alloys for Dental Amalgam

Type		Approximate percentage of composition by weight
Low-copper	Silver	65-72
	Tin	26-29
	Copper	2-4
	Zinc	Up to 2
High-copper	Silver	40-60
	Tin	27-30
	Copper	13-30

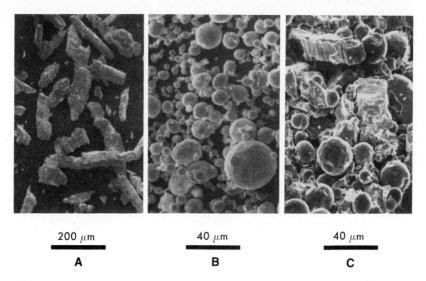

200 μm   40 μm   40 μm

A   **B**   **C**

Fig. 5-1. Micrographs of alloy particles. **A,** Comminuted. **B,** Spherical. **C,** Admixed with comminuted and spherical particles.

AMALGAMATION

The two main types of amalgam alloy compositions are silver-tin alloys with and without significant amounts of copper. The setting reactions with mercury are different. The silver-tin alloys with low copper form a silver-mercury phase and a weak tin-mercury **phase.** However, the high-copper alloys eliminate the tin-mercury phase by forming a copper-tin phase resulting in superior properties.

A phase is an identifiable region of distinct composition.

The reaction that occurs between mercury and amalgam alloy is called **amalgamation.** More specifically, the chemical reaction of a comminuted or spherical low-copper alloy is the following:

Mercury + Silver-tin alloy (excess) → Silver-tin phase (unreacted) +
Silver-mercury phase + Tin-mercury phase

The silver-tin phase is called the **gamma** (γ) **phase** and is composed of the unreacted alloy particles. The silver-mercury phase is called **gamma-1** (γ_1), whereas the tin-mercury phase is called **gamma-2** (γ_2). Because amalgamation is a surface reaction, amalgam can be thought of as particles of γ surrounded by, or bonded together by, a continuous matrix of γ_1 and γ_2. The manipulation and properties of amalgam are determined by the relative amount of each phase.

The hardening of amalgam is the result of two phenomenon—solution and crystallization. When mercury initially comes into contact with the alloy, the particles are wet by the mercury and they begin to absorb it. The diffusion of mercury into the alloy particles leads to the formation at their surfaces of silver-mercury and tin-mercury phases. It is the crystallization of the γ_1, and γ_2 phases and their subsequent growth that cause amalgam to harden.

The setting reaction of the high-copper alloys forms a copper-tin phase, rather than a tin-mercury phase, as shown in the following:

Mercury + Silver-tin-copper → Silver-mercury + Copper-tin + Silver-tin-copper (unreacted alloy)

Since the tin-mercury (γ_2) phase is weak and corrodes easily, its elimination leads to an amalgam restoration with superior properties. The original dispersed alloys containing the silver-copper eutectic formed the tin-mercury (γ_2) phase initially, which in turn was eliminated by a reaction with copper to form the copper-tin alloy. The final result with all high-copper alloys is an amalgam with the superior properties that result from the elimination of the tin-mercury (γ_2) phase.

It should be clearly understood from the preceding discussion that once amalgamation occurs, for all practical purposes, no free (unreacted) mercury is associated with the amalgam restoration. The mercury in an amalgam is alloyed with silver or tin and no longer has the toxic properties of unreacted mercury. If, however, amalgam is heated beyond approximately 80° C, liquid mercury can form on the surface of the amalgam, and its vapor can present a health hazard.

PROPERTIES

The clinical behavior of an amalgam restoration is based on the properties developed by the amalgam as a result of its manipulation. Properties of clinical importance include dimensional change, strength, creep, tarnish, and corrosion.

Dimensional change

As amalgam hardens, dimensional changes occur that may cause the amalgam to expand or contract, depending on its manipulation. Either expansion or contraction, if excessive, is undesirable. Too much expansion in a Class I preparation can result in postoperative sensitivity in the tooth or a protrusion of the restoration from the cavity. Excessive contraction in a Class I preparation can cause the amalgam to pull away from the cavity walls and permit leakage to occur. The current ANSI–ADA Specification No. 1 for alloy for dental amalgam states that at the end of 24 hours the dimensional change (either expansion or contraction) should be no more than 20 micrometers*/centimeter (μm/cm).

---

*1 μm = 0.00004 inch.

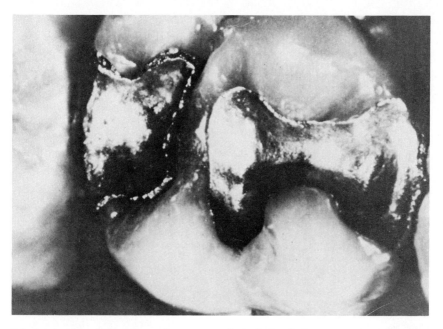

Fig. 5-2. Amalgam restoration from a low-copper spherical alloy *(left)* and an amalgam from a high-copper admixed alloy *(right)* after 3 years of service. (Courtesy Dr. GT Charbeneau, University of Michigan School of Dentistry, Ann Arbor, Mich.)

Improper manipulation of amalgam can lead to excessive dimensional change as a result of either excessive solution or excessive crystallization. The diffusion of mercury into alloy particles causes a contraction or decreased expansion, whereas the growth of γ_1 and γ_2 causes an expansion. Normally both dimensional changes occur, but they compensate for each other, with the result that the net dimensional change is not excessive.

Strength

Amalgam does not develop sufficient strength to resist the forces of mastication without proper enamel support. For this reason the cavity should be designed (if possible) to provide a certain bulk of amalgam wherever stress may be applied. In addition, the manipulation of amalgam should be done properly. Insufficient strength in amalgam may be manifested by marginal breakdown, as shown in Fig. 5-2. A summary of properties measuring the strength of five types of amalgam is shown in Table 5-2.

The strength of amalgam is determined by the presence of the γ, γ_1, and γ_2 phases and by voids. Studies have given the following information on the relative strength of these four phases: (1) the unreacted alloy particle (γ) is the

Table 5-2. Properties of Five Types of Amalgam

Property	Type of amalgam				
	Comminuted low-copper	Comminuted high-copper	Admixed high-copper	Spherical low-copper	Spherical high-copper
Dimensional change (μm/cm)	8	5	-3	2	-5
30-minute compressive strength					
(MPa)	53	59	67	105	111
(psi)	7680	8550	9710	15,200	16,100
1-hour compressive strength					
(MPa)	89	97	109	169	188
(psi)	12,900	14,100	15,800	24,500	27,300
1-day compressive strength					
(MPa)	430	477	402	341	451
(psi)	62,300	69,200	58,300	49,400	65,400
Tensile strength					
(MPa)	52	45	50	50	54
(psi)	7540	6520	7250	7250	7830
Creep (%)	2.05	0.17	0.44	0.79	0.15
Knoop hardness, kg/mm^2	146	174	143	106	166

Adapted from Greener EH, Vrijhoef MMA: Dental amalgams. In O'Brien WJ, ed: *Dental materials: properties and selection,* Chicago, 1989, Quintessence.

strongest phase of hardened amalgam, and (2) the silver-mercury phase is the second strongest, followed by (3) the tin-mercury phase and (4) voids. Thus manipulative technics should be followed that result in sufficient formation of matrix to bond together the unreacted particles and to reduce the presence of voids, the most influential parameter in reducing strength. The compressive strength of amalgams made from admixed or spherical high-copper alloys is superior to that of the comminuted or spherical low-copper amalgams because of the elimination of the weak γ_2 phase. The current ANSI–ADA Specification No. 1 requires that amalgam made from a certified alloy have a compressive strength of at least 11,600 psi (80 MN/m^2 or 80 MPa) after 1 hour. **The tensile strength of dental amalgams is substantially less than the compressive strength** (Table 5-2). The substantially higher tensile strength at 1 hour for the spherical amalgams should be noted.

The rate at which amalgam develops strength is an important clinical characteristic. If an amalgam restoration is subjected to forces of mastication too soon after insertion, it may be seriously damaged by being sufficiently overloaded to cause fracture of the amalgam mass. The development of compressive strength of comminuted, spherical low-copper, admixed, and spherical high-copper types of amalgam is compared in Table 5-2 for times of 30 minutes, 1 hour, and 1 day.

Comminuted and spherical low-copper amalgams have particularly poor resistance to marginal fracture. The term **edge strength** has been applied to this property. The result of marginal fracture is an increased susceptibility to corrosion and marginal leakage. Recent clinical and laboratory studies have shown that the resistance of amalgam to marginal fracture can be indicated by measurement of the creep. The admixed and spherical high-copper amalgams have low values of creep and superior resistance to marginal fracture clinically.

Creep

The **creep** of amalgam is a dimensional change that occurs under load as a result of the viscoelastic properties of amalgam. Excessive creep that occurs under normal masticatory forces results in distorted cuspal portions of the restoration or in an increased incidence of marginal fracture, as already discussed. Creep of a 7-day-old specimen under a static stress of 36 MN/m^2 at 37° C is a property tested in the ANSI–ADA specification for dental amalgam alloys. The maximum value of creep allowed for a certified product is 3% between 1 and 4 hours after specimen loading. Values of creep of several types of amalgam are compared in Table 5-2.

> **Creep is the gradual flow of a material under an applied stress.**

Tarnish and corrosion

Amalgam restorations are subject to the effects of **tarnish** and **corrosion** when exposed to conditions present in the oral cavity. Slight tarnish or corrosion that results in a discolored restoration is often not objectionable. In their later stages, however, tarnish and corrosion can lead to an unesthetic restoration and may even cause the restoration to fail by altering its mechanical properties. The rate of failure of amalgam restorations by processes of tarnish and corrosion can be greatly reduced by using a careful finishing and polishing sequence. A comparison of corroded and polished amalgam restorations is shown in Fig. 5-3.

> **Tarnish is surface discoloration. Corrosion is loss of surface caused by chemical attack.**

Tarnish, which was discussed in Chapter 2, is a deposit of surface film that produces a discoloration. The film may be from sulfide formation or may be a hard or soft deposit such as calculus or plaque that becomes darker the longer it remains on the surface of the restoration. Tarnish is more likely to occur on amalgams that are poorly polished and that provide a retentive surface. The discoloration resulting from tarnish can be easily removed by polishing procedures.

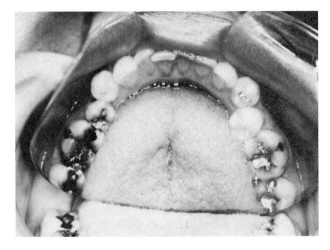

Fig. 5-3. Comparison of corroded *(left)* and polished amalgam restorations *(right)*. (Courtesy Dr. GT Charbeneau, University of Michigan School of Dentistry, Ann Arbor, Mich.)

Corrosion, which was also discussed in Chapter 2, is a surface and subsurface deterioration of the restoration by chemical or electrochemical action. Tin hydroxychloride has been identified as a corrosion product. Chemical corrosion also is likely to occur on poorly polished amalgams, in which case pits and scratches on the surface act to entrap debris that attacks the amalgam. Electrochemical corrosion occurs where dissimilar metallic restorations such as gold and amalgam on adjacent teeth come into contact. Unlike tarnish, the process of corrosion can take place beneath the surface of the amalgam, thereby weakening the restoration and possibly causing fracture to occur.

Of the three phases present in amalgam, the γ_2 phase is most susceptible to corrosion, followed by γ and then the γ_1 phase. **Manipulation of amalgam to minimize the formation of the γ_2 phase is therefore desirable.** The admixed and spherical high-copper amalgams are less susceptible to corrosion than the comminuted and spherical low-copper amalgams, which contain a continuous γ_2 phase.

MANIPULATION

The clinical success of most amalgam restorations is highly dependent on the correct manipulation of the alloy. If an established technic is strictly adhered to, the properties of amalgam made from modern alloys are adequate. The following areas of manipulation are discussed to explain the role of manipulation in obtaining optimum properties of dental amalgam: selection of product, proportioning of mercury and alloy, methods of mixing, factors in mixing, condensation, and finishing.

Table 5-3. Examples of Commercial Silver Alloys for Amalgams

Product	Manufacturer
Spherical type	
Indiloy	Shofu Dental
Sybraloy	Kerr Manufacturing
Tytin	Kerr Manufacturing
Admixed type	
Contour	Kerr Manufacturing
Dispersalloy	Johnson & Johnson
Valiant PH.D.	L.D. Caulk

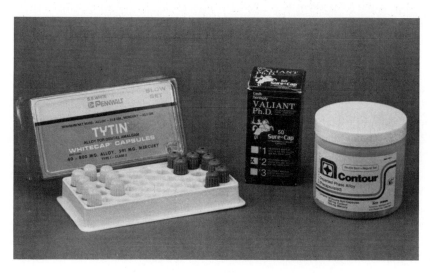

Fig. 5-4. Examples of silver alloys for dental amalgams.

Selection of product

The selection of a particular amalgam should be based on the clinical requirements of the restoration and the physical and mechanical properties of the amalgam. For restorations subjected to occlusal forces, for example, an amalgam with high resistance to marginal fracture would be desirable. Handling characteristics are often important in the selection of a product also. A list of a few alloys is given in Table 5-3. Amalgam alloy should be chosen from products certified to meet or exceed the properties listed in ANSI–ADA Specification No. 1 for dental amalgam alloy.

The particles of alloy are prepared for packaging in two basic forms: powder and tablets (Fig. 5-4). The manufacturer can form both comminuted and spherical powders into tablets. The tablets are supplied either in bulk or in plastic

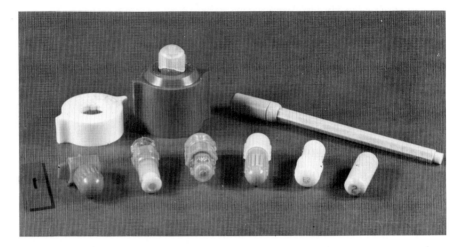

Fig. 5-5. Various commercial disposable capsules containing amalgam alloy and mercury.

tubes that are inserted conveniently into the manufacturer's alloy dispenser. The powdered alloys are supplied either in bulk packages containing 284 gm (10 ounces) of alloy or now most commonly in a disposable capsule that contains enough alloy and mercury for a single or a double mix (Fig. 5-5). In the disposable capsule, the alloy and mercury are kept separate by a thin membrane of plastic before use. This latter form of packaging is convenient and accurate but is more expensive.

Proportioning of mercury and alloy

The amount of mercury and alloy that is to be mixed is described by the mercury-alloy ratio. A mercury-alloy ratio of 1:1, for example, would indicate that 1 part of mercury is to be mixed with 1 part of alloy by weight. If the amount of mercury were represented as a percentage of the total weight, a mercury-alloy ratio of 1:1 would indicate a mix with 50% mercury. The mercury-alloy ratio is used most commonly when determining the proper setting of a volumetric dispenser of mercury. Several mercury dispensers are shown in Fig. 5-6.

The mercury-alloy ratio is a unique characteristic of a particular amalgam alloy. The mercury must wet the alloy particles before the two components can react. The physical process of wetting of an alloy by mercury is dependent on a number of factors, such as alloy composition, surface condition, and particle size and shape. These factors are different for every alloy; therefore the manufacturer's recommended mercury-alloy ratio should be followed. Comminuted, spherical low-copper, and admixed alloys commonly require 46% to 54% mer-

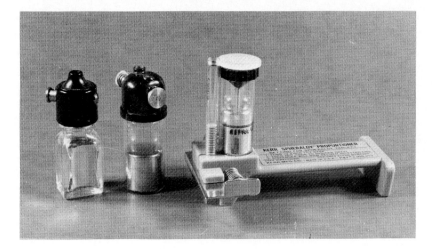

Fig. 5-6. Mercury dispensers. The dispenser on the right also serves as a tablet dispenser.

cury for proper mixing, whereas the spherical high-copper alloys require as little as 43% mercury. The spherical low-copper alloys generally require less mercury for mixing than do the comminuted alloys.

Mercury is most commonly dispensed by volume. Because mercury is a liquid, it can be dispensed accurately if the dispenser is used properly. It should be held vertically and kept at least half full to ensure uniform spills. If the mercury in the dispenser becomes contaminated, the dispenser should be cleaned and the mercury replaced. The contaminated mercury can be recycled by returning it to the manufacturer.

Powdered alloy in bulk form may be dispensed by either weight or volume. The volumetric dispensers are generally accurate if the manufacturer's operating instructions are followed. Because this type of dispenser is gauged to the particle size and shape of a particular alloy, proper dispensing may not be obtained with other alloys.

From clinical observations it has been determined that the mass of amalgam necessary for an average restoration can be produced from a double mix (about 800 mg of alloy mixed with the proper amount of mercury). Mixes that are oversized or undersized in relation to the particular container in which they are mixed may not be properly amalgamated and thus may have inferior properties. When larger quantities of amalgam are required, more than one mix is preferable. When smaller quantities are desired, a single mix (about 600 mg of alloy) can be made and the unused portion sacrificed. Scrap amalgam can be recycled by the alloy manufacturers or by various refining companies.

Methods of mixing

Mechanical amalgamators are used to **triturate** amalgam alloy and mercury; examples of mechanical amalgamators are listed in Table 5-4 and are shown in Fig. 5-7. These units contain a timing device that measures a desired interval of time, after which the motor is stopped. The alloy and mercury are placed in a plastic capsule that is rotated eccentrically or with a reciprocating motion during trituration. Often a small rod or pellet made of metal or plastic, known as a **pestle,** is included in the capsule to improve the mixing and to shorten the mixing time. The pestle is required in the

> Trituration is the process of mixing mercury with the amalgam alloy.

Table 5-4. Examples of Motor-Driven Amalgamators

Product	Manufacturer
Medium-speed	
Capmaster	Mission White Dental
Wig-L-Bug DS-80	Crescent Dental Manufacturing
Variable speed	
Vari-Mix II	L.D. Caulk
Wig-L-Bug LP-602E	Crescent Dental Manufacturing
High-speed	
Silamat	Vivadent

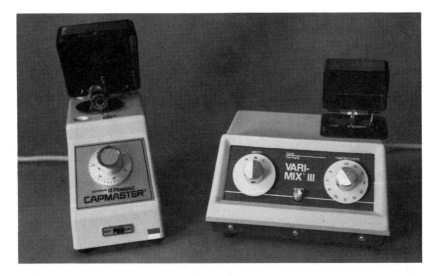

Fig. 5-7. Mechanical amalgamators for triturating amalgam. (From Craig RG: *Restorative dental materials,* ed 8, St. Louis, 1989, Mosby–Year Book.)

capsule if an alloy tablet is to be amalgamated, although it may be omitted if a powdered alloy is used.

The operating speed of different mechanical amalgamators varies. Both medium- and high-speed units, as well as variable-speed units, are available. Because of the differences in speed, the operating performance of all amalgamators is not identical for a given alloy and mercury combination. **Not only must the correct mixing time be chosen with a particular unit, but the proper capsule and pestle also must be determined for the type of alloy to be triturated.**

Contamination of a freshly mixed amalgam mass by hardened amalgam can readily occur if the capsule and pestle are not cleaned thoroughly after each mix. In addition, capsules should be replaced periodically, since the interior surfaces of capsules become scarred from the abrasive action of the alloy particles during trituration. Worn capsules leak mercury during trituration and can present a health hazard in the dental operatory. Of the various reusable capsules, those having screw-type caps best prevent leaking of droplets of mercury during trituration. Two types of reusable capsules are shown in Fig. 5-8. The disposable capsules should not be reused.

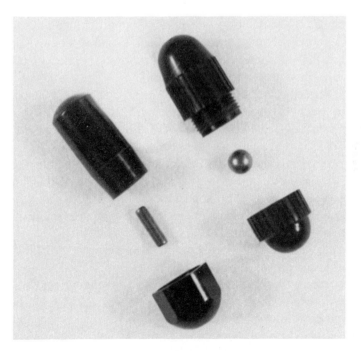

Fig. 5-8. Types of capsules and pestles used with mechanical amalgamators. (From Craig RG: *Restorative dental materials,* ed 8, St. Louis, 1989, Mosby–Year Book.)

Factors in mixing

Trituration. The quality of an amalgam mass is controlled by the factors of time, speed, and force applied during trituration. These interrelated factors determine the work of trituration, factors that must remain constant from one mixing operation to another if uniform results are expected for a given alloy and mercury combination. Controlling these factors requires an understanding of the performance of the mechanical amalgamator.

The time of trituration is the easiest factor to vary and will range from 6 to 20 seconds for different combinations of alloy and mercury, speed and action of the amalgamator, weight of the pestle and size of the capsule, and size of the mix. For example, the time of trituration for a disposable capsule mixed on a variable-speed amalgamator (medium setting) might vary from 10 to 20 seconds for a comminuted or spherical low-copper alloy, but from 6 to 10 seconds for a spherical high-copper alloy. If available, the manufacturer's recommendations should be followed as a guideline for determining the proper mixing time for a particular situation. Variations of 2 to 3 seconds from the ideal mixing time are sufficient to produce what might be considered an overmixed or undermixed mass. Increasing the size of the mix can dramatically increase the time necessary for trituration.

As was mentioned, the speed and action of amalgamators vary. Speed can be controlled only on the variable-speed units, although the medium setting is normally used. As an amalgamator becomes worn, however, changes in speed occur that are sufficient to alter the degree of trituration. For this reason the efficiency of a unit must be periodically checked.

The force applied during mechanical amalgamation is a function of the weight of the pestle, the size of the capsule, and the design of both. Pestles frequently vary in weight from 0.2 to over 1 gm. The manufacturer's recommendations for the selection of a capsule and pestle should be followed.

Undermix, normal mix, and overmix. Variations in the conditions of trituration of alloy and mercury can lead to undermixing, normal mixing, and overmixing. These three mixes have different appearances (Fig. 5-9), respond differently to subsequent operations of manipulation, and have characteristically different properties.

The undermixed mass is dull in appearance and crumbly, making it inconvenient to manipulate during insertion. Of greater importance is the reduction in strength observed in undermixed amalgams. The undermixed mass may be considered synonymous with a mass that is underworked. The conditions of trituration should be changed accordingly.

The normal-mixed mass responds well to subsequent operations of insertion into the cavity and requires only a minimum of mulling to develop a smooth, homogeneous mass. The normally mixed mass is shiny in appearance. Its

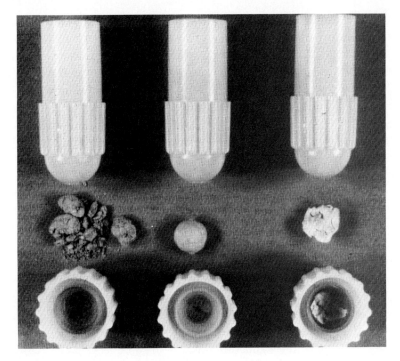

Fig. 5-9. Amalgam. *Left,* Undermixed; *center,* normal mixed; *right,* overmixed. (Courtesy Dr. K Asgar, University of Michigan School of Dentistry, Ann Arbor, Mich.)

strength is less than that of the overmixed mass for comminuted alloys but is higher than the overmixed mass for spherical alloys. However, the normal mix can be managed with greater ease during condensation into the cavity.

The overmixed mass is difficult to remove from the capsule and pestle. It has a soupy appearance and is difficult to handle because it has little tendency to hold its form. The overmixed mass may be considered synonymous with an overworked mass.

Condensation

The objectives of condensation are adaptation of the amalgam to prepared cavity walls, matrix (if used), and margins; development of a uniform, compact mass with minimum voids; and reduction of excess mercury content. Triturated comminuted alloys contain a higher mercury concentration than spherical alloys, and as much excess mercury as possible should be removed during condensation using adequate force on the appropriate condenser. Spherical alloys are mixed with less mercury (42% to 46%), and less or no excess mercury is removed during condensation; lower condensation force and larger condensers are used to place the amalgam. In general, if more mercury is left in the amalgam during condensation, the restoration will change more dimensionally during setting and will exhibit higher creep under the forces of mastication. An increase in final mercury content that reflects the presence of an excessive amount of matrix phases will result in a decrease in strength of the amalgam. The properties of the high-copper amalgams are less sensitive to excess mercury content than the conventional amalgams because the alloys are mixed with less mercury initially and the γ_2 phase is not present. Selection of a condensing instrument and technic must be based on their effectiveness in removing excess mercury and in applying the force necessary for adaptation.

Hand condensing instruments are available with a variety of geometrically shaped tips, such as circular, triangular, oval, and crescent, and with several different cross-sectional areas. A condenser tip that is too small in cross section is inadequate in condensing a reasonable quantity of amalgam. One that is too large exerts a low pressure that results in poor adaptation. In general, an optimum size for condensing comminuted alloys appears to be a circular, smooth-surfaced condenser tip with a diameter of 2 or 3 mm. **Spherical alloys are somewhat more plastic than the comminuted ones and therefore require a tip with larger diameter.**

The force applied to the hand condenser should be as great as possible under the existing clinical conditions and should be applied evenly, firmly, and uniformly to small increments of amalgam. Laboratory studies have shown that a force of 8 to 10 pounds on a condenser tip is sufficient for adequate condensation of amalgams made from comminuted and spherical alloys. Since the pressure exerted by the condenser has its greatest effect on the amalgam immediately beneath the tip, condensation of small increments of amalgam is essential for adequate condensation with a minimum of excess mercury. The surface of the restoration should be obtained by carving an overpacked restoration, since the surface layer of the amalgam contains excess mercury.

Mechanical condensing instruments, which are shaped to resemble a contra-angle handpiece instrument, are available. Some of these condensers develop a tapping or malleting action during condensation, whereas others are based on the principle of vibration. As with the hand instruments, force must be applied to the instrument to obtain satisfactory condensation. **Ultrasonic condensers are not recommended because of mercury contamination.**

Condensation of the amalgam mass into the cavity must occur promptly after the mercury and alloy are mixed. Delay in condensation makes effective removal of remaining excess mercury difficult because the mass is partially hardened. The resulting amalgam will show reduced strength and increased creep because of the increased mercury content. **Moisture contamination of the**

amalgam must also be prevented before and during condensation of the mass into the cavity. Delayed expansion of several hundred micrometers per centimeter will occur in the zinc-containing alloys if they are exposed to moisture. It is also undesirable, for other reasons, to contaminate nonzinc amalgams with saliva. Moisture contamination can be minimized by various dry-field procedures.

Finishing

A properly condensed amalgam made from a modern alloy sufficiently hardens within a few minutes to permit the start of carving with sharp instruments. Burnishing, or rubbing, of the newly condensed amalgam with a metal instrument having a broad surface can be employed to smooth the surface after the initial carving. Burnishing over margins, however, should be avoided, since thin areas susceptible to fracture can easily be formed. **Final finishing and polishing procedures are usually done at least 24 hours after the initial carving operation. For spherical high-copper alloys that develop their strength rapidly, finishing and polishing may be done at the same appointment.** The amount of time it takes depends on the particular products.

Clinical observations have shown that a well-finished and well-polished amalgam restoration retains its shiny metallic appearance for a longer time, is easier to keep clean at home, and undergoes less corrosion. It is thought that a smooth surface provides for less retention of acids, small food particles, plaque, and materials that promote tarnish; thus it retards the corrosion process.

It is desirable that the final polish be developed through a series of finishing and polishing steps after the carving operation. The initial sequence includes the use of green stones, finishing burs, and abrasive disks. The final polish is developed by the application of a suitable polishing agent such as extra fine silex, followed by a thin slurry of tin oxide applied with a rotating soft brush. Care should be taken to polish in the presence of water, since dry polishing can cause the vaporization of mercury from the amalgam and a consequent reduction in strength properties.

Dental amalgam restorations can last for many years if the manipulation is carefully done. The mercury-alloy ratio needs to be carefully proportioned according to the manufacturer's instructions to give the correct plasticity for handling and strength when set. Trituration and condensation also need to be carefully done for the best properties. Polishing is important for minimizing tarnish in service.

Self-test questions

In the following multiple choice questions, one or more responses may be correct.

1 The vapor pressure of mercury increases with:
  a. Increasing temperature
  b. Decreasing size of mercury droplets
  c. Contamination by dust

2 Which of the following office conditions serve to minimize the health hazard from spilled mercury?
  a. Baseboard heating
  b. Floor carpeting
  c. Tile flooring without seams
  d. Amalgam scrap stored in a closed container

3 Which of the following represents the maximum safe concentration of mercury vapor in the breathing zone for a 40-hour work week?
  a. 0.05 ng Hg/m3 of air
  b. 30 ng Hg/m3 of air
  c. 100 ng Hg/m3 of air
  d. 0.05 mg Hg/m3 of air

4 For each of the following types of alloys, list which of the phases (Ag-Sn, Ag-Cu, Ag-Sn-Cu, Hg, Ag-Hg, Sn-Hg, Cu-Hg, Cu-Sn) are present after amalgamation and complete reaction.
  a. Spherical low-copper
  b. Spherical high-copper

5 Once amalgamation has occurred, mercury:
  a. Is combined primarily with silver
  b. Has the toxic properties of unreacted mercury
  c. Can form at the surface of amalgam restorations if heated to 60° C

6 For each of the following properties, list which of the phases (Ag-Sn, Ag-Hg, Sn-Hg) has the lowest value for the following properties:
  a. Corrosion resistance
  b. Strength
  c. Marginal fracture

7 Which of the following types of amalgam (comminuted low-copper, spherical low-copper, admixed high-copper, and spherical high-copper) have the highest value for each of the three properties?
  a. 1-hour compressive strength
  b. Tensile strength
  c. Creep

8 Which of the following conditions are necessary for accurate dispensing of mercury?
  a. The dispenser should be held vertically upside down during dispensing.
  b. The dispenser should be kept at least one-fourth full.
  b. The dispenser should be kept at least one-fourth full.
  c. The surface of the mercury in the dispenser should be clean and bright.

9 Which of the following statements are true with respect to amalgam capsules?
  a. Worn capsules can leak mercury droplets during mechanical trituration.
  b. Residual hardened amalgam inside a capsule has no significant effect on subsequent mixes of amalgam.

c. Disposable capsules contain amalgam alloy and mercury and, after use, may be implemented as a reusable capsule.

d. Each alloy usually requires a specific capsule and pestle.

10 Which of these statements are correct in terms of preparing a correctly triturated mass of amalgam?

a. An undertriturated mass is crumbly and dull.

b. A correctly triturated mass is smooth, homogeneous, and dull.

c. An overmixed mass is removed readily from the capsule but is soupy in appearance.

11 The objectives during condensation of amalgam are:

a. Adaptation to cavity walls, margins, and matrix

b. Development of a compact mass free from voids

c. No change in mercury concentration from that used in the mix

12 Which of these statements apply to condensation of amalgam?

a. Amalgam should be condensed in small increments with uniform force applied.

b. A condenser is selected on the basis of its ability to remove excess mercury and to apply pressure needed for adaptation.

c. Too large a condenser tip results in low condensation pressure and poor adaptation.

d. A force of 8 to 10 pounds on a condenser is satisfactory for adequate condensation of comminuted and spherical alloys.

13 In the finishing of an amalgam restoration:

a. Final finishing and polishing are done just after the amalgam hardens, regardless of the type of alloy.

b. Burnishing over margins should not be done, since thin areas of amalgam susceptible to fracture can be formed.

c. Polishing should be done in the presence of water.

d. A correct finishing and polishing sequence would include finishing burs, green stone, silex, and tin oxide.

Suggested supplementary readings

Council on Dental Materials and Devices: Recommendations in dental mercury hygiene, *J Am Dent Assoc* 96:487, 1978.

Council on Dental Materials, Instruments, and Equipment: *Recommendations in dental mercury hygiene*, Chicago, 1981, American Dental Association.

Dodes JE: Amalgam toxicity: a review of the literature, *Oper Dent* 13:32, 1988.

Farah JW, Powers JM, editors: Amalgams, *Dent Advis* 1(3):1, 1984.

Mahler DB: Dental amalgam. In Craig RG, editor: *Dental materials review*, Ann Arbor, Mich, 1977, University of Michigan School of Dentistry.

Mantyla DC, Wright OD: Mercury toxicity in the dental office: a neglected problem, *J Am Dent Assoc* 92:1189, 1976.

O'Brien WJ, Greener E, Mahler DB: Dental amalgam. In Reese JA, and Valega TM, editors: *Restorative dental materials*, vol 1, London, 1985, Quintessence.

chapter six

Finishing, Polishing, and Cleansing Materials

Finishing and polishing technics are meant to remove excess material and to smooth roughened surfaces. A rough surface on a restoration may be uncomfortable and make oral hygiene difficult because food debris and plaque can easily cling to it. In cases in which a restoration is located in proximity to the gingiva, surface roughness can cause painful irritation and eventual recession of the soft tissue. It is well established that roughness of metallic restorative materials is responsible for accelerating corrosion. The finishing and polishing of restorative dental materials are important steps in the fabrication of clinically successful restorations.

Cleansing technics are meant to remove food and other debris from a surface without damaging it. Polishing and cleaning are routine procedures for maintaining the health of the natural dentition. These procedures, however, can lead to roughened enamel surfaces by the use of excessively abrasive dentrifices at home or coarse prophylactic slurries at the dental office. Some restorative materials can also be abraded by dentifrices and prophylactic pastes during a cleansing procedure.

The materials used for finishing and polishing are primarily abrasives. Most cleansing materials are also abrasives, although a number of chemical cleansing agents for denture bases exist. An understanding of the properties of these materials and the process of abrasion can lead to improved clinical usage of finishing, polishing, and cleansing materials.

ABRASION

Abrasion results when a hard, rough surface, such as a sandpaper disk, or hard, irregularly shaped particles, such as those present in an abrasive slurry, plow grooves in a softer material and cause material from such grooves to be removed from the surface. The action of an abrasive is essentially a cutting action. Abrasive tools or slurries, however, differ from dental cutting instruments in that the cutting edges or points of the abrasive are not arranged in any particular pattern. Each point or edge of an abrasive acts as an individual cutting blade and removes some material from the surface being abraded.

Abrasion is a wear process.

The process of abrasion is affected by the physical and mechanical properties of the material being abraded. Properties such as hardness, strength, ductility, and thermal conductivity are important. These properties are discussed with respect to the abrasion of individual restorative materials later in this chapter.

Rate

The rate of abrasion of a given material by a given abrasive is determined primarily by three factors: the size of the abrasive particle, the pressure of the abrasive against the material being abraded, and the speed at which the abrasive particle moves across the surface being abraded. All these factors can be clinically controlled.

The size of an abrasive particle is an important factor in the rate at which the surface is abraded. **Larger particles cause deeper scratches in the material and wear away the surface at a faster rate.** The use of a coarse abrasive is indicated on a surface with many rough spots or large nodules. The scratches caused by the coarse abrasive must then be removed by finer ones.

A second important factor is the pressure of the abrasive against the surface being abraded. **Heavy pressure applied by the abrasive causes deeper scratches and more rapid removal of material.** However, heavy pressure may also cause the abrasive to fracture or to dislodge from the grinding wheel, thereby reducing cutting efficiency. Operator control of the abrasion process is lessened when excessive pressure is exerted because material is worn away too rapidly to keep the abrasion from occurring uniformly over the entire surface of the material. Judgment must be exercised in the amount of force applied to the dental handpiece or to the surface that is against a grinding wheel to avoid excessive pressure.

A third factor that controls the rate of abrasion is the speed at which the abrasive travels across the surface being abraded. The higher the speed, the greater the frequency per unit of time the particle contacts the surface. **Thus increasing the speed increases the rate of abrasion. In a clinical situation it is easier to**

control speed than pressure to vary the rate of abrasion. Varying the speed has the additional advantage of using low pressure while still maintaining a high cutting efficiency.

Types of abrasives

The three types of abrasives used in dentistry can be classified as finishing, polishing, and cleansing abrasives. Finishing abrasives are generally hard, coarse abrasives that are used primarily for developing desired contours of a restoration or tooth preparation and for removing gross irregularities on the surface. Polishing abrasives have finer particle sizes and are generally less hard than abrasives that are used for finishing. The polishing abrasives are used to smooth surfaces that have been roughened typically by finishing abrasives or wear particles encountered in the mouth. Cleansing abrasives are generally soft materials with small particle sizes and are intended to remove softer materials that adhere to enamel or restorative material substrates.

Dental abrasives are applied by means of a number of tools, shown in Fig. 6-1. The abrasive particles may be glued onto plastic or paper disks that can be attached to a dental handpiece or attached to strips for finishing of interproximal areas. Paper disks are preferable for finishing contoured surfaces because

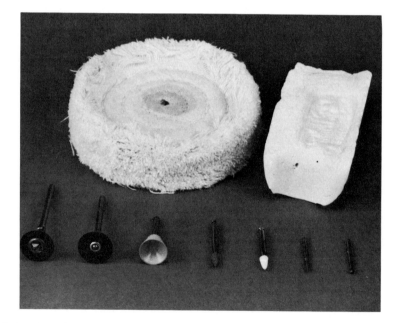

Fig. 6-1. A variety of cutting, finishing, and polishing tools. *Top,* Rag wheel and Bendick polish. *Bottom, left to right,* Silicon carbide disk, aluminum oxide disk, rubber polisher, green stone, white stone, diamond bur, and carbide bur.

they are more flexible than plastic disks. The waterproof variety of paper disks is more durable. In the case of diamond rotary instruments, diamond chips are attached to steel wheels, disks, and cylinders. With grinding wheels and dental stones, the abrasive particles are bonded by a matrix material that is molded to form tools of desired sizes and shapes. The abrasive tools just described are used only for finishing.

Abrasives may also be mixed with water, glycerin, or some other medium to produce slurries or pastes. The use of glycerin as a medium prevents the change in consistency that occurs when water, which evaporates, is used to mix a slurry. The slurry or paste is then rubbed over the surface of the material being abraded with a cloth or felt wheel, brush, or rubber cup. Abrasive slurries and pastes are most commonly used in dentistry for polishing and cleaning.

The following is a brief discussion of the abrasive agents commonly used for finishing. Values of hardness and grades of abrasives used on some commercial disks are listed in Table 6-1.

Table 6-1. Hardness and Grade of Various Types of Finishing Disks

| Product* | Abrasive | Hardness | | Grade |
		Mohs value	Knoop value	
Emery, coarse	Silicon carbide	9+	2480	100
Emery, medium				120
Emery, fine				220
Waterproof, fine	Silicon carbide	9+	2480	320
Waterproof, extra fine				400
Waterproof, double extra fine				600
Adalox, coarse	Aluminum oxide	9	2100	150
Adalox, medium				220
Adalox, fine				320
Garnet, extra coarse	Garnet	6.5-7	1360	60
Garnet, coarse				80
Garnet, medium				120
Garnet, fine				180
Garnet, extra fine				240
Sand, coarse	Flint (quartz)	7	820	60
Sand, medium				100
Sand, fine				220
Cuttle, coarse	Flint (quartz)	7	820	150
Cuttle, medium				220
Cuttle, fine				400
Crocus	Iron oxide	—	—	—

From Charbeneau GT: Unpublished data, University of Michigan School of Dentistry, Ann Arbor, Mich.
*E.C. Moore Co., Inc., Dearborn, Mich.

Aluminum oxide (Al_2O_3) is an abrasive manufactured from bauxite, an impure aluminum oxide, and produced in various particle sizes. The particles are most commonly applied to paper or plastic disks in coarse, medium, and fine grits. The disks are reddish brown.

Cuttle is an abrasive manufactured from the bones of fish, although this form is no longer used as a dental abrasive. Presently cuttle is a trade name that refers to a fine grade of quartz (SiO_2). The particles are applied to a paper disk in coarse, medium, and fine grits. The medium cuttle grit is similar in abrasive action to a fine sand grit. Cuttle disks are beige.

Diamond is the hardest known substance. Diamond chips are normally impregnated in a binder to form diamond "stones" and disks.

Garnet is an abrasive that is mined. In pure form it has the chemical composition $Al_2O_3 \cdot 3FeO \cdot 3SiO_2$. Garnet is available on paper or plastic disks in extra coarse, coarse, medium, fine, and extra fine grits and is red.

Sand is a form of quartz (SiO_2) used as an abrasive agent. It is available on plastic or paper disks in coarse, medium, and fine grits and is beige. Sand disks should not be used interchangeably with cuttle disks, although also of quartz, since the particle sizes of the coarse, medium, and fine grits are not the same for both abrasives.

Silicon carbide (SiC) is the second hardest of the dental abrasives and is usually applied to paper or plastic disks. The disks are available in fine, extra fine, and double extra fine grits and are black.

The abrasive agents commonly used in dentistry for polishing and cleaning follow.

Calcite is a form of calcium carbonate ($CaCO_3$). It is available in various grades as used in prophylactic pastes. Another physical form of calcium carbonate is chalk, which is used in dentifrices as a polishing agent.

Kieselguhr is a polishing agent and is composed of the siliceous remains of minute aquatic plants known as *diatoms*. The coarse form of kieselguhr is known as diatomaceous earth.

Pumice is a highly siliceous volcanic glass that when ground is useful as a polishing agent in prophylactic pastes and for finishing acrylic denture bases in the laboratory.

Rouge is a fine red powder composed of iron oxide (Fe_2O_3) that is usually employed in cake form. It may be impregnated in paper or fabric known as *crocus cloth*. It is an excellent laboratory polishing agent for gold and other precious metal alloys.

Silex refers to siliceous materials such as quartz or tripoli that are used as polishing abrasives in the mouth.

Tin oxide (SnO_2) is a pure white powder used extensively as a final polishing agent for teeth and metallic restorations in the mouth. It is mixed with water, alcohol, or glycerin and used as a paste.

Tripoli is a polishing agent that originates from certain porous rocks found in North Africa. It is often confused with kieselguhr.

Zirconium silicate ($ZrSiO_4$) is a hard abrasive that, in small particle sizes, is used as a polishing agent.

In addition to the abrasive agents already cited, several other abrasives are found in prophylactic pastes, including quartz, anatase (TiO_2), feldspar, montmorillonite, aluminum hydroxide, kaolinite, and talc. Further information on prophylactic materials is presented later in this chapter.

The abrasives found in dentifrices include calcium carbonate, dibasic calcium phosphate dihydrate, anhydrous dibasic calcium phosphate, tricalcium phosphate, calcium pyrophosphate, sodium metaphosphate, hydrated alumina, and silica. These are mainly cleansing and polishing abrasives that are not meant to severely abrade enamel.

Finishing and polishing technics

The finishing and polishing technics for most restorative dental materials follow similar principles. Initial contouring and smoothing of the surface are done with a coarse abrasive or bur. The large scratches produced are then removed by successively finer abrasives. The use of too fine an abrasive after a coarse one is time consuming and does not give a properly finished surface. **A key to successful finishing and polishing is strict adherence to a recommended abrasive sequence.**

Finishing abrasives are coarse, hard particles, whereas polishing abrasives are fine particles.

With each successive change in abrasive, the area being finished and polished should be rinsed to remove the previously used abrasive particles. One remaining particle of coarse abrasive can mar a well-polished surface. Care must also be taken not to allow the abrasive tool or slurry to be used in a dry condition. The efficiency of the abrasive may be dramatically reduced by dry polishing, and the danger of overheating the surface is increased.

The abrasives chosen to finish and polish various restorative materials depend to a great extent on the properties of the particular restorative material. The discussion that follows considers the surface roughness that is caused by various abrasive agents, a recommended finishing and polishing sequence, and the precautions that should be taken in finishing and polishing some common restorative materials.

Amalgam. The average surface roughness produced by various methods of instrumentation on amalgam is listed in Table 6-2. A suggested abrasive sequence for finishing and polishing an occlusoproximal restoration is indicated therein.

When an amalgam restoration has been properly manipulated, it will be sufficiently hardened within a few minutes to permit carving with a sharp instrument. Then carving to the margins should be done to remove all excess amal-

Table 6-2. Average Surface Roughness of Dental Amalgam Produced by Various Methods of Instrumentation

Method of instrumentation	Micrometers
Carved	4.6*
Carved and immediately smoothened (burnished)	0.36*
Condensed against uncontoured matrix band	0.61
Rotating finishing instruments	
S.S. White green stone	0.64-1.0*
Finishing bur	0.46-0.64*
Moore's Adalox fine	0.81
Fine sand	0.76
Waterproof (silicon carbide) fine	0.58*
Fine cuttle	0.30
Rotating polishing instruments	
Robinson soft cup brush	
With flour of pumice	0.30
With extra fine silex	0.18*
With tin oxide	0.10*
Interproximal finishing strips	
Moyco "Evenwet" extra fine sand	0.30*
Extra fine sand + Dentotape with silex + tin oxide	0.10*

Modified from Charbeneau GT: *J Mich Dent Assoc* 47:320, 1965.
*Suggested abrasive sequence for finishing and polishing an occlusoproximal amalgam restoration.

gam. Burnishing with a metal instrument that has a broad surface can be employed to smooth the surface. After this initial carving operation, the restoration should be left undisturbed for an appropriate period before finishing and polishing with rotating instruments or interproximal strips. Most amalgams can be polished the day after their placement. The time delay allows the amalgams to develop strength. Only amalgams that have high early strengths can be finished and polished at the first appointment.

Polishing, in these cases, is done through the application of a sequence of operations that includes the use of fine stones and abrasive disks or strips. The final polish is developed, as indicated in Table 6-2, by the application of extra fine silex, followed by the application of a thin slurry of tin oxide, with a rotating soft brush. During this final polishing operation the restoration should be kept moist to avoid overheating.

Some of the fast-setting high-copper amalgams (Chapter 5) can be polished about 8 to 12 minutes after placement because of their rapid development of strength. Polishing is done with a creamy paste of extra fine silex and water that is gently applied in an unwebbed rubber cup with a slow-speed handpiece for 30 seconds per surface.

Gold alloy. The average surface roughness produced by various methods of in-

Table 6-3. Average Surface Roughness of a Type II Gold Casting Produced by Various Methods of Instrumentation

Method of instrumentation	Micrometers
Polished wax, pickled casting	0.43*
Electropolished casting	0.33
Finishing instruments	
Moore's	
Fine sand	0.86
Medium cuttle	0.46
Fine cuttle	0.23*
Polishing instruments	
Disks	
Moore's Crocus	0.08*
Impregnated wheels	
Burlew	0.13
Cratex extra fine	0.10
Rag wheel	
Radoff	0.09
Sureshine	0.05*
Bendick	0.05
Chamois	
Rouge	0.04-0.05*

From Charbeneau GT: Unpublished data, University of Michigan School of Dentistry, Ann Arbor, Mich.
*Suggested abrasive sequence for finishing and polishing.

strumentation on a Type II gold casting, as well as a suggested abrasive sequence for finishing and polishing, is listed in Table 6-3.

Gold restorations made by the indirect technic are finished and polished on the die after the occlusion and margins have been properly adjusted. Gold restorations made by the direct technic are polished on the tooth when the surfaces are accessible. Finishing of the pickled casting and polishing of proximal surfaces are done in the laboratory. **The overfinishing of margins and contours must be avoided by careful control of the direction and force of the polishing action.** The casting is generally scrubbed with alcohol to prepare its surface for cementation.

Denture base. The acrylic denture base is ready for finishing and polishing once it has been processed and deflasked. Any gypsum material that remains on the denture can be removed by light scraping or with a **"shell blaster."** Feathered edges of acrylic can be smoothed and rounded with an acrylic finishing bur. A rag wheel and felt cone with a pumice slurry are used to finish the tongue side of a maxillary base. A single-row brush wheel and a rag wheel about ¼ inch in width are used with a pumice slurry to smooth the labial and buccal surfaces on the tongue side of a mandibular denture without destroying the contour. A final high polish is given to all non-tissue-bearing surfaces by a rag wheel with tripoli, Bendick, or a paste of tin oxide and water.

A shell blaster sprays finely divided nut shells against the surface under high velocity.

Overheating during the polishing of an acrylic denture base can occur because of the low thermal conductivity of the plastic and must be avoided. **Overheating affects the appearance of the denture and may cause warpage to occur. Plastic denture teeth must be protected from the pumice because they are easily abraded.** After the polishing, the denture should be washed with soap and water and stored in water until delivery to the patient.

To maintain infection control, separate polishing burs, rag wheels, and pumice pans should be used for each prosthesis. Pumice can be mixed with a liquid disinfectant (5 parts sodium hypochlorite to 100 parts distilled water) and green soap (3 parts) to keep the pumice suspended. Pumice should be changed daily. Rag wheels can be sterilized in a steam autoclave or by ethylene oxide.

Composite restorative materials. The average surface roughness produced by various methods of instrumentation on blended and microfilled composite restorative materials, as well as a suggested sequence for finishing, is listed in Table 6-4.

Composite restorative materials in the past presented a problem in finishing and polishing because of the hard filler particles in a soft resin matrix. The smoothest surface on a composite resin is produced by allowing polymerization

Table 6-4. Average Surface Roughness of Composites Produced by Various Methods of Instrumentation

Method of instrumentation	Roughness, μm	
	Hybrid	Microfilled
Mylar matrix	0.12*	0.09*
Diamond stones		
Medium grit	1.41*	—
Superfine grit	0.67*	—
Carbide finishing burs	0.65	—
Abrasive disks		
Coarse	2.02	1.87*
Medium	0.6*	0.71*
Fine	0.3*	0.25*
Superfine	0.11*	0.09*
Polishing paste	0.1*	0.1*

Modified from Herrgott AML, Ziemiecki TL, Dennison JB: *J Am Dent Assoc* 119:729, 1989.
*Suggested sequence for finishing and polishing.

of the freshly inserted resin to occur against a Mylar matrix. An acceptable finishing procedure for current fine-particle, hybrid, or microfilled composite resins includes the use of diamond stones or 12-blade carbide burs for removal of gross excesses that are not near enamel margins. This step should be followed by the use of abrasive disks for the finishing of accessible areas or by the use of white stones of suitable shape for the finishing of more inaccessible areas. Fine and microfine diamonds and diamond polishing pastes are suitable for the final finishing of composites.

PROPHYLACTIC PASTES

Routine dental prophylaxis for the removal of exogenous stains, pellicle, materia alba, and oral debris is a widely used procedure in the dental office. Prophylaxis should precede the application of a fluoride gel or solution to make the enamel accessible and more reactive to the fluoride. **Ideally a dental prophylactic paste should be sufficiently abrasive to remove effectively all types of accumulation from the tooth surface without imparting undue abrasion to the enamel, dentin, or cementum.** In addition to acting as a cleansing agent, the paste should have the quality of endowing the hard tissue with a highly polished, esthetic appearance. Certain prophylactic pastes contain sodium fluoride or stannous fluoride either mixed with the abrasive or in a more complex, buffered system.

Composition. The abrasives in various commercial prophylactic pastes are listed in Table 6-5.

Properties. Laboratory and clinical studies of cleaning and polishing have compared the efficiency of various prophylactic pastes. Products containing predominantly pumice and quartz show higher cleansing values but generally result in a greater abrasion to both enamel and dentin. In fact, abrasion data have indicated that some prophylactic pastes may be unnecessarily destructive to enamel. The products containing coarse pumice are generally the most abra-

Table 6-5. Abrasives in Various Commercial Prophylactic Pastes

Prophylactic paste	Abrasive	Manufacturer
Coral Plus Fluoride Treatment	Recrystallized kaolinite	Lorvic
Luride Acidulated Phosphate Fluoride	Silicon dioxide	Colgate-Hoyt
Nupro Fine	Diatomaceous silicon dioxide	Johnson & Johnson
Preventodontic APF	Pumice	Mynol
Pro Care	Sodium-potassium aluminum silicate	Young Dental
Zircate	Zirconium silicate	Dentsply/Caulk

Modified from Putt MS, Kleber CJ, Muhler JC: *Dent Hygiene* 56:38, 1982.

sive. Zirconium silicate is a particularly effective cleansing and polishing agent, but the polishing properties of zirconium silicate are markedly influenced by the distribution of particle sizes of the material in various commercial products. In clinical study, prophylactic pastes with silicate abrasives produced higher polishing scores for enamel with lower abrasion of enamel than did pastes with other abrasives (Table 6-5). Abrasion of dentin has been measured to be five to six times greater than abrasion of enamel, regardless of the product used.

Prophylaxis pastes that contain fluoride have been subjected to several clinical trials. Results have varied from no benefit to benefits as high as 35% reduction in caries after 3 years. The design of some of these studies makes it difficult to assess the effects of the prophylaxis agent alone.

During a prophylactic procedure, care must be exercised to avoid excessive abrasion of any restorative material present. Polymeric materials such as denture base and artificial tooth resins, acrylic veneering materials, and composite restorative resins are particularly susceptible to wear because of their low hardness. The result of such wear can be possible reduction in contours and increased surface roughness, both of which are undesirable.

DENTIFRICES

The primary function of a dentifrice is to clean and polish the surfaces of the teeth accessible to a toothbrush. In addition to enhancing personal appearance by maintaining cleaner teeth, brushing with a dentifrice may reduce the incidence of dental caries, help maintain a healthy gingiva, and reduce the intensity of mouth odors. During the process of cleaning, extraneous debris or deposits to be removed, given in order of increasing difficulty of removal from the tooth surface, are food debris; plaque—a soft, mainly bacterial film; acquired pellicle—a proteinaceous film of salivary origin; and calculus.

Composition and role of ingredients. Dentifrices are prepared in various forms, including paste, powder, and liquid. Of these, the paste and powder forms are the most common. The liquids have not gained prominence because they are not sufficiently abrasive to maintain clean teeth. Tooth powders contain an abrasive, a surface-active detergent, flavoring oils, and sweetening agents. In addition to the powder ingredients, toothpastes contain water, a humectant (to prevent dehydration), a binder, and a preservative. Some dentifrices contain fluoride (Table 6-6) in the form of sodium fluoride, sodium monofluorophosphate, or stannous fluoride to help prevent dental caries. The composition of a dentifrice containing stannous fluoride is given in Table 6-7. Soluble pyrophosphates (3.3%) may be added to reduce the rate of formation of supragingival calculus, thus providing a cosmetic benefit.

The abrasives that are used in various dentifrice preparations are listed earlier in this chapter. **Ideally the abrasive should exhibit a maximum cleansing effi-**

Table 6-6. Examples of Dentifrices Containing Fluoride

Product*	Therapeutic ingredient	Manufacturer
Aqua-Fresh	Sodium monofluorophosphate	Beecham
Colgate with MFP	Sodium monofluorophosphate, 0.76%	Colgate-Palmolive
Crest	Sodium fluoride, 0.24%	Procter & Gamble
Macleans Fluoride	Sodium monofluorophosphate, 0.76%	Beecham

Modified from *Handbook of nonprescription drugs*, ed 8, Washington, DC, 1986, American Pharmaceutical Association.
*Accepted fluoride dentrifrices of Council on Dental Therapeutics, American Dental Association.

Table 6-7. Composition of a Therapeutic Dentifrice

Major ingredients	Percent
Abrasives	40
Water	29.6
Sorbitol (70% solution)	20
Glycerin	10
Stannous fluoride	0.4

Modified from Council on Dental Therapeutics: *Accepted dental therapeutics*, Chicago, 1979, American Dental Association.

ciency with minimum tooth abrasion. In addition, an abrasive should be present to polish the teeth. Some toothpastes advertised as able to whiten or brighten teeth contain the harsher abrasive agents such as silica, calcium carbonate, or anhydrous dibasic calcium phosphate. The only satisfactory method of determining the abrasiveness of a dentifrice appears to be a test on teeth, although laboratory data have been published.

Abrasion of enamel by modern dentifrices is generally not a problem unless unusual oral conditions exist; however, **exposed dentin and cementum are susceptible to abrasion.** An example of cervical abrasion resulting from excessive use of a toothbrush and dentifrice is shown in Fig. 6-2. Patients having exposed cementum or dentin should avoid regular use of dentifrice powders or highly abrasive pastes.

Polymeric restorative materials are also susceptible to abrasion from toothbrush and dentifrice use. A patient should be cautioned not to use dentifrices for cleansing denture bases or acrylic denture teeth.

The remaining ingredients in dentifrices serve to increase the effectiveness of the cleansing and polishing agents or to make the dentifrice more appealing to use. A surface-active agent, generally a detergent, is added to improve the wettability of the enamel by the dentifrice, thereby improving contact with enamel

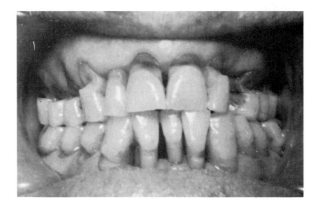

Fig. 6-2. Cervical abrasion from excessive use of toothbrush and dentifrice. (Courtesy Dr. RE Buchholz, University of Michigan School of Dentistry, Ann Arbor, Mich.)

by the abrasives. Flavoring oils and sweetening agents, usually saccharin, are added to make the dentifrice more appealing. Additional ingredients are added to pastes. To keep the paste from drying out, a humectant such as sorbitol, propylene glycol, or glycerin is used. Sorbitol is also a sweetening agent. To aid in controlling consistency and to keep the abrasives in suspension, a binder, such as sodium alginate, is used. Sodium carboxymethyl cellulose may serve as a stabilizer for the alginate binder. A foaming agent is added to favor the formation of a stable foam when the paste is used.

A therapeutic dentifrice contains some drug or chemical that, by reason of its bactericidal, bacteriostatic, enzyme-inhibiting, or acid-neutralizing qualities, reduces the incidence of dental caries or aids in the control of periodontal disease. Among the chemicals and drugs that have been added to dentifrices are urea, dibasic ammonium phosphate, water-soluble copper chlorophyllins, penicillin, fluorides, sodium N-lauroyl sarcosinate, and sodium dihydroacetate. There is no general agreement that any one of these compounds except fluorides contributes to dental health beyond that attained with a well-formulated cleansing dentifrice.

Effect of toothbrush. A number of studies have examined the influence of the toothbrush and its variables on abrasion. **When compared with the abrasion of common dentifrices, the bristles have little abrasive power.** Properties of the bristles, such as geometry, hardness, stiffness, and number, generally do not influence abrasion by themselves, although they do affect the abrasion caused by the dentifrice. Mechanical toothbrushing devices generally cause less abrasion of enamel and dentin than does manual brushing because the force applied to the mechanical devices is usually less.

Selection of toothbrush and dentifrice. The best available guidelines to follow in selecting a dentifrice for a patient are based on evaluation of the following factors: (1) degree of staining of the dentition, (2) force exerted on the brush, (3) method of brushing, and (4) amount of exposed dentin or cementum. Choice of a dentifrice for appropriate abrasion can then be based on the ranking of the abrasivity of dentifrices reported by the American Dental Association. Even so, comparison of products with similar abrasivity scores is not possible because of the experimental error associated with measuring the abrasion data. Selection of a toothbrush should be based on the requirements of the patient's soft tissue. In particular, **abrasion of the soft tissue by hard, stiff bristles should be avoided.**

DENTURE CLEANSERS

Denture base materials and denture teeth collect deposits in the same manner as do natural teeth. Soft food debris that clings to a denture can be removed easily by light brushing followed by rinsing. Hard deposits of calculus and stains, such as those that occur from tobacco tars, are much more difficult to remove. Two methods are commonly used to remove both stains and calculus: (1) professional repolishing of the denture and (2) soaking or brushing of the denture on a daily basis at home.

The first method, repolishing the surfaces of the denture at extended time intervals, is not suitable for home care of dentures. Repolishing is a technic that follows much the same sequence recommended for the initial finishing and polishing of denture base materials described earlier. The technic can alter the surface of a denture made of plastic appreciably if it is applied too vigorously or too often because denture base plastics have a relatively poor resistance to abrasion.

The second method, soaking a denture in a solution or brushing it with a powder or paste, is suitable for home care. If these denture cleansers are properly used, the accumulation of dental plaque and stains can be effectively controlled.

Requirements. An ideal denture cleanser should be (1) nontoxic and easy to remove, leaving no traces of irritant material; (2) able to attack or dissolve both the organic and inorganic portions of denture deposits; (3) harmless to all materials used in the construction of dentures, including denture base polymers and alloys, acrylic and porcelain teeth, and resilient lining materials; (4) not harmful to eyes, skin, or clothing if accidentally spilled or splashed; (5) stable during storage; and (6) preferably bactericidal and fungicidal.

Types. The five major types of denture cleansers for use at home are (1) alkaline perborates, (2) alkaline peroxides, (3) alkaline hypochlorites, (4) dilute acids, and (5) abrasive powders and creams. The properties of these cleansers and examples of available commercial products are listed in Table 6-8.

Table 6-8. Types of Commercial Denture Cleansers

Type of cleanser	Commercially available products	Active ingredients	Disadvantages
Alkaline perborate	K.I.K. (K.I.K. Co.)	Sodium perborate or derivative Potassium monopersulfate	Does not easily remove heavy deposits
	Efferdent tablets* (Warner–Lambert) Effervescent tablets (Rexall) Kleenite (Vicks) Polident tablets* (Block Drug) Polident powder* (Block Drug)		May be harmful to soft lining materials
Alkaline peroxide	Denalan (Whitehall)	Sodium percarbonate	Harmful to soft lining materials
Alkaline hypochlorite	Mersene (Colgate-Palmolive)	Sodium perborate Trisodium phosphate Troclosene potassium	May cause bleaching Can corrode stainless steel and cobalt-chromium alloys May leave an odor on denture
Dilute acid	Denclenz (Creighton)	Hydrochloric acid	May corrode some alloys
Abrasive powder or cream	Complete* (Vicks) Dentu-Creme* (Block Drug)	Calcium carbonate	Can abrade denture polymers and plastic teeth

Modified from *Handbook of nonprescription drugs*, ed 8, Washington, DC, 1986, American Pharmaceutical Association.
*Acceptable product according to ADA Acceptance Program.

Certain denture cleansers contain sodium perborate ($NaBO_2 \cdot H_2O_2 \cdot 3H_2O$), which is a source of peroxide (H_2O_2). The decomposition of peroxide in water is favored in a basic solution. The pH of several perborate cleansers ranges from 7 to 11.5. Cleansing presumably results from the oxidizing ability of the peroxide decomposition and from the effervescing action of evolved oxygen. Some of these cleansers also contain chloride ions that can cause corrosion of base metal components.

Effectiveness. The brushing of a denture surface is an effective means of improving denture cleanliness and maintaining a healthy mucosa beneath a removable denture. Chemical cleansers may be useful alternatives to brushing among geriatric or disabled denture patients. **Daily overnight immersion of dentures in an alkaline peroxide solution provides a safe and relatively effec-**

tive means of cleansing; however, customary 15-minute soaking is neither effective on mature plaque nor completely effective on stains and deposits. Ultrasonic vibration is not an efficient method for removal of denture plaque.

Experimental work has been done on a denture cleanser containing enzymes (mutanase and protease). After 6 weeks of daily 15-minute denture soaking, a significant reduction in denture plaque was observed. Improvements of the clinical condition of the palatal mucosa among the patients also was seen. Disinfectants not available commercially, such as chlorhexidine gluconate and salicylate, have also been studied experimentally to treat yeast infections beneath dentures and to reduce denture plaque. Some success was observed.

Recommended technics and precautions. Several technics for cleaning dentures can be recommended. One effective technic requires immersion in a solution of one part of 5% sodium hypochlorite in three parts of water followed by light brushing. Another technic for cleaning plastic dentures is immersion in a solution containing 1 teaspoon of a hypochlorite (Clorox) and 2 teaspoons of a glassy phosphate (Calgon) in one-half glass of water. This cleanser is not recommended for use on prosthetic appliances fabricated from base metals such as cobalt-chromium alloy because chlorine solutions tend to darken these metals. **Dentures should never be soaked in hot water because the heat may cause the plastic to distort.**

Although light meticulous brushing is a recommended method of cleaning the denture, brushing with hard, stiff bristles should be avoided because these bristles produce scratches on the surface of the denture. **Dentifrices generally should not be used to aid in cleaning a denture at home,** although pastes with gentle abrasives (acrylic resin, sodium bicarbonate, or a $ZrSiO_4$-ZrO_2 system) can be used. Organic solvents such as chloroform should not be used, since these chemicals may dissolve or craze an acrylic denture. If the denture is not worn after cleaning, it should be stored in water to retain its dimensional accuracy. **Some soaking types of denture cleansers may cause soft liners to change color.** A procedure for cleaning a denture with a soft liner is to clean the external and tooth surfaces of the denture with a soft brush and denture paste and the soft lining material with cotton under cold water.

BLEACHING

In-office bleaching technics may be effective for lightening teeth stained by fluorosis, tetracycline, and acquired superficial discolorations. Recently, bleaching technics have been combined with composite bonding and porcelain veneering as a procedure in esthetic dentistry. Bleaching teeth outside the dental office was introduced in 1989 and received immediate acceptance, although clinical and laboratory data to support home bleaching are inadequate.

Composition. Bleaching agents used in the office commonly contain 30% to

35% hydrogen peroxide. One system mixes 35% hydrogen peroxide with silica to form a gel. Another system contains calcium, phosphate, and fluoride ions to allow remineralization during treatment. A microabrasion system (Prema, Premier) contains a low concentration of hydrochloric acid and fine abrasive particles suspended in a water-soluble paste.

Home bleaching products typically contain 10% carbamide peroxide or 1.5% to 6% hydrogen peroxide. The pH of these products ranges from 4.6 to 6.7 when undiluted and from 4.3 to 6.6 when diluted 1:2 with water.

Properties. Bleaching is often the primary treatment to improve esthetics. The effects may last a year, and retreatment is simple. Yellow, orange, or light brown stains, often associated with aging, are treated most successfully. If no major improvement in color occurs within a reasonable time, bonding or laminating should be considered.

Bleaching agents do not adversely affect gold alloys, amalgam, microfilled composites, or porcelain. Some hybrid composites have been roughened slightly by bleaching gels. Bleach should not come in contact with dentin, since the smear layer may be removed by some products.

Side effects are uncommon but include tooth hypersensitivity, soft tissue lesions or sloughing, nausea, temporomandibular joint syndrome from the tray, and sore throats from swallowing the bleach. Gels with a higher viscosity are less likely to be diluted or swallowed during application.

Technics. Three major methods of in-office bleaching involve the use of heat, light, and gels, and microabrasion. Heat and light systems typically use a powerful bleaching light or wand that is calibrated to control bleaching temperatures. Three in-office treatments or one in-office treatment combined with a home program is needed to produce satisfactory results.

The gel technic is a more conservative chairside approach. The gel is placed on tooth enamel in a 2-mm thick layer for 20 to 30 minutes. Patients with dark tetracycline stains usually require three to four 30-minute appointments. The gel technic works faster if combined with the use of a composite curing light or bleaching unit for 10 minutes.

The microabrasion compound is applied using a slow speed (10:1 gear reduction) handpiece with a special mandrel. Discolored superficial enamel is polished away.

Home bleaching technics require plaque removal followed by use of a tray of gel for 3 to 4 hours once or several times a day. The gel should be replenished each hour. Bleaching effectiveness is related to the number of hours the tray is worn. Construction of a 2-mm plastic application tray is similar to that of a custom-made mouth protector (see Chapter 3), except that gauze may be used to outline areas of the tray where bleach is to be applied.

Dentists should follow universal bleaching guidelines: comprehensive clinical examination, full-mouth radiographs, photographs, evaluation of existing restorations and pathology, prophylaxis, rubber dam, eyewear and glove protection, no anesthesia, and constant patient monitoring. When using gels it is important to follow additional guidelines: avoid breathing silica dust, refrigerate stored 35% hydrogen peroxide activator, never use anesthesia, never leave the patient unattended, and protect the patient's eyes.

Finishing and polishing technics are important in preparing clinically successful restorations. The process of abrasion is affected by properties of the abrasive and the material being abraded. Finishing and polishing begin with coarse abrasives and end with fine ones. Clinically, it is easier to control the rate of abrasion by speed rather than pressure. Care must be taken to avoid overfinishing margins and contours of restorations and to avoid overheating denture plastics and other restorations. The use of prophylactic pastes and dentrifices also must not unduly abrade tooth structure or restorative materials.

Self-test questions

In the following multiple choice questions, one or more responses may be correct.

1 A rough surface on a restoration is undesirable for which of the following reasons:
   a. Food debris and plaque can easily cling to it.
   b. Irritation and recession of soft tissues can occur in proximity to it.
   c. It is responsible for acceleration of corrosion of metallic restorations.
2 The rate of abrasion is increased by use of:
   a. A finer particle size
   b. An abrasive tool with rounded cutting surfaces
   c. Greater pressure on the abrasive tool
   d. Greater speed on the tool
3 Indicate which of the following are finishing abrasives and which are polishing abrasives:
   a. Tin oxide
   b. Sand
   c. Rouge
   d. Alumina
   e. Silicon carbide
   f. Diamond
   g. Silex
   h. Zirconium silicate
4 Final polishing of a dental amalgam to the smoothest surface is achieved by:
   a. Burnishing
   b. Carving

    c. Use of tin oxide

    d. Use of fine silicon carbide

5 Final polishing of cast gold alloy to the smoothest surface is achieved by:

    a. Pickling

    b. Electropolishing

    c. Use of rouge

    d. Use of Bendick on a rag wheel

    e. Use of fine cuttle

6 Final polishing of non-tissue-bearing surfaces of a denture resin is achieved by:

    a. Shell blasting

    b. Use of Bendick on a rag wheel

    c. Use of fine pumice

    d. Use of an acrylic finishing bur

7 The best surface for a hybrid composite resin is achieved by:

    a. Allowing polymerization to occur against a Mylar matrix

    b. Use of a green stone

    c. Use of an extra-fine silicon carbide disk

    d. Use of a white stone

8 Which of the following statements about prophylactic pastes are true?

    a. The abrasion of enamel is about twice that of dentin for a given product.

    b. Zirconium silicate is an effective cleansing and polishing agent, independent of its particle-size distribution.

    c. Use of a prophylactic paste should precede the application of a fluoride gel to make the enamel accessible and more reactive to the fluoride.

    d. Composites are not susceptible to abrasive wear by a prophylactic paste because of their hardness.

9 Desirable effects of toothbrushing are:

    a. Reduction of incidence of dental caries

    b. Maintenance of a healthy gingiva

    c. Reduction in intensity of mouth odors

    d. Enhancement of personal appearance

10 The components in a dentifrice may include:

    a. An abrasive such as insoluble sodium metaphosphate

    b. A therapeutic agent such as stannous fluoride

    c. A humectant such as glycerin

    d. A sweetening agent such as sorbitol

11 Which of the following surfaces are particularly susceptible to abrasion by dentifrices?

    a. Cementum

    b. Dentin

    c. Enamel

    d. Gold alloys

    e. Acrylic facings

    f. Denture resins

    g. Composite resins

12 Which of the following statements about denture cleansers are true?
  a. Dentures should not be soaked in hot water because the heat may cause the plastic to distort.
  b. A dentifrice should be used with a stiff-bristled brush.
  c. Customary 15-minute soaking of a denture with chemical cleansers is effective neither on mature plaque nor on some stains and deposits.
  d. Some chemical denture cleansers may cause corrosion of base metal components of a denture.

Suggested supplementary readings

Budtz-Jorgensen E: Materials and methods for cleaning dentures, *J Prosthet Dent* 42:619, 1979.

Council on Dental Materials, Instruments, and Equipment and Council on Dental Therapeutics: Accepted dental products, *J Am Dent Assoc* 116:249, 1988.

Council on Dental Therapeutics and Council on Prosthetic Services and Dental Laboratory Relations: Guidelines for infection control in the dental office and the commercial dental laboratory, *J Am Dent Assoc* 110:969, 1985.

Farah JW, Powers JM, editors: Finishing and polishing, *Dental Advis* 5(3):1-6, 1988.

Gershon SD, Pader M: Dentifrices. In Balsam MS, and Sagarin E, editors: *Cosmetics science and technology,* vol 1, ed 2, New York, 1972, John Wiley & Sons.

Handbook of non-prescription drugs, ed 8, Washington, DC, 1986, American Pharmaceutical Association.

Nygaard-Østby P, Edvardsen S, and Spydevold B: Access to interproximal tooth surfaces by different designs and stiffness of toothbrushes, *Scand J Dent Res* 87:424, 1979.

Nygaard-Østby P, Spydevold B, Edvardsen S: Suggestion for a definition, measuring method and classification system of bristle stiffness of toothbrushes, *Scand J Dent Res* 87:159, 1979.

Sulong MZAM, Aziz RA: Wear of materials used in dentistry: a review of the literature, *J Prosthet Dent* 63:342, 1990.

chapter
seven

Cements

Cements are generally hard, brittle materials that are formed by mixing a powdered oxide with a liquid. When mixed to a primary or luting consistency, dental cements are used to hold restorations such as gold crowns on prepared teeth. When mixed to a secondary consistency, cements are used as temporary filling materials or to provide thermal insulation and mechanical support to teeth restored with other materials, such as amalgam or gold. Cements classified as low-strength bases or liners provide protection to the pulp from irritants or serve therapeutically as pulp-capping agents. Varnishes are not cements but are used in conjunction with cements to provide pulpal protection from irritants. Some other cements are used for special purposes in endodontics, periodontics, oral surgery, and orthodontics. Cements are classified according to function in Table 7-1.

CEMENTATION

The retention of restorations on prepared teeth is a major function of dental cements. Long-term cementation is required for permanent restorations such as crowns and bridges (Figs. 1-5 and 1-8). Strong cements such as zinc phosphate, reinforced zinc oxide–eugenol, zinc polycarboxylate, or glass ionomer would be used. Often a bridge must be cemented temporarily to allow adjustments in fit, occlusion, and esthetics, or a temporary restoration such as an aluminum or acrylic crown must be cemented for 4 to 8 weeks until the permanent restoration is ready. In these cases, zinc oxide–eugenol and noneugenol zinc oxide cements would be used because of their low strength and good handling characteristics. Cements used for retention of restorations are mixed to a primary or luting consistency.

Table 7-1. Summary of Uses of Cements in Restorative Dentistry

Functions	Cements
Final cementation of cast crowns and bridges	Composite resin (self-cured), glass ionomer, reinforced zinc oxide–eugenol, zinc phosphate, zinc polycarboxylate
Temporary cementation of cast crowns and bridges or cementation of temporary restorations	Noneugenol zinc oxide, zinc oxide–eugenol
High-strength bases	Glass ionomer, reinforced zinc oxide–eugenol, zinc phosphate, zinc polycarboxylate
Temporary fillings	Reinforced zinc oxide–eugenol, zinc oxide–eugenol, zinc polycarboxylate
Low-strength bases	Calcium hydroxide (self- and light-cured), glass ionomer (self- and light-cured), resin, zinc oxide–eugenol
Liners	Calcium hydroxide in a suspension
Varnishes	Resin in a solvent
Special applications:	
Cementation of ceramic or composite inlays and onlays	Adhesive resin, composite resin (dual-cured)
Cementation of ceramic veneers	Composite resin (dual-cured or light-cured)
Cementation of orthodontic bands	Glass ionomer, zinc phosphate, zinc polycarboxylate
Cementation of resin-bonded bridges	Adhesive resin, composite resin (self-cured)
Direct bonding of orthodontic brackets	Acrylic resin, composite resin
Gingival tissue pack	Zinc oxide–eugenol
Periodontal dressing	Zinc oxide–eugenol, zinc oxide preparation
Root canal sealer	Zinc oxide–eugenol

Zinc phosphate cement

Zinc phosphate cement (Type I) is used primarily for final cementation in which high strength is necessary. Because of its acidity at the time of placement into a tooth, pulpal protection is needed. The cement is formed by mixing a powdered oxide with an acidic liquid. Examples of commercial products are listed in Table 7-2.

Composition and reaction. The zinc phosphate cement powder is primarily zinc oxide with additions of magnesium oxide and pigments. The liquid is a solution of phosphoric acid in water buffered by aluminum and zinc ions to help slow the setting reaction during mixing.

A chemical reaction begins when the cement powder is incorporated into the liquid. The surface of the alkaline powder is dissolved by the acidic liquid, resulting in an **exothermic** reaction. **The cement is mixed in such a way as to minimize the temperature rise from the heat given off.**

An exothermic reaction gives off heat as the components react.

Table 7-2. Examples of Cements Suitable for Final Cementation of Cast Crowns and Bridges

Cement	Product	Manufacturer
Composite resin	Biomer	Dentsply/Caulk
Glass ionomer	Fuji Type I*	G-C
	Ketac–Cem*	ESPE/Premier
Zinc oxide–eugenol (Type II)		
EBA-alumina-reinforced	Alumina Super EBA†	Bosworth
Polymer-reinforced	Fynal	Dentsply/Caulk
Zinc phosphate (Type I)	Fleck's Extraordinary†	Mizzy
	Modern Tenacin†	Dentsply/Caulk
	Zinc Cement Improved†	Mission White
Zinc polycarboxylate	Durelon†	ESPE/Premier
	Hy-Bond†	Shofu
	Tylok Plus	Dentsply/Caulk

*Provisionally acceptable product according to ADA Acceptance Program.
†Certified product according to ANSI–ADA Specification Nos. 8, 30, or 61.

The set cement is essentially a hydrated amorphous network of zinc phosphate that surrounds incompletely dissolved particles of zinc oxide. The cement is very porous.

Properties. Some important properties of zinc phosphate cement include viscosity and setting time of the setting cement, mechanical properties, film thickness, solubility, and acidity of the set cement. Requirements for certified products are described by ANSI–ADA Specification No. 8.

Viscosity of zinc phosphate cement is affected by time and temperature (Fig. 7-1). **Cooling the mixing slab increases the working time.** Cement normally sets in the mouth within 5 to 9 minutes from the start of mixing. **Factors such as a higher powder-liquid ratio, faster incorporation of powder into the liquid, and a warmer slab cause the cement to set faster.** Cementation should be completed promptly after mixing; delays can result in higher film thicknesses and insufficient seating of restorations.

The mechanical properties of zinc phosphate cement are compared with other high-strength cements in Table 7-3. The high compressive strength and modulus of zinc phosphate cement can be adversely affected by a low powder-liquid ratio, improper mixing, and premature exposure to oral fluids. The strength develops rapidly, with two thirds of final strength being reached in 1 hour. The low tensile strength of zinc phosphate cement compared with its compressive strength indicates the brittle nature of this cement. **The retention of zinc phos-**

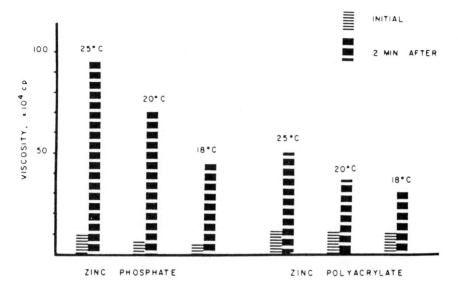

Fig. 7-1. Viscosity of zinc polycarboxylate and zinc phosphate cements as a function of time and temperature. (Modified from Vermilyea S, Powers JM, Craig RG: *J Dent Res* 56:762, 1977.)

Table 7-3. Mechanical Properties of Cements for Final and Temporary Cementation*

Cement	Compressive strength (psi [MN/m²])	Tensile strength (psi [MN/m²])	Modulus of elasticity (10⁶ psi [GN/m²])†
Cements for final cementation			
Composite resin	23,000 (160)	—	0.5 (3.5)
Glass ionomer	13,500-32,700 (90-220)	650 (4.5)	0.8 (5.4)
Zinc oxide–eugenol (Type II)			
Ethoxybenzoic acid-alumina-reinforced	9000 (64)	1000 (7)	0.8 (5.4)
Polymer-reinforced	5400 (37)	550 (4)	0.4 (3.0)
Zinc phosphate	14,000-19,000 (96-130)	450-660 (3-5)	1.3-1.9 (9-13)
Zinc polycarboxylate	8000-14,000 (55-96)	500-900 (3-6)	0.6 (4.4)
Cements for temporary cementation			
Noneugenol zinc oxide	400-700 (2-5)	60-140 (0.4-1.0)	0.03 (0.18)
Zinc oxide–eugenol (Type I)	400-2000 (2-14)	—	—

*Properties measured at 24 hours.
†10^6 psi = 1,000,000 psi, and GN/m² = 1000 MN/m².

Table 7-4. Effects of Manipulative Variables on Selected Properties of Zinc Phosphate Cement

	Property				
Manipulative variables	**Compressive strength**	**Film thickness**	**Solubility**	**Initial acidity**	**Setting time**
Decreased powder-liquid ratio	Decrease	Decrease	Increase	Increase	Lengthen
Increased rate of powder incorporation	Decrease	Increase	Increase	Increase	Shorten
Increased mixing temperature	Decrease	Increase	Increase	Increase	Shorten
Water contamination*	Decrease	Increase	Increase	Increase	Shorten

*Water contamination should not be confused with water incorporated in the frozen slab method.

phate cement is caused by mechanical interlocking with the surfaces of the tooth and restoration.

The film thickness (25 μm maximum) and solubility in water (0.2% maximum weight loss after 24 hours) are within clinically acceptable limits. The pH of zinc phosphate cement is initially low (pH 4.2) but increases to nearly neutral after 48 hours. The initial acidity may have a deleterious effect on the pulp, particularly on one that is traumatized already. **Pulpal protection is recommended.**

The properties of zinc phosphate cement are sensitive to variations in manipulation. A summary of effects of manipulation on selected properties is shown in Table 7-4.

Manipulation. Materials and instruments for mixing and placement of zinc phosphate cement are shown in Fig. 7-2, A. The bottle of powder is gently shaken and the bottle of liquid swirled before the contents are dispensed. The cement powder normally is dispensed with a scoop supplied by the manufacturer. The powder is divided in one corner of the glass slab into four to six portions, depending on the product (Fig. 7-2, B). The amount of liquid, given by drops as directed in the instructions, is dispensed to an area of the slab away from the powder. A typical powder-liquid ratio is 2.6 gm of powder:1.0 ml* of liquid for a primary consistency of cement. Before the powder and liquid are dispensed, the slab is cooled under cold water to about 21° C (70° F) and dried. **Any moisture left on the slab or condensed onto the slab because it was too cold will have a deleterious effect on the properties of the cement.**

The powder is added to the liquid in portions at 15-second intervals for a total mixing time of 60 to 120 seconds depending on the product. The cement is mixed over a large area of the slab with broad strokes of a flexible metal spatula. The consistency of the cement should be tested before the last portion of pow-

*1 ml = 20 drops.

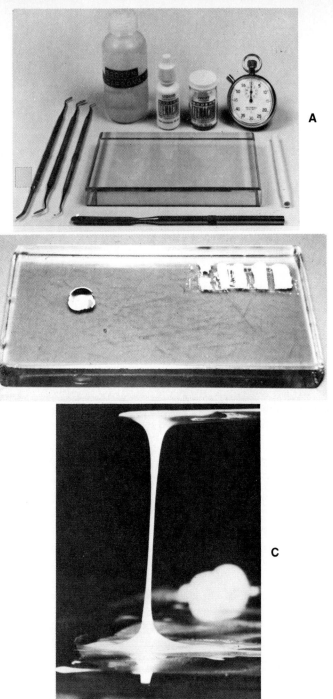

Fig. 7-2. A, Materials and instruments for mixing and placement of zinc phosphate cement. **B,** Zinc phosphate cement liquid and powder dispensed on the glass slab; the smaller portions of powder are mixed first. **C,** Primary or luting consistency strings about an inch above the mixing slab. (**A** and **C** from Charbeneau GT, et al: *Principles and practice of operative dentistry,* ed 2, Philadelphia, 1981, Lea & Febiger.)

der is added. Only part of that portion of powder may be necessary to reach the desired consistency. **The luting consistency strings about an inch above the slab** (Fig. 7-2, C).

Frozen slab method. The normal mixing procedure, as described, results in mixes with adequate working and setting times for cementation of crowns and inlays. **The frozen slab method provides longer working times** that are necessary for cementation of orthodontic bands and multiunit bridges. A glass slab is cooled in a refrigerator at 6° C (42° F) or in a freezer at −10° C (14° F). Moisture that condenses on the slab during mixing is incorporated into the cement mix along with 50% to 75% more powder than is used in the normal mixing procedure. The powder is added to the mix within 30 seconds until the correct consistency is reached.

Normal and frozen slab mixes are the same in strength and solubility. The frozen slab mix does have a longer working time of up to 11 minutes for a slab temperature of −10° C but a shorter setting time in the mouth of 20% to 40% compared with a normal mix made at 23° C.

Zinc oxide–eugenol cements

Zinc oxide–eugenol cements have a sedative effect on the pulp and are especially useful for cementation on prepared teeth with exposed dentinal tubules. The addition of reinforcing agents to zinc oxide–eugenol cement has resulted in permanent luting cements (Type II, Table 7-2). Temporary cements (Type I, Table 7-5) are not as strong but are useful for short-term cementation of temporary stainless steel crowns and permanent restorations. Noneugenol zinc oxide cements (Table 7-5) are used for short-term cementation of temporary acrylic crowns and completed cast restorations. They are weak and easily cleaned from the casting.

Composition and reaction. The zinc oxide–eugenol cement powder (Type I) contains zinc oxide (69%); rosin (29%), to reduce brittleness; and zinc acetate,

Table 7-5. Examples of Cements Suitable for Temporary Cementation of Completed Restorations or Cementation of Temporary Restorations

Cement	Product	Manufacturer
Zinc oxide–eugenol (Type I)	Flow-Temp	Premier
	Temp-Bond*	Sybron/Kerr
	ZOE 2200	Dentsply/Caulk
Noneugenol zinc oxide	Freegenol	G-C
	Nogenol	Coe/G-C
	Temp-Bond NE	Sybron/Kerr

*Certified product according to ANSI–ADA Specification No. 30.

an accelerator. The liquid is eugenol or a mixture of eugenol and other oils. The powder reacts with the eugenol in
the presence of moisture to form an amorphous **chelate** of
zinc eugenolate. The noneugenol zinc oxide cements
(Type I) are formulated with oils other than eugenol for patients sensitive to eugenol.

**A chelate is a ringlike
compound formed from
the organic groups and
the zinc oxide.**

The polymer-reinforced zinc oxide–eugenol cements (Type II) contain 80%
zinc oxide and 20% acrylic resin in the powder, and eugenol in the liquid. The
ethoxybenzoic acid-(EBA) alumina-reinforced cements contain 70% zinc oxide
and 30% alumina in the powder. The liquid is 62.5% EBA and 37.5% eugenol.
The EBA in the liquid promotes the formation of a stronger, crystalline matrix.
Water and heat accelerate the setting reaction of these cements.

Properties. The strength and pH of the zinc oxide–eugenol cements are important properties. Requirements for certified products are described by ANSI–
ADA Specification No. 30.

The compressive strengths of the permanent and temporary zinc oxide–eugenol cements are listed in Table 7-3. The permanent zinc oxide–eugenol cements are not as strong as zinc phosphate cements but have been shown to be
clinically successful for final cementation of crowns and bridges that have good
retention. The temporary cements are weaker, a desirable feature for cementation of temporary crowns or for temporary cementation of completed crown and
bridge restorations that must be easily removed.

The pH of the zinc oxide–eugenol cements is neutral. Because of the sedative nature of these cements, they do not require a protective varnish or cavity
liner.

Manipulation. The permanent zinc oxide–eugenol cements (Type II) are powder-liquid systems. The bottles are shaken gently; then the powder is dispensed
with the supplied scoop, and the liquid with a dropper. The mixing is done on a
glass slab with a metal spatula. The powder is incorporated into the liquid all at
once and is mixed for 30 seconds. The mix initially is like putty, but continued
mixing for an additional 30 seconds causes the polymer-reinforced cement mix
to become fluid. Therefore the EBA-alumina-reinforced cement must be
stropped for 60 seconds with broad strokes of the spatula after the initial 30-
second mixing to obtain a suitable consistency. The working time of the EBA-
alumina cements is long (about 22 minutes), unless moisture is present on the
slab. In the mouth the zinc oxide–eugenol cements set quickly because of the
moisture and heat.

The temporary cements (Type I) are typically two-paste systems. Equal
lengths of the accelerator and base pastes are dispensed on a paper pad or glass
slab (Fig. 7-3). The pastes are colored differently. Mixing should continue until
a uniform color is achieved.

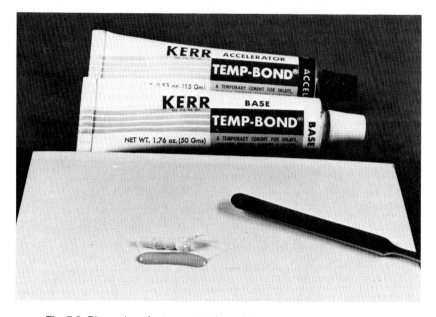

Fig. 7-3. Dispensing of a two-paste zinc oxide–eugenol temporary cement.

Zinc oxide–eugenol cements are difficult to remove from the tissues and mixing surfaces after setting. Thus the patient's lips and adjacent teeth should be coated with a silicone grease before application of the cement. Glass slabs and spatulas should be wiped clean before the cement sets. **Oil of orange is a solvent useful in removing set cement.**

Zinc polycarboxylate cements

Zinc polycarboxylate cements of a luting consistency are used as final cements for retention of crowns and bridges. They are not as strong as zinc phosphate cements but are less irritating to the pulp. Examples of commercial products are listed in Table 7-2.

Composition and reaction. Zinc polycarboxylate cements are supplied usually as a powder and liquid, although several products, such as Tylok Plus (Dentsply/Caulk), are supplied as powders to be mixed with tap water. The powder is mainly zinc oxide, and the liquid is a viscous solution of polyacrylic acid in water. The viscosity and reactivity of the liquid are controlled by the manufacturer by adjustment of the pH with sodium hydroxide, by control of the molecular weight of the polyacrylic acid between 25,000 and 50,000, and by the addition of other polycarboxylic acids. The powder of the products mixed with water consists of zinc oxide coated with solid polyacrylic acid.

The zinc oxide and the polyacrylic acid react to form a zinc polyacrylate that surrounds the partially reacted zinc oxide powder particles. The reaction is accelerated by heat but to a lesser extent than zinc phosphate cement is accelerated.

Properties. The important properties of zinc polycarboxylate cements are viscosity, strength, bonding to enamel, and pH. Requirements for certified products are described by ANSI–ADA Specification No. 61.

The viscosity of polycarboxylate cement initially is slightly higher than zinc phosphate cement (Fig. 7-1), but its viscosity is less affected by temperature. **The mixed polycarboxylate cement appears to be too thick, but it flows readily when applied to the surfaces to be cemented.**

The compressive strength of polycarboxylate cement (Table 7-3) is less than that of zinc phosphate cement and is similar to the reinforced zinc oxide–eugenol cements. It provides clinically satisfactory retention for well-fitting restorations. The slightly higher tensile strength of the polycarboxylates is caused by the test method.

In laboratory studies the polycarboxylate cements show chemical bonding (adhesion) to properly prepared human enamel and dentin. The cements bond well to sandblasted or electrolytically etched gold alloys, although clinical studies have not demonstrated improved retention with these cements.

Zinc polycarboxylate cements are slightly more acidic (lower pH) than zinc phosphate cements when first mixed, but the acid is weakly dissociated. Histological reactions are similar to those of zinc oxide–eugenol cements, but more reparative dentin is observed with the polycarboxylates.

Manipulation. The powder bottle should be shaken gently. The powder is dispensed with a scoop onto a disposable paper pad or a glass slab, which can be cooled to permit a longer working time. The viscous liquid is dispensed from the dropper bottle in uniform drops. Durelon liquid (ESPE-Premier) is supplied in a calibrated syringe to improve the accuracy of dispensing the liquid. The powder-liquid ratio is typically 1.5 gm of powder:1.0 gm of liquid for a luting consistency.

About 90% of the powder is added immediately to the liquid and mixed for 30 to 60 seconds, depending on the product. The remainder of the powder is added to adjust the consistency. The mixture is made over a small area of the mixing surface with a stiff spatula. The proper consistency is creamy but slightly more viscous than zinc phosphate cement. The cement should be used immediately because the working time is short (about 3 minutes after mixing at 22° C). **The cement is no longer usable when it loses its luster and becomes stringy or starts to "cobweb."**

Glass ionomer cements

The glass ionomer cements are used for final cementation of crowns and bridges. A cement with a thicker consistency is used for Class V restorations as described in Chapter 4. Core materials such as Ketac-Silver (ESPE-Premier) and Miracle Mix (G-C) contain finely divided silver added to the glass ionomer composition to produce a contrasting shade. Clinical data on the glass ionomer cements are limited, but properties measured in the laboratory are promising. Examples of commercial products are listed in Table 7-2.

Composition. The cement powder is a finely ground aluminosilicate glass, and the viscous liquid is a polycarboxylate copolymer in water. One product, Ketac-Cem (ESPE-Premier), supplies a powder coated with polyacrylic acid copolymers. It is mixed with a low-viscosity liquid to form the cement. The components of glass ionomer cements react to form a cross-linked gel matrix surrounding the partially reacted powder particles. **Chelation between the polycarboxylate molecules and calcium on the surface of the tooth results in a chemical (adhesive) bond.**

Properties. Requirements for certified products are described by ANSI–ADA Specification No. 66. The compressive and tensile strengths of glass ionomer cements are similar to those of zinc phosphate cements (Table 7-3). The cement has the nonirritating qualities of zinc polycarboxylate cements; however, a calcium hydroxide base is recommended for pulpal protection when the ionomer cement is used in a deep cavity. Because of fluoride incorporated in the powder, the cement has an anticariogenic effect as it is leached out. The ionomer cements have a relatively high early solubility compared with other cements, and the complete setting reaction takes about 1 day; thus **cement exposed at the margins of a restoration must be protected during the first 24 hours.**

Manipulation. The bottle of powder is tumbled gently before dispensing. The powder and liquid are dispensed onto a paper pad or glass slab. The powder-liquid ratio is 1.25 gm of powder to 1.0 gm of liquid. The powder is divided into two equal portions. The first portion of powder is mixed with a stiff spatula into the liquid before the next portion is added. The mixing time should be 30 to 60 seconds, depending on the product. One product (Ketac-Cem Maxicaps, ESPE-Premier) is encapsulated and requires a 10-second mechanical mixing. The cement must be used immediately because the working time after mixing is about 2 minutes at 22° C. **The cement should not be used once a "skin" forms on the surface or when the consistency becomes noticeably thicker.** During application, contact with water must be avoided; thus the field must be completely isolated. The cement sets in the mouth in about 7 minutes from the start of mixing. A coating agent supplied with the cement should be applied immediately to exposed cement margins.

Table 7-6. Examples of High- and Low-Strength Bases

Cement	Product	Manufacturer
High-strength bases		
Glass ionomer (self-cured)	Ketac–Bond Aplicap	ESPE/Premier
	Glasionomer base cement	Shofu
	Dentin cement	G-C
Polymer-reinforced zinc oxide– eugenol (Type III)	B & T	Dentsply/Caulk
Zinc phosphate	Modern Tenacin*	Dentsply/Caulk
Zinc polycarboxylate	Durelon*	ESPE/Premier
Low-strength bases		
Calcium hydroxide (light-cured)	Prisma VLC Dycal†	Dentsply/Caulk
Calcium hydroxide (self-cured)	Life†	Sybron/Kerr
Glass ionomer (light-cured)	Vitrabond	3M
	XR Ionomer	Sybron/Kerr
Glass ionomer (self-cured)	Gingival Seal	Parkell
	Zionomer	Den-Mat
Resin	Timeline	Dentsply/Caulk
Zinc oxide–eugenol (Type IV)	Cavitec*	Sybron/Kerr

*Certified product according to ANSI–ADA Specification Nos. 8, 30, or 61.
†Accepted preparation of Council on Dental Therapeutics.

HIGH-STRENGTH BASES

High-strength bases are used to provide mechanical support for a restoration and thermal protection for the pulp. Bases may be prepared from a secondary (puttylike) consistency of a zinc phosphate or zinc polycarboxylate cement, examples of which are listed in Table 7-6. A polymer-reinforced zinc oxide–eugenol cement and glass ionomer bases are also available.

The composition and reaction of the cements used for high-strength bases are discussed under the section "Cementation."

Properties. Some important properties of cements used as high-strength bases are strength, modulus of elasticity, and thermal conductivity.

The compressive and tensile strengths of high-strength bases are listed in Table 7-7. The base consistency is generally stronger than the luting consistency (see Table 7-2) because the base is mixed at a higher powder-liquid ratio. The strength must develop quickly because the base may be required to support the condensation forces during the insertion of a dental amalgam. **The ability of the base to resist occlusal forces and to support the restoration is affected by**

Table 7-7. Mechanical Properties of High- and Low-Strength Bases*

Cement	Compressive strength (psi [MN/m²])	Tensile strength (psi [MN/m²])	Modulus of elasticity (10⁶ psi [GN/m²])†
High-strength bases			
Glass ionomer (self-cured)	10,200-30,700 (70-210)	560-1200 (3.9-8.3)	0.5-1.3 (3.7-9.0)
Polymer-reinforced zinc oxide–eugenol (Type III)	5500 (38)	500 (3.4)	0.3 (2.1)
Zinc phosphate	19,000-23,000 (130-160)	1200 (8)	3.0 (22)
Zinc polycarboxylate	12,000 (80)	2400 (16)	0.7 (5.0)
Low-strength bases			
Calcium hydroxide (light-cured)	14,000 (96)	5500 (38)	—
Calcium hydroxide (self-cured)	1800-3800 (12-26)	150 (1.0)	0.06 (0.4)
Glass ionomer (light-cured)	9500 (66)	1400-3000 (9.6-20)	0.2-0.3 (1.5-2.2)
Glass ionomer (self-cured)	5800-25,400 (40-175)	—	0.25-0.40 (1.8-2.8)
Resin	23,000 (160)	—	0.3 (2.2)
Zinc oxide–eugenol (Type IV)	800 (5.5)	60 (0.4)	0.04 (0.3)

*Properties measured at 24 hours.
†10^6 psi = 1,000,000 psi, and GN/m² = 1000 MN/m².

its modulus of elasticity. Zinc phosphate cement provides the best support for amalgam because it has the highest modulus (Table 7-7).

The base must provide thermal protection to the pulp. As indicated in Chapter 2 (Table 2-2), the thermal conductivity of metallic restorations is high compared with tooth structure. The thermal conductivity of cement bases is similar to tooth structure; thus the base can protect the pulp from thermal changes. **Effective protection requires the base be at least 0.5 mm thick.**

Glass ionomer bases are used as structural bases for posterior composites and porcelain or composite inlays and onlays and for crown buildups when adequate tooth support is available. These bases are viscous and are best placed with a syringe. One product (Ketac–Bond Aplicap) is encapsulated and requires mechanical mixing.

Manipulation. A zinc phosphate or zinc polycarboxylate high-strength base is mixed by first reaching the luting or primary consistency of the cement as discussed. Additional powder is then added to achieve the puttylike base consistency. The powder-liquid ratio of zinc phosphate cements for luting consistency increases from 2.6 to 4.8 gm of powder per milliliter of liquid for the base consistency. Unlike the other bases, the glass ionomer bases are mixed directly to their final consistency.

TEMPORARY FILLINGS

Certain cements mixed to a base consistency may be used successfully as temporary fillings. The temporary filling protects the pulp, reduces pulpal inflammation, and maintains tooth position while restoring esthetics until a permanent restoration can be placed. Zinc oxide–eugenol cements are used most frequently. For shorter term fillings, an unmodified zinc oxide–eugenol cement such as TemPak (Westward Dental) is mixed to a puttylike consistency. Several cotton fibers may be added to the mix. Setting of this mix is accelerated by patting the surface of the filling with a cotton pellet saturated with hot water. For longer-term fillings, a modified zinc oxide–eugenol cement such as B & T or IRM (Dentsply/Caulk) or a zinc polycarboxylate cement can be used.

LOW-STRENGTH BASES

Low-strength bases harden when mixed and form a cement layer usually with minimum strength and low rigidity. These bases function as a barrier to irritating chemicals and provide a therapeutic benefit to the pulp. Examples of calcium hydroxide, glass ionomer, resin, and zinc oxide–eugenol (Type IV) low-strength bases are listed in Table 7-6. Their properties are summarized in Table 7-7. Low-strength bases are often called liners and should be distinguished from the cavity-liner suspensions described in the next section.

Calcium hydroxide cement

A calcium hydroxide cement is used for direct and indirect pulp capping and as a protective barrier beneath composite restorations. It does not interfere with the polymerization of these materials.

Composition and reaction. The base paste of one calcium hydroxide cement contains calcium tungstate, calcium phosphate, and zinc oxide in glycol salicylate. The catalyst paste contains calcium hydroxide, zinc oxide, and zinc stearate in ethylene toluene sulfonamide. Setting results from the formation of an amorphous calcium disalicylate. The cements usually contain a radiopaque filler.

The light-cured product is a urethane dimethacrylate resin with calcium hydroxide and barium sulfate fillers and a low-viscosity monomer.

Properties. Calcium hydroxide cements have low mechanical properties (Table 7-7) compared with cements used as high-strength bases, but they are stronger than zinc oxide–eugenol cement (Type IV). The cements have a low thermal conductivity but usually are not used in thick enough layers to provide thermal protection. The cements stimulate the formation of reparative dentin under an indirect pulp cap or at the site of a direct pulp cap. The pH of the cements is basic and varies from 11 to 12. Setting times vary from 2 to 7 minutes, with faster-setting cements being more desirable. Solubility in water and in acid varies considerably among products. Products with low-acid solubility can be placed in conjunction with acid-etched composites.

Manipulation. Most calcium hydroxide cements are a two-paste system. Equal lengths of each paste are dispensed on a paper pad and mixed to a uniform color. The light-cured cement should be cured by a visible-light source for 20 seconds for each 1-mm layer.

Glass ionomer cement

The glass ionomer low-strength bases are used primarily as liners under amalgam and composite restorations and are available in self-cured and light-cured formulations (Fig. 7-4 and Table 7-6).

Composition and reaction. The self-cured glass ionomer liners are similar in composition to the luting cements and bases described previously only more fluid. The light-cured liners are resin-based systems in which curing is accelerated by visible light.

Properties. The glass ionomer liners are the strongest and most rigid of the low-strength bases (Table 7-7). **The liners, however, are less rigid than the glass ionomer high-strength bases and should not be used to provide sole mechanical support for amalgam or composite restorations.** Because the pH is acidic, the use of calcium hydroxide for pulpal protection is recommended. The glass ionomer liners release fluoride, although the long-term, clinical benefit of that release has not been established. These liners also bond to conditioned dentin, with values as high as 700 psi (4.9 MN/m^2) being reported. Dentin conditioners are described for use with Class V glass ionomer restorations in Chapter 4.

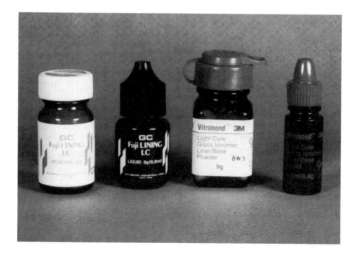

Fig. 7-4. Examples of light-cured glass ionomer low-strength bases (liners).

Manipulation. The self-cured glass ionomer liners are powder-liquid systems. One scoop of powder is mixed rapidly with one drop of liquid. The liner is applied to moist dentin with a small burnisher. Most self-cured liners set within 2 to 3 minutes.

Resin cement

The resin low-strength base is used primarily with composite restorations and is light-cured. It is a urethane dimethacrylate resin with barium glass, barium sulfate fillers, and dispersed sodium fluoride. This liner is strong but has a low rigidity.

Zinc oxide–eugenol cement

A nonmodified zinc oxide–eugenol cement is used in a deep cavity to retard penetration of acids and reduce possible discomfort to the pulp. Because it is used in thin layers, the base provides little thermal insulation. The strength and modulus of a Type IV zinc oxide–eugenol cement are low (Table 7-7). The base should be limited to small or non-stress-bearing areas but normally will support forces associated with placement of a restoration. The eugenol has a sedative (obtundent) effect on pulpal tissue.

The cement is supplied as a two-paste system (Fig. 7-5). Equal lengths of the different colored pastes are dispensed on a paper pad and are mixed to a uniform color. The cement should not be used when an unfilled resin or composite is to be placed because the eugenol inhibits the polymerization. **Often a high-strength base is placed over the zinc oxide–eugenol low-strength base to provide strength, rigidity, and thermal protection.**

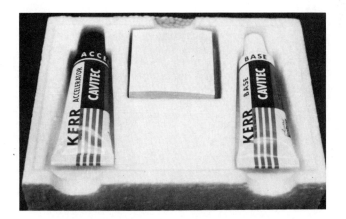

Fig. 7-5. Zinc oxide–eugenol low-strength base cement.

CAVITY LINERS AND VARNISHES

Cavity liners and varnishes function as a protective barrier between dentin and the restorative material, minimize the ingress of oral fluids at the restoration-tooth interface, and may provide some therapeutic benefits to the tooth. They are applied in thin films, and the solvent evaporates. They have no significant mechanical strength and provide essentially no thermal insulation.

Liners

Cavity liners are suspensions of calcium hydroxide in water or in an organic liquid (Table 7-8). The suspension may be thickened with methyl or ethyl cellulose. In addition, some liners contain fluoride. The film serves as a barrier and may neutralize acids. These liners are susceptible to solubility and disintegration in oral fluids and thus should be restricted to coverage of dentin. **Some liners may be disrupted by the monomers in resin or composite restorations.**

Varnishes

Cavity varnishes (Table 7-9) are solutions of resins, such as copal or nitrated cellulose, contained in organic liquids (e.g., chloroform or alcohol). When ap-

Table 7-8. Examples of Cavity Liners

Product*	Composition	Manufacturer
Hydroxyline	Calcium hydroxide and acrylic polymer in methyl ethyl ketone	George Taub
Accu-Spense	Calcium hydroxide, barium sulfate, and hydroxypropyl cellulose in ethyl alcohol	Cadco Dental
Hypo-Cal	Calcium hydroxide and barium sulfate in aqueous hydroxyethyl cellulose solution	Ellman
Pulpdent Cavity Liner	Calcium hydroxide in aqueous methyl cellulose solution	Pulpdent

*Accepted preparations of Council on Dental Therapeutics.

Table 7-9. Examples of Cavity Varnishes

Product	Manufacturer
Cavi-Line	Dentsply/Caulk
Copalite	Bosworth
Handi-Liner	Mizzy

plied to the tooth, the solvent evaporates leaving a porous, resinous film that may be 2 to 40 μm thick depending on the product. More than one layer of the thinner films may be necessary to act as an effective barrier. Varnishes are insoluble in oral fluids. They reduce leakage around margins and walls of the restoration-tooth interface and appear to prevent penetration of corrosion products from amalgam into dentin. **Varnishes may be disrupted by monomers of resin or composite restorations and are not used under a therapeutic base.**

Varnish solutions are usually applied by means of a small cotton pledget at the end of a wire or root canal reamer. Thin layers of the varnish should be applied with a partially saturated pledget. A gentle stream of air may be used for drying, but care must be taken to avoid forming ridges. A new layer is added only to a previously dried one. Two thin layers have been found to be more protective than one heavy layer. To prevent contamination of the cavity varnish, a new cotton pledget should be used for each application. Varnish solutions should be tightly capped immediately after use to minimize loss of solvent. Most varnishes are supplied with a separate bottle of pure solvent, which may be used to keep the varnish from becoming too thick. The bottle should be kept half full by dilution with the solvent. Eventually the solvent will be exhausted and a new supply should be purchased. The solvent is also useful for removing varnish from external tooth surfaces.

SPECIAL APPLICATIONS OF CEMENT

Cements have many special applications in dentistry as indicated in Table 7-10.

Root canal sealer. If the dental pulp is removed, the root canal can be sealed by cementation of a gutta-percha point or by filling with a paste. Many root canal sealers are formulated from zinc oxide and eugenol. Some important properties of root canal sealers are setting time, flow, film thickness, strength, solubility, and radiopacity. Biological properties have been studied extensively.

Gingival tissue pack. Temporary displacement of the gingival tissues is desirable during certain restorative procedures. An effective method of reflecting tissues combines fine cotton twills with a slow-setting zinc oxide–eugenol cement. The cement is mixed to a thin, creamy consistency, and cotton twills of an appropriate size are rolled into the mass (Fig. 7-6). The pack is held in place in the gingival sulcus for 2 to 7 days by an interim dressing of zinc oxide–eugenol cement.

Periodontal dressings. Dressings may be applied to the gingiva following surgical periodontal procedures. These dressings typically contain zinc oxide and eugenol with modifiers such as tannic acid, rosin, and various oils. Several commercial preparations are listed in Table 7-10. The products are generally paste-paste or powder-liquid systems that are mixed to a paste or puttylike consistency.

Table 7-10. Examples of Cements Used for Special Applications

Application	Product	Manufacturer
Cementation of ceramic or composite inlays and onlays		
Adhesive resin	CR Inlay Cement	Kuraray
Composite resin (dual-cured)	Porcelite Dual Cure	Sybron/Kerr
Cementation of ceramic veneers		
Composite resin (dual-cured)	Insure	Cosmedent
	Optec	Jeneric/Pentron
	Ultra-Bond	Den-Mat
Composite resin (light-cured)	Luminbond	Vident
Cementation of orthodontic bands		
Glass ionomer	Ketac–Cem	ESPE-Premier
Zinc phosphate	Ormco Gold	Sybron/Ormco
Zinc polycarboxylate	Durelon	ESPE-Premier
Cementation of resin-bonded bridges		
Adhesive resin	Panavia	Kuraray
	Super-Bond C&B	Sun Medical
Composite resin (self-cured)	Resin Bonded Bridge Cement	Sybron/Kerr
Direct bonding of orthodontic brackets		
Acrylic resin	Bond-eze	Unitek
Composite resin (paste-primer)	Mono-Lok2	Rocky Mountain
Composite resin (self-cured)	Concise Orthobond	3M
	Endur	Sybron/Ormco
Gingival tissue pack	WondrPak	Westward Dental
Periodontal dressings		
Zinc oxide–eugenol	PCA Periodontal Pack*	Pulpdent
Zinc oxide preparation	Coe-Pack*	Coe/G-C
	Perio-Putty*	Cadco Dental
Root canal sealer		
Zinc oxide–eugenol	Roth Cements	Roth Drug

*Acceptable preparation of Council on Dental Therapeutics.

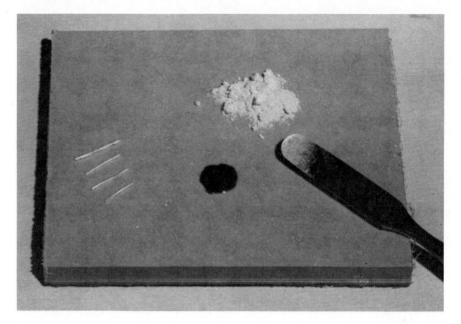

Fig. 7-6. Materials dispensed for making a mechanical tissue pack of zinc oxide–eugenol cement. (From Charbeneau GT, et al.: *Principles and practice of operative dentistry,* ed 2, Philadelphia, 1981, Lea & Febiger.)

Cementation of orthodontic bands. Orthodontic bands are cemented to the teeth most frequently with zinc phosphate cement, but zinc polycarboxylate and glass ionomer are also used. The compositions of these cements have been described earlier. Some zinc phosphate cements formulated specifically for orthodontics may contain fluoride to provide protection from caries. To achieve longer working times, the zinc phosphate cement is routinely mixed using the cold or frozen slab technic. The zinc phosphate cement bonds to the enamel by mechanical interlocking with the surface. Demineralization of the tooth surface, which occurs with zinc phosphate cement, is minimized with glass ionomer cement.

Direct bonding of orthodontic brackets. Recently, direct bonding of orthodontic brackets (Fig. 7-7) has been accomplished with the use of acrylic resin and composite resin cements. The composition of these cements is similar to that of the restorative materials described in Chapter 4. The surfaces of the teeth to be bonded are carefully acid etched. The cement is mixed and applied to the etched enamel, and the bracket (without a band) is positioned. Paste-primer and light-cured resin cements also are available (Table 7-10). With the former cement, the primer is applied to the enamel and the paste is applied to the

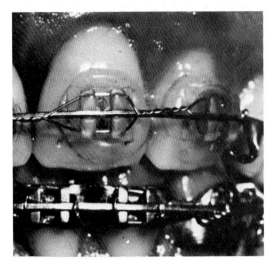

Fig. 7-7. Orthodontic brackets bonded directly to the enamel of maxillary teeth without bands by a resin cement. Mandibular teeth are banded using a zinc phosphate cement.

bracket. Setting occurs when the bracket is pressed into the primer on the tooth. **The film thickness should be less than 0.25 mm to ensure proper setting.** Plastic brackets are bonded successfully with acrylic cements and also with composite cements if conditioned with a bracket primer. Metal brackets are bonded best with a composite cement. When properly applied, the cements bond tenaciously to enamel. **Removal of the brackets and cement after treatment requires care to minimize damage to enamel.** Use of a 12-fluted finishing but without water and then pumice is recommended for efficient removal of cement, as well as a fiber-optic handpiece to keep the area well lit.

Cementation of resin-bonded bridges. Cast retainers such as Maryland bridges are bonded to acid-etched enamel with adhesive resin or composite resin cements. Before cementation, nickel-chromium alloy retainers are **electroetched** or sandblasted. The bond to the sandblasted alloy is stronger than the bond to enamel. The adhesive resin bonds better than the composite resin under conditions of in vitro thermocycling. The cements are characterized by short working times, low film thicknesses, and high strengths. Translucent and opaque cements are available.

Electroetching is a process in which the surface of the metal is deplated in an electrolytic solution under the influence of an electric current.

Cementation of ceramic or composite inlays and onlays. Esthetic inlays and onlays are cemented with strong, radiopaque composite resins capable of dual-curing (can be light-cured and chemically cured). For cementation of an inlay, the cement must be wear resistant at exposed margins. An adhesive cement (CR Inlay Cement) based on an organic phosphonate that bonds to tooth structure is now available.

Cementation of ceramic veneers. Ceramic veneers (Cerestore, Den-Mat, Mirage, and Chameleon) require strong cements, which are available with a variety of shades, tints, and opaquers. Nonsetting try-in pastes of matching shades are a convenient accessory.

Cements are used for luting of restorations and as bases. The most common cements (zinc phosphate, zinc oxide–eugenol, zinc polycarboxylate, and glass ionomer) are composed of a zinc oxide or glass powder and have an acidic liquid or eugenol, which are usually mixed by hand. Adhesive and composite resin cements composed of dimethacrylate resin and filler are used for special dental applications. Important properties include working time, film thickness, tensile and compressive strengths, modulus of elasticity, and biocompatibility. These properties are best when manipulative technics are followed precisely.

Self-test questions

In the following multiple choice questions, one or more responses may be correct.
1 Zinc phosphate cement is used:
   a. As a base for thermal and mechanical protection of the pulp
   b. For cementation of orthodontic bands
   c. For retention of cast metallic restorations
   d. As a liner
2 Which of the following statements are true?
   a. The marginal adaptation of a casting to the tooth is affected by the film thickness of the cement.
   b. Typical values of film thickness and compressive strengths of zinc phosphate cement are 25 μm and 17,000 psi, respectively.
   c. The retaining action of zinc phosphate cement is one of mechanical bonding between surface irregularities of the tooth and casting by the cement.
   d. Zinc phosphate cement is as strong in tension as it is in compression.
3 Which of the following statements are true for zinc phosphate cements?
   a. The powder is added to the liquid in small increments to minimize the amount of temperature rise in the mixture.
   b. Total mixing time varies between 30 and 120 seconds.
   c. Moisture on the mixing slab accelerates the setting reaction.
   d. Once the cementing or primary consistency is obtained, the base consistency is achieved by the addition of powder to the mix.
4 An increased amount of powder in a cementing consistency mix of zinc phosphate cement:
   a. Decreases the solubility   **c.** Decreases the film thickness
   b. Increases the strength   **d.** Increases the setting time

5 The components of zinc oxide–eugenol cement may include:
   a. Ethoxybenzoic acid (EBA) in the eugenol to improve strength
   b. Alumina or acrylic polymer in the powder to improve strength
   c. Zinc acetate in the powder as an accelerator
   d. Zinc oxide and eugenol formulated as pastes in separate tubes
6 Which of the following statements are true for zinc oxide–eugenol cements?
   a. Zinc oxide powder is added to the eugenol liquid on a treated paper pad in six equal increments.
   b. Equal lengths of the base paste and the accelerator paste are mixed together until the mix has a uniform color.
   c. Increases in temperature and humidity shorten the setting time.
   d. A mix appears thick at the start of mixing, but, after 30 seconds of additional spatulation, it becomes more fluid.
   e. Water accelerates, but heat retards the setting of zinc oxide–eugenol cements.
7 Which of the following statements about zinc oxide–eugenol cements are true?
   a. The permanent zinc oxide–eugenol cements are clinically successful for final cementation of crowns and bridges having good retention.
   b. The tensile strength of zinc oxide–eugenol cements increases with the addition of EBA and alumina reinforcers but does not exceed about 1000 psi.
   c. The compressive strength of an EBA-alumina-reinforced zinc oxide–eugenol cement is about 9000 psi.
   d. The compressive strengths of polymer-reinforced zinc oxide–eugenol cements are as high as EBA-alumina-reinforced zinc oxide–eugenol cements.
8 The components of zinc polycarboxylate cements include:
   a. Zinc polyacrylate crystals in water
   b. A solution of polyacrylic acid in water
   c. Zinc oxide powder
   d. A paste of zinc oxide and one of acrylic acid
9 Which of the following statements are true?
   a. The pH of the mix of zinc polycarboxylate cement is initially acidic and increases to neutrality in several days.
   b. The pulpal reaction to zinc polycarboxylate cement is similar to that of zinc phosphate cement.
   c. Zinc polycarboxylate cement acts as an obtundent like zinc oxide–eugenol cement.
10 Which of the following statements are true for zinc polycarboxylate cements?
   a. The powder is incorporated into the liquid within 30 seconds.
   b. The working time can be extended by use of a cooled glass mixing slab.
   c. After a cement loses its luster and becomes stringy, it is ready to be used.
   d. The correct consistency for cementation is about one and one-half parts powder to one part liquid by weight.
   e. Cementation consistency of zinc polycarboxylate cement is similar to that of zinc phosphate cement.

11 Which of these statements apply to the comparison of zinc polycarboxylate and zinc phosphate cement?

   a. The viscosity of zinc polycarboxylate cement increases more rapidly with temperature than that of zinc phosphate cement.

   b. Zinc polycarboxylate cements provide superior clinical retention of crowns compared with zinc phosphate cements.

   c. Both cements depend primarily on mechanical bonding for retention clinically.

   d. When first mixed, zinc polycarboxylate cements are slightly more acidic than zinc phosphate cements.

12 Two characteristics of light-cured resin cements for cementation of ceramic veneers are:

   a. High strength

   b. Variety of stains and shades

   c. Chemical bonding to dentin and ceramics

   d. Fluoride content

13 Which of the following statements about glass ionomer cements are true?

   a. The cement powder is an aluminosilicate glass, whereas the liquid is a polycarboxylate copolymer in water.

   b. The cement must be protected from exposure to water during setting.

   c. Pulpal protection is not necessary for use of a glass ionomer cement in a deep cavity.

   d. The cement is mixed by the addition of increments of powder to the liquid within 45 seconds.

14 Which of the following cement bases has the highest elastic modulus to best support an extensive amalgam restoration?

   a. Zinc phosphate

   b. Polymer-reinforced zinc oxide–eugenol

   c. Zinc polyacrylate

   d. Glass ionomer

15 Which of the following materials are used over pulp exposures?

   a. Zinc phosphate

   b. Polymer-reinforced zinc oxide–eugenol

   c. Calcium hydroxide

   d. Zinc polycarboxylate

16 Which of the following statements are true?

   a. Calcium hydroxide bases are supplied with a powder and a liquid catalyst, which is colored.

   b. A small spatula is used to mix equal lengths of the two pastes of a calcium hydroxide base on a paper pad.

   c. Some cavity liners that contain calcium hydroxide harden quickly by evaporation when dried by air.

   d. Varnishes form resin films usually less than 40 μm thick by evaporation of the solvent.

Suggested supplementary readings

Council on Dental Materials, Instruments and Equipment: Biocompatibility and postoperative sensitivity, *J Am Dent Assoc* 116:767, 1988.

Council on Dental Materials, Instruments and Equipment: Using glass ionomers, *J Am Dent Assoc* 121:181, 1990.

Council on Dental Materials, Instruments and Equipment and Council on Dental Therapeutics: Accepted dental products, *J Am Dent Assoc* 116:2498, 1988.

Farah JW, Powers JM: Cements, *Dent Advis* 2(1):1, 1985.

Farah JW, Powers JM: Resin cements, *Dental Advis* 5(1):1, 1985.

Farah JW, Powers JM: Glass ionomers and electric laboratory handpieces, *Dental Advis* 7(2):1, 1990.

O'Keefe K, Powers JM: Light-cured resin cements for cementation of esthetic restorations, *J Esthet Dent,* in press.

Powers JM, Craig RG: A review of the composition and properties of endodontic filling materials, *J Mich Dent Assoc* 61:523, 1979.

Impression Materials

The function of an impression material is to record the dimensions of oral tissues and their spatial relationships accurately. In making an impression, a material in the plastic state is placed against the oral tissues to set. After setting, the impression is removed from the mouth and is used to make a replica of the oral tissues. The impression gives a negative reproduction of these tissues. A positive reproduction is obtained by pouring dental stone or other suitable material into the impression and allowing it to harden. The positive reproduction is called a **model** or cast when large areas of the oral tissues are involved or a **die** when single or multiple tooth preparations are recorded.

The relationships between a tooth, an impression of the tooth, and a die are illustrated in two dimensions in Fig. 8-1. Note that when examined from the anterior side, the various parts of the tooth and the impression are in the same relationship to each other, although the highest portions of the tooth are the deepest parts of the impression. When the maxillary die is examined with the occlusal portion downward, the die is a positive reproduction of the tooth preparation. If the die is examined with the occlusal surface upward, the buccal surface (B) is on the left rather than the right. A similar relationship is shown in Fig. 8-1 for a cross section of a mandibular left molar, its impression, and the die made from it. The impression of the mandibular molar, when examined from the anterior side, is inverted for ease of examination and the buccal (B) and lingual (L) surfaces are reversed with respect to the tooth. The cusp (C) is the highest area on the tooth and the lowest area of the impression, and the position of C for the tooth is on the left but on the right for the impression. The die of the mandibular molar, however, is a positive duplication of the tooth.

Impressions may be taken of portions of a tooth, a single tooth, several teeth, a quadrant of the mouth, or an entire dentulous or edentulous arch. Examples

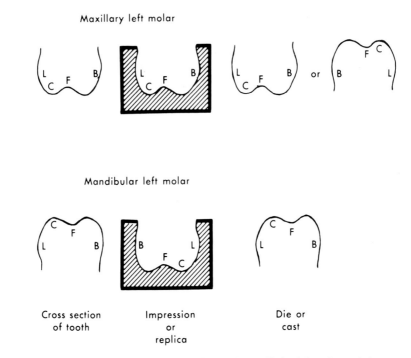

Fig. 8-1. Two-dimensional sketches of a maxillary and mandibular left molar and the corresponding impressions and dies.

of some of these types of impressions and the corresponding dies or casts are shown in Fig. 8-2.

A variety of impression materials are described in this chapter, indicative of the fact that no single material is ideal for all applications. The following list of properties for an ideal impression material emphasizes the many demands placed on these materials. Not surprisingly, none of the current materials completely satisfies these requirements.

1. Ease of manipulation and reasonable cost
2. Adequate flow properties
3. Appropriate setting time and characteristics
4. Sufficient mechanical strength not to tear or permanently deform during removal
5. Good dimensional accuracy
6. Acceptability to the patient
7. Safety (not toxic or irritating)
8. Compatibility with die and cast materials
9. Good keeping qualities (no deterioration of unused material in the dental office)

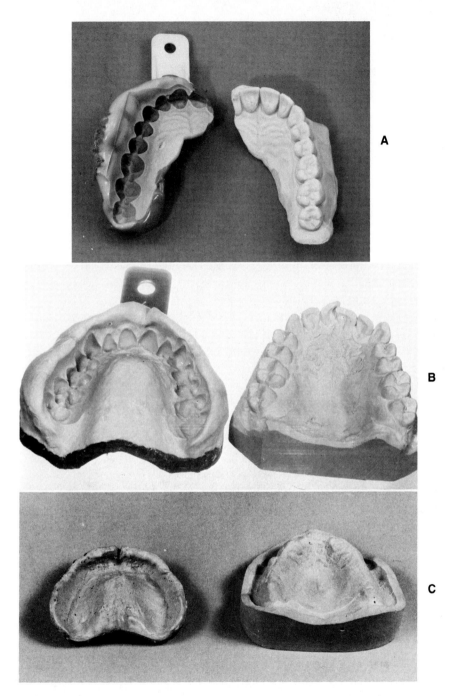

Fig. 8-2. Examples of impressions with the corresponding gypsum dies or casts. **A,** Quadrant impression in addition silicone rubber. **B,** Full-arch impression in alginate. **C,** Edentulous zinc oxide–eugenol impression.

Table 8-1. Classification of Dental Impression Materials

Rigid	Flexible
Dental compound	Agar hydrocolloid
Impression plaster	Alginate hydrocolloid
Zinc oxide–eugenol	Polysulfide rubber
	Silicone rubber
	Polyether rubber

Nine classes of impression materials are discussed, and several means of classifying them may be used. They can be divided into those that set as a result of a chemical reaction and those that set as a result of a change in temperature, or they can be classified as those that are flexible and those that are rigid at the time of removal from the mouth. The latter method of classification will be used since their rigidity places much more restriction on their use than does the method of setting.

A rigid impression material is restricted to applications in areas where no undercuts exist. A rigid impression material could not be used on the teeth shown in Fig. 8-1, since, on setting, it would be locked in place and could not be removed over the bulge of the tooth without fracturing. A rigid material can be removed from a tooth prepared for a full crown or from an edentulous arch, as shown in Fig. 8-2, C, since no undercut areas are present. However, a flexible impression material could make these two impressions, as well as impressions of single teeth or a full dentulous arch. It is not surprising that impression materials that are flexible when set are used most frequently.

Impression materials discussed are listed in Table 8-1 and are classified as rigid or flexible.

DENTAL IMPRESSION COMPOUND

Dental impression compound is sometimes called simply impression compound, which is a little confusing because it is available in two distinctly different types, identified as **tray compound** and **impression compound.** To avoid this confusion, the term **dental compound** will be used to refer to the general class of materials and tray or impression compound to denote the specific type. Tray compound is used to prepare a custom-made preliminary impression or tray that will later hold a second impression material, which will record the final impression, commonly referred to as a **corrective wash** (Fig. 8-2, C). Impression trays are more commonly made from tray-type acrylic described in Chapter 13. Impression compound may be used to make a final impression of a tooth preparation, or it may be used as a check impression to evaluate the adequacy of a cavity preparation.

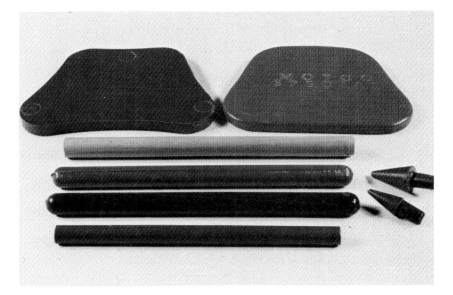

Fig. 8-3. *Top,* Two cakes of tray compound. *Bottom,* Sticks and cones of impression compound.

Composition

Dental compound contains about 40% resins, 7% waxes, 3% organic acids, 50% fillers, and small amounts of coloring agents. Dental compound has the quality of being **thermoplastic.** Stearic acid functions as a **plasticizer,** besides making the material tougher and less brittle. The addition of fillers decreases the flow of the material and reduces the adhesiveness of the softened material to the oral tissues. The filler may be talc, chalk, or iron oxide, and various pigments may be added. The most common colors for dental compound are brown, gray, or green, but they have also been supplied in black and white.

> A thermoplastic material reversibly softens on heating and hardens on cooling.

> A plasticizer is a material that is added to increase the flow.

Dental compound is supplied in various shapes and sizes, as shown in Fig. 8-3. Tray compound is sold in larger pieces and usually is in the general shape of a tray, whereas impression compound is provided in smaller quantities in the form of sticks and cones. Impression compound may be labeled as low or high fusing, with the former having greater flow at mouth temperature and above.

Properties

Minimum flow is required at mouth temperature, but sufficient flow is needed at a temperature only 8° C above mouth temperature to record the detail in the impression. The oral tissues will not be burned at this temperature.

Table 8-2. Requirements for Flow of Dental Compound

Dental compound	Flow	
	37° C	45° C
Impression	<6%	>85%
Tray	<2%	70%-85%

Therefore these materials are hard at mouth temperature (37° C) but plastic and capable of recording an impression at 45° C. The flow requirements differ for tray and impression compound and are reflected by separate requirements of ANSI–ADA Specification No. 3 for dental compound listed in Table 8-2. The higher flow required of the impression compound at 45° C is based on its use as a final impression material, whereas the tray compound is used only for the initial impression (tray), and a second impression material such as zinc oxide–eugenol is used in the tray to record the final impression.

Dental compound has **low thermal conductivity.** During heating, the outside of the material becomes soft, whereas the inside may still be hard and have lower flow properties than desired. During cooling the reverse condition exists. **Time must be allowed during heating or cooling to allow dental compound to come to a uniform temperature.**

Thermal conductivity measures the rate of heat transfer.

Since pressure is applied during the formation of an impression, residual stress exists in the cooled impression. Storage in a warm environment or for extended periods causes dimensional changes and a warpage. Dental compound may be heated over a flame or in hot water. Precautions should be taken to avoid burning the compound, since this will alter its composition and flow. Extended storage in hot water will extract some components, and the flow properties will be altered. Since the transfer of heat in dental compound is slow, it has become a common practice to knead the material after it has been heated in water to ensure its being at a uniform temperature. Kneading in water for 1 minute nearly doubles the flow allowed at 37° C.

The manufacturer is required to supply instructions on the method of softening, the working temperature, and a curve of the shrinkage from 40° to 20° C. A typical contraction of an impression compound from mouth to room temperature is −0.3%. Additional properties required by the ANSI–ADA specification are (1) homogeneity; (2) smooth, glossy surface after flaming; and (3) firm, smooth margins after trimming with a knife at room temperature. A further requirement of impression, but not tray, compound is that at 45° C a series of V-shaped grooves 0.2 mm apart be recorded.

Manipulation

Tray compound. The trays are made by softening the compound in water, usually in a special thermostatically controlled bath, and then adapting the compound in the mouth or occasionally to a dental stone cast that has been prepared from a preliminary alginate impression of the edentulous arch. The tray compound may be supported in an aluminum tray. When the compound has hardened, the borders of the tray are trimmed with a knife and then flamed to produce a smooth, nonirritating surface. The aluminum tray containing the tray compound is then used to hold a mix of zinc oxide–eugenol impression material that would be too fluid to be self-supporting (see Fig. 8-2, C). Casts should be prepared promptly, since the compound can deform during storage. Because of this possibility and also because the compound is brittle, it has become more popular to fabricate custom trays from acrylic plastics.

Impression compound. The two principal applications of impression compound are for check impressions and final impressions. For a check impression, a stick or cone of the material (Fig. 8-3) is heated over a flame until the end is thoroughly softened. The softened end is then pressed into the area of the cavity preparation and held firmly until it cools thoroughly. A water spray in the temperature range of 16° to 18° C (60° to 65° F) may be used to aid in the cooling. It is then removed and the impression checked for indications of fracture or deformation, which would indicate undesirable undercut areas in the cavity preparation.

Impression compound may be used for final impressions, and in these instances the softened compound is placed in a suitably adapted copper band used for indirect inlay and crown technics. These copper bands are supplied in a variety of diameters and have thin walls. They can be adapted by trimming with scissors and bending. The copper band confines the compound to areas with no undercuts. The softened compound in the band is pressed into the impression area and is held firmly until it cools. Again, 16° to 18° C water spray, which is not uncomfortable to the patient, may be used. The compound is removed when it is sufficiently cooled, and a dental stone or copper die can be prepared.

IMPRESSION PLASTER

Impression plaster is rarely used to take impressions, since it is rigid and fractures easily. However, because of its short setting time and accuracy, it is primarily used to mount casts on an articulator or to record occlusal bite registrations.

Impression plaster is supplied as a finely divided powder that is added to water and sets as a result of the hydration reaction described in Chapter 9 for model plaster. The calcium sulfate hemihydrate has been modified by the addition of inorganic salts, such as potassium nitrate or sulfate, to adjust the setting time to 3 to 5 minutes and the dimensional change during setting to +0.06%. If the powder is stored so it is exposed to moisture in the air, it will absorb water, and some material will react to form calcium sulfate dihydrate. If the powder is kept in an airtight container, it should be usable for at least a year.

ZINC OXIDE–EUGENOL IMPRESSION MATERIAL

Zinc oxide–eugenol impression material is mixed to the consistency of a thin paste and is used in a custom-made compound or acrylic tray to record impressions of completely or partially edentulous arches. It has been largely replaced by light-bodied rubber impression materials. The zinc oxide–eugenol impression material sets to a brittle solid (see Fig. 8-2, C). When used as a thin layer in a tray, the impression is sometimes referred to as a wash impression.

Composition and reaction

Zinc oxide–eugenol is supplied as two pastes in collapsible tubes, as shown in Fig. 8-4. One tube contains zinc oxide, oils, and additives and the other tube contains eugenol, oils, resin, and additives. The two pastes are of contrasting colors with the zinc oxide paste being white and the eugenol paste being amber or some other contrasting color. The tube containing eugenol is easily identified by the characteristic odor of oil of cloves.

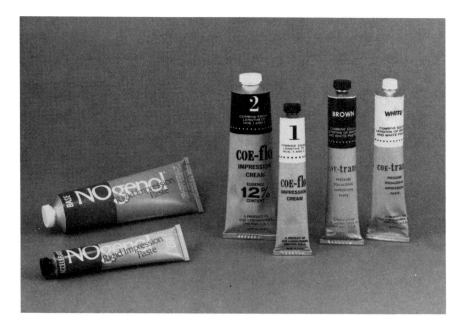

Fig. 8-4. Zinc oxide–eugenol and a substitute impression material supplied as two pastes.

Some patients find eugenol irritating to the soft tissues, and a comparable product, shown in the lower left of Fig. 8-4, is available that substitutes lauric acid for eugenol that reacts with zinc oxide in a similar manner.

The two pastes, usually in equal lengths, are thoroughly spatulated on an oil-resistant paper pad. Setting results from the reaction of the eugenol with the zinc oxide, as indicated by the following:

Zinc oxide (excess) + Eugenol → Zinc eugenolate + Zinc oxide (unreacted)

The set material consists of a matrix of amorphous **chelate,** zinc eugenolate, which holds the unreacted zinc oxide particles together. The manufacturers incorporate several percent of water, which is necessary for the material to set. Incorporation of or contact with water during the mixing accelerates the setting reaction and shortens the setting time. Once mixed, the material is sticky until set.

A chelate is a compound formed from an organic molecule and an inorganic atom such that a ring structure is formed.

Properties

Zinc oxide–eugenol impression materials are available in two types identified as **hard-** and **soft-set.** The principal difference between the two types is that the soft-set material is tougher and not as brittle; however, both types are classed as rigid materials and cannot be used to record undercut areas. The hard-set material generally has a more fluid consistency when mixed, a shorter final setting time (maximum of 10 minutes compared with 15 minutes for the soft-set), and a higher resistance to penetration when set. These setting times are much shorter at mouth temperature and humidity. The soft-set material has a buttery consistency when mixed, but the initial setting time is in the same range as the hard-set material, 3 to 5 minutes. **The setting time is shortened by the presence of water, high humidity, and increases in temperature.** The contrasting colors of the pastes provide a guide to when thorough mixing has been accomplished. Zinc oxide–eugenol impression materials are accurate, with dimensional changes during setting of about −0.1%.

The mixed materials have adequate adhesion to tray compound or acrylic tray material; therefore adhesives do not need to be applied to the tray in clinical usage. **The model materials used with zinc oxide and eugenol impression materials are restricted to the gypsum type** (model plaster or dental or high-strength stone). The model is easily separated from the impression.

Strength is not a critical requirement for this impression material, since the material is supported by a tray and is not used in areas where it would be required to withstand extensive deformation and stress during removal from the mouth.

Manipulation

Equal lengths of the two pastes are squeezed from the tubes, making sure that the extruded strips have about the same diameter as the orifices of their respective tubes. An oil-resistant paper pad is generally used, although a glass slab would serve as well except that the use of a disposable piece of paper is more convenient than cleaning the glass slab. A stiff-bladed spatula is recommended for mixing, one type of which is shown in Fig. 8-5.

The pastes should be mixed with broad strokes in a sweeping motion. The mixing can readily be accomplished in 30 to 45 seconds. The mix is then spread in a thin layer over the dry tissue-bearing surface of the tray, and the tray containing the zinc oxide–eugenol mix is placed in the mouth.

Under oral conditions the material usually sets in 3 to 5 minutes and can be checked by probing. After the material has set, the impression is removed, thoroughly rinsed under cold running water, shaken to dispose of excess water, and disinfected. No separating medium is needed before the stone model is poured. After the stone has set, it can be separated from the impression by immersion in hot water at 49° to 60° C (120° to 140° F) for 5 to 10 minutes.

Removal of zinc oxide–eugenol from the patient's lips and face can be readily accomplished by using oil of orange. The use of a light coating of facial cream or petrolatum (Vaseline) on the patient's lips before taking the impression makes the cleaning process much easier.

If the mixed impression paste sets too slowly, setting may be accelerated by incorporating a drop or two of water or ethyl alcohol into the eugenol paste before it is mixed with the zinc oxide paste. In the event that the mix sets too fast, a drop or two of glycerin will retard the setting time.

Temperature and humidity are the critical conditions controlling the setting

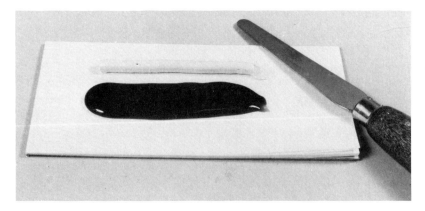

Fig. 8-5. Dispensed paste type of zinc oxide–eugenol impression material with mixing spatula.

time. Storage of the materials in the dental office should be done with these factors in mind. Keeping the tubes closed when not in use and storage in a cool location are important considerations.

ALGINATE IMPRESSION MATERIAL

Alginate is one of the most widely used dental impression materials. The wide use of alginates results from (1) the ease of mixing and manipulating them, (2) the minimum equipment necessary, (3) the flexibility of the set impression, (4) their accuracy if properly handled, and (5) their low cost. One of their principal disadvantages is that they restrict the choice of model and die materials to those of the gypsum type and rule out the preparation of metal dies, which have a higher resistance to abrasion than does gypsum. Also, they do not transfer to gypsum dies as much surface detail as agar or rubber impressions do.

Alginates are used extensively to prepare study models of either the entire dental arch or a segment of it. They are also used to prepare gypsum models of patients for the preparation of athletic mouth protectors. They are not recommended for making impressions of cavity preparations.

Packaging

Alginate is supplied by the manufacturers as a powder that is packaged in bulk or in preweighed individual containers, shown in Fig. 8-6. The bulk material is packaged in a sealed screw-top plastic container or in a hermetically sealed metal can, such as that used to package coffee. The preweighed packages are constructed of plastic and metal foil and contain enough material for a single full-arch impression. These packages minimize moisture contact with the powder and extend the storage life of the alginate.

A plastic scoop (Fig. 8-6) is provided for dispensing the bulk powder, and a plastic cylinder is supplied for measuring the water. A wide-bladed, reasonably stiff spatula is used to mix the powder and water.

Composition

The alginate powder may contain the ingredients that are shown along with their functions in Table 8-3. When water is mixed with the alginate powder, a smooth plastic mass is formed, which becomes an irreversible gel a few minutes after mixing. The overall simplified reaction is as follows:

$$\text{Paste} \rightarrow \text{Gel}$$
$$\text{Sodium alginate} + CaSO_4 + H_2O \rightarrow \text{Calcium alginate} \downarrow + Na^+ + SO_4^= + H_2O$$

The manufacturer controls the time of setting by the amount of sodium phosphate present in the alginate powder. As long as any sodium phosphate is present, it will react preferentially with the soluble calcium ions. After all the

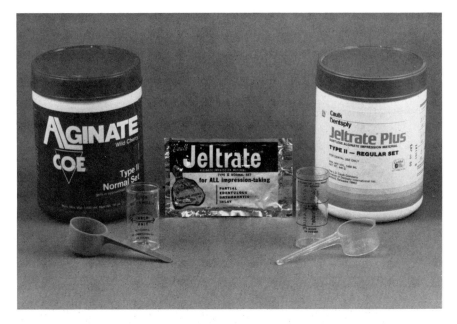

Fig. 8-6. Alginate powders supplied in bulk or in preweighted hermetically sealed packages, together with powder and water dispensers.

Table 8-3. Ingredients and Their Function in Alginate Powder

Ingredient	Function
Sodium or potassium alginate salt	To dissolve in water
Calcium sulfate	To react with dissolved alginate to form insoluble calcium alginate
Sodium phosphate	To react preferentially with calcium sulfate and serve as a retarder
Diatomaceous earth or silicate powder	To control consistency of mix and flexibility of impression
Potassium sulfate or potassium zinc fluoride	To counteract inhibiting effect of alginate on setting of gypsum model or die material
Organic glycol	To coat the powder particles to minimize dust during dispensing
Quaternary ammonium compounds	To provide self-disinfection

sodium phosphate has reacted, the soluble sodium alginate will react with the remaining calcium ions, and calcium alginate will precipitate. The sodium phosphate is therefore called **a retarder.** The calcium alginate precipitates into a fibrous network, with water occupying the intervening capillary spaces. This type of structure is called a **gel** or more specifically, since water is the liquid, a **hydrogel.** At least one of the dimensions of the network is colloidal (<0.5 μm), and this material has been traditionally named **alginate hydrocolloid.** The reaction is driven by the lower solubility of calcium alginate compared with sodium alginate. These materials are frequently referred to as **irreversible hydrocolloids,** since the process cannot be reversed once the paste sets to a gel.

A gel is a colloidal system in which the solid and liquid phases are continuous.

Properties

The ANSI–ADA Specification No. 18 for alginates established requirements for odor, flavor, lack of irritation, uniformity, mixing and setting times, permanent deformation (alteration in shape) at the time of removal from the mouth, flexibility at the time of pouring the model or die, compressive strength, reproduction of detail, compatibility with gypsum, and deterioration of the packaged powder during storage.

Mixing and setting times. Alginates, when properly mixed by hand, should develop a smooth, creamy consistency free of graininess in less than 1 minute for the normal set material and should be suitable for making impressions in the mouth. The setting time of the alginate is indicated as normal or fast by the manufacturer. An alginate sold as a normal-setting material should set in no less than 2 minutes or more than 4½ minutes after the start of the mix and be workable for up to 2 minutes. The setting time of fast-setting alginate is between 1 and 2 minutes and workable for at least 1¼ minutes. The mixing time of fast-setting alginate is 30 to 45 seconds.

Since the setting occurs as a result of a chemical reaction, **an increase in the temperature of the water used to prepare the mix shortens the working and setting times.** The proportions of powder and water also affect the setting times, with **thinner mixes increasing the time required for the material to set.** The usual range of setting times for normal-setting mixes of commercial alginate impression materials is from 2½ to 5 minutes.

Permanent deformation. Since the set alginate is held between the impression tray and the tissues, it is important to know the extent of any permanent deformation during the removal of the impression. The ANSI–ADA specification requires less than 3% permanent deformation when the alginate is compressed 10% for 30 seconds, simulating removal of the impression from the mouth. Many commercial alginates have actual values of 1.5% permanent deformation. Thus **alginate impression material is flexible but not perfectly elastic.** The

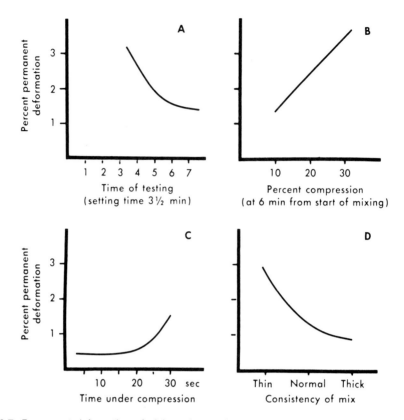

Fig. 8-7. Permanent deformation of alginate impressions as a function of, **A,** time of testing; **B,** amount of compression; **C,** time under compression; **D,** consistency of mix.

amount of permanent deformation is increased when the time before testing is shortened, when the amount of deformation during removal is increased, when the time that it is held under compression is increased, and when the water-powder ratio is increased. These effects are shown in Fig. 8-7.

Flexibility. The ANSI–ADA specification sets limits of 10% to 20% in compression at the time a model or die is prepared in the impression (10 minutes after the start of mixing). The compression is measured between a stress of 100 and 1000 gm/cm². Typical values for commercial alginates are between 11% and 15%, but a few manufacturers supply "hard set" alginates, which have values of about 3%.

The relative amounts of water and powder influence the flexibility of the set alginate. **Lower water-powder ratios (thicker mixes) result in lower flexibility.**

Strength. The strength of alginates in compression and resistance to tearing are important requirements, although the tear strength is the more critical. The

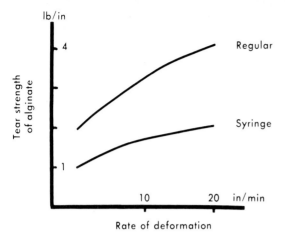

Fig. 8-8. Effect of rate of deformation (removal) on the tear strength of alginate impressions.

compressive strength, however, is frequently used to estimate the tear resistance. The ANSI–ADA specification requires a minimum compressive strength of 3500 gm/cm^2 at a time when the material is removed from the mouth. Most commercial products have compressive strengths substantially higher than this limit, with values ranging from 5000 to 7000 gm/cm^2.

The tear strength of alginates used for most impressions varies from 2 to 4 lb/in (358 to 716 gm/cm). Since most sections of an impression are much less than an inch in thickness, tearing may result from a rather small applied force. Alginates formulated for a syringe technic, however, have lower values of about 1 lb/in (179 gm/cm).

It should be emphasized that the **strength of alginates is a function of the rate at which the impression is deformed, with higher rates of deformation (removal) resulting in higher compressive and tear strengths.** An example of the effect of rate of deformation on tear strength is shown in Fig. 8-8, which illustrates that alginate impressions are less likely to tear during removal from the mouth when they are removed rapidly.

Again the strength of alginate impression materials is increased if thick rather than thin mixes are used. The advantage of using increasingly thicker mixes is limited because the consistency becomes too thick and the flow during seating of the impression so low that an adequate impression cannot be obtained.

The tear and compressive strengths at the time of removal of the impression increase if the time of removal is delayed. The effect of the consistency of the mix and of the time of removal on the tear strength is shown in Fig. 8-9. Again only limited advantage can be taken of the increase in tear strength with time because of the inconvenience of leaving the impression in the mouth for longer periods.

Fig. 8-9. Effect of consistency of the mix of alginate and time of testing on the tear strength of alginate impressions.

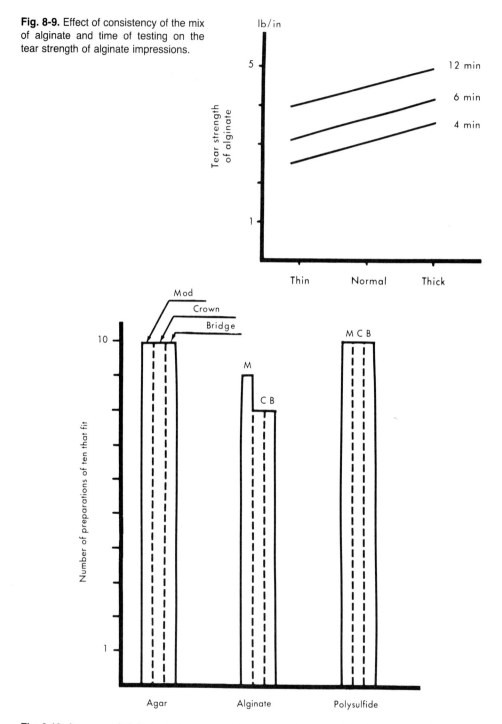

Fig. 8-10. Accuracy of alginate, agar, and polysulfide impression materials. (Modified from Myers GE, Stockman DG: *J Prosthet Dent* 10:525, 1960.)

Dimensional change. The accuracy of an impression material is of prime importance, and alginates are no exception. Their accuracy has been studied by numerous investigators. The bar graphs in Fig. 8-10 summarize the relative accuracy of alginate compared to agar and polysulfide impressions. The study was a simulated clinical one, done with highly critical preparations (nearly parallel walls). Alginate is shown to be slightly less accurate than agar and polysulfide impressions.

A problem with alginate impressions is loss of accuracy with increased time of storage. The set alginate is a hydrocolloid gel that contains large quantities of water. This water evaporates if the impression is stored in air, and the impression shrinks. If the impression is placed in water it absorbs water and expands. Therefore **storage in either air or water results in serious changes in dimensions and a loss of accuracy. Storage in humid air approaching 100% relative humidity results in the least dimensional change.** Alginate gels, however, shrink even under conditions of 100% relative humidity as a result of a process called **syneresis.** Fortunately, syneresis occurs rather slowly, and alginate impressions can usually be stored under conditions of 100% relative humidity for about an hour without serious dimensional changes.

Syneresis is the formation of an exudate on the surface of the gel.

Studies of the dimensional change of alginates during storage all emphasize that they should be stored for as short a period as possible and that the preparation of the model or die should proceed directly after the impression has been made. If the immediate preparation of the model or die is not possible, the next most appropriate procedure is to store the impression in an atmosphere of 100% relative humidity for the shortest possible time.

Reproduction of detail. It is important for the impression material to record the detail of the oral tissues, but this detail must also be transferred to the model or die. The products certified by the American Dental Association must have the minimum capabilities of transferring a line only 0.075 mm wide to a gypsum model or die material. A number of products have properties that exceed this minimum value.

Disinfection. Guidelines recommend that all impressions be rinsed and disinfected. Sodium hypochlorite, iodophor, and glutaraldehyde, and phenylphenol solutions have been used, and some manufacturers have added disinfectants to the alginate powder. Studies have shown that test viruses have been inactivated in alginate impressions by (1) a 10-minute soak in 0.5% sodium hypochlorite or a 10-minute wait after spraying the impression with this solution, (2) a 10-minute immersion in an iodophor solution diluted 1:213, and (3) a 20-minute immersion in 2% glutaraldehyde diluted 1:4, and (4) a 20-minute immersion in phenylphenol diluted 1:32. The incorporation of disinfectants in the alginate powder was also found to be effective. Measurements of dimensional changes showed that immersion of alginate impressions for 30 minutes did not affect their clinical accuracy.

Manipulation

The facilities needed to mix alginates are shown in Figs. 8-6 and 8-11, and their simplicity is noteworthy. The only items needed are (1) a powder-dispensing cup, (2) a water-dispensing cup, (3) a rubber mixing bowl, and (4) a spatula with a reasonably wide and flexible blade. If one is using preweighed packages of alginate rather than bulk, the first item is not needed.

Dispensing. The water-dispensing cup usually has three marks indicating the amount of water to be used for a one-, two-, or three-scoop mix of alginate powder. The appropriate amount of water at 21° C (70° F), room temperature, is measured into the rubber mixing bowl. **The temperature should be checked, since cold or hot water will lengthen or shorten the time for setting.**

The alginate powder in the closed screw-top or metal can is aerated, or fluffed up, by inverting the can several times. The top of the can should be taken off carefully to prevent the very fine particles being distributed around the room (not necessary with dustless alginates). The powder-dispensing cup should be slightly overfilled without the powder's being compacted and should be tapped

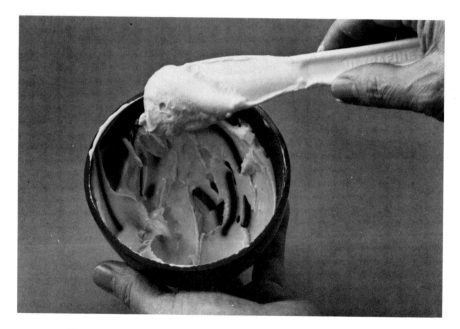

Fig. 8-11. Proper consistency of a mixed alginate impression material.

lightly with the spatula to fill any large voids. Then, using the blade of the spatula, the excess should be scraped from the top of the cup. One scoop of powder should be used for each mark on the water-dispensing cup. Even with care in dispensing the powder, a variation of 10% from the average amount is not unusual, but 10% variation will not affect the clinical results. Since the ratio of powder to water affects the setting time, permanent deformation, flexibility, and strength, **care should be taken to dispense alginate correctly.**

Mixing. The powder is added to the water in the rubber mixing bowl and is mixed with a stirring action to wet the powder. Once the powder has been moistened, the alginate should be mixed with a vigorous stropping action that squeezes the material between the blade of the spatula and the side of the mixing bowl. Mixing is continued for 1 minute for normal-setting and 30 to 45 seconds for fast-setting alginate and should result in a mix with a smooth, creamy consistency that does not drip off the spatula when held as shown in Fig. 8-11. Inadequate mixing of alginates results in grainy mixes and poorer detail in an impression.

Loading of impression tray. The proper size tray should be selected before mixing the alginate powder and water. Trays come in a multitude of designs, and a few of the more popular varieties are shown in Fig. 8-12. Some of the trays are perforated to retain the set impression during removal from the mouth. Other trays have rim locks around the periphery to accomplish this purpose. In some instances it may be necessary to extend the depth or length of the tray. This

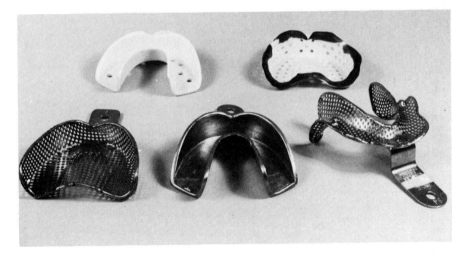

Fig. 8-12. Examples of impression trays. *Left to right: Top,* Perforated plastic mandibular and maxillary trays with wax beading. *Bottom,* Metal perforated maxillary, rim lock mandibular, and perforated mandibular trays.

may be accomplished by adding utility wax to the periphery of the tray, as shown in Fig. 8-12, *top right*. The wax is soft and can be adapted to the tray at room temperature without heating.

The mixed alginate is transferred to the tray by the mixing spatula and is generally added to the posterior portion of the tray and pushed toward the anterior part. It is wise to have less alginate in the posterior than in the anterior part of the tray, since this reduces the amount of alginate in the posterior palatal area and minimizes gagging by the patient. The surface of alginate in the filled impression tray may be smoothed out by moistening the finger with water and running it over the surface of the alginate. The loaded impression tray should be offered with the handle toward the dentist. **Loading of the tray should be done quickly,** since 1 minute has been used to mix the material and a material with a setting time of 3 minutes will set 2 minutes from the time that one starts loading the tray.

Making the impression. Impression procedures are described in many textbooks, and only a superficial description is given here. The posterior portion of the tray is usually seated first and then the anterior portion (Fig. 8-13), making sure that sufficient alginate is present to record the adjacent soft tissues. The tray is held gently but firmly in position until the alginate sets. The setting is determined by noting when the surface of the alginate is no longer tacky. It is advisable to allow the impression to remain in the mouth for 2 additional minutes because the physical properties improve sharply during this period, with increases in tear strength and decreases in permanent deformation.

During the insertion and setting of the alginate, the patient should be in an upright position or leaning slightly forward to reduce the flow of alginate in a posterior direction.

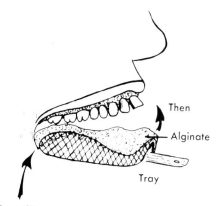

Then

Alginate

Tray

Seat this
end first

Fig. 8-13. Schematic sketch illustrating the insertion of an alginate impression material in a tray.

Removal of the impression. The seal between the impression and the periph-eral tissues is broken by moving the cheek or lips with the finger. After the seal has been broken, the impression and tray are removed with a single firm mo-tion. **The rapid removal takes advantage of the fact described earlier that the more rapidly alginates are deformed, the higher tear strength and lower per-manent deformation (more accuracy) they have.** The probability that tearing will occur in a thin section is reduced by rapid removal of the impression.

A reasonable bulk of alginate between the tissues and the tray (about 6 mm or ¼ inch) also reduces the chances of rupture of the alginate impression, since more force is required to rupture a thick than a thin section. Also, a reasonably thick section is subjected to less percentage compression from an undercut area than a thin section, and will result in a more accurate impression. An example of an acceptable maxillary alginate impression is shown in Fig. 8-14.

Preparing the impression for model or die material. The impression should be rinsed with water to remove any saliva or blood, since these fluids will interfere with the setting of the gypsum model and die materials. After the impression is thoroughly washed, it is disinfected, rinsed with water, and the excess water is removed, first by shaking the impression, and second by using a mild stream of air. Water tends to collect in the depressed areas of the impression, such as the cusps of teeth, and, if not removed, it will cause the gypsum model or die to be weak and have low resistance to abrasion in these areas. **Care should be taken, however, to avoid dehydrating the surface of the impression,** since this will result in shrinkage and consequent inaccuracy. When the excess water has been removed, the surface becomes dull in appearance.

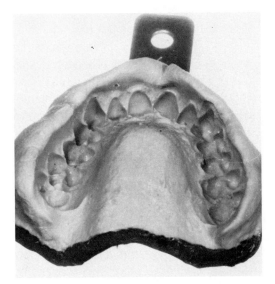

Fig. 8-14. Acceptable alginate impres-sion. (From Craig RG, editor: *Restor-ative dental materials,* ed 8, St. Louis, 1989, Mosby–Year Book.)

The impression is now ready for pouring of the gypsum model or die, which is described in Chapter 9.

Storage of the impression. No storage of alginate impressions is the best procedure; however, this is not always practical. Thus the following alternatives and problems should be considered.

The impression should never be placed alginate side down on the bench. Although the material is flexible, the weight of the tray can result in compression of the alginate, and permanent deformation of portions of the impression may occur; thus the impression should be placed with the tray against the bench top.

Alginate not supported by the tray should be cut away, since the weight of this excess material can cause deformation of alginate in this area and inaccuracy in the impression.

As indicated earlier, storage for short periods causes no serious problems if the impression is stored in a humid environment. A few simple methods can be used. First, a paper towel may be soaked with water and the excess squeezed out. The impression may be wrapped in this towel and then covered with a mixing bowl. Again care should be taken to avoid wrapping the impression tightly so that the alginate is not placed under stress. In addition, if a large excess of water is left in the towel, the excess may be absorbed by the alginate impression, and inaccuracy can result.

A plastic bag is convenient for storing alginate impressions under humid conditions. In no instance should impressions be stored, even under humid conditions, for longer than 1 hour.

AGAR HYDROCOLLOID IMPRESSION MATERIAL

Agar hydrocolloid was the first successful elastic impression material used in dentistry. The flexibility of the material at the time that it is removed from the mouth allows impression of undercut areas and thus fully dentulous impressions of the entire arch. Although agar hydrocolloid is an excellent impression material and yields accurate impressions, it has been largely replaced by alginate hydrocolloid and rubber impression materials. The preference for these latter materials has been a result of the minimum equipment required in their clinical application and of the possibility of obtaining metal and epoxy dies from rubber impressions. A combination agar-alginate technic has simplified the use of agar impression material.

Composition

The agar impression material is supplied as a gel in a collapsible tube or as a number of cylinders in a glass jar, as shown in Fig. 8-15. The first form is used with a water-cooled impression tray and the second with a syringe, examples of

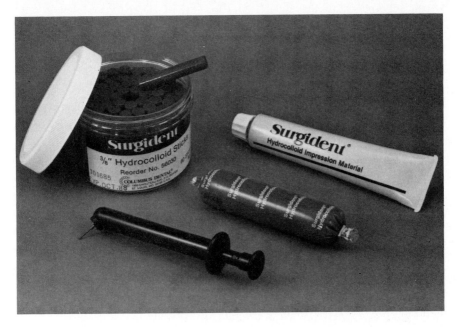

Fig. 8-15. Various forms in which agar impression material is supplied.

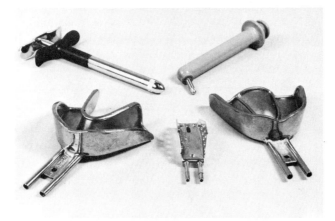

Fig. 8-16. Agar impression trays and syringes.

which are shown in Fig. 8-16. The syringe material may be used in combination with a tray material or a copper-band technic as with impression compound.

The gel of the tray material consists of 12% to 15% agar, 0.2% borax as a strength improver, 1% to 2% potassium sulfate to ensure proper setting of the gypsum model and die materials against the agar, 0.1% benzoates as preservatives, other additives to control the flow of the material when heated, the flavoring, and 80% to 85% water as the balance. The syringe materials have the same components but a lower concentration of agar (~6% to 8%).

Properties

The agar gel consists of a network of agar molecules, which holds the water in the intervening capillary spaces. When heated, the network breaks up, and agar particles are dispersed in water, which is termed a sol. The agar gel is converted to a sol by heating in water, usually boiling (100° C [212° F]), and becomes a gel again by cooling to 43.3° C (110° F). Once the gel has been converted to a sol, it will remain fluid for extended periods (all day) by being stored at 65.7° C (150° F). The phenomenon of the gel's having a liquefaction temperature different from the solidification temperature of the sol is termed hysteresis and has important clinical significance. Agar hydrocolloid impression material frequently is called **reversible** hydrocolloid, since the transformation of the gel to the sol is reversible with respect to heat.

A sol is a colloidal system in which the dispersed phase is solid and the continuous phase is liquid.

Agar impressions are highly accurate at the time of removal from the mouth but shrink when stored in air or 100% relative humidity and expand when stored in water, as shown in Fig. 8-17. **The least dimensional change occurs when the impressions are stored in 100% humidity; however, prompt pouring of plaster or stone models is recommended.**

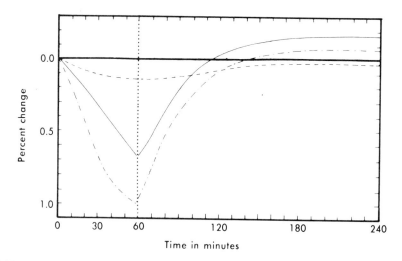

Fig. 8-17. Dimensional change of three different agar impression materials after 60 minutes when stored first in air and then in water. (Modified from Skinner EW, Cooper EN, Beck FE: *Am Dent Assoc* 40:196, 1950.)

The agar gel must transform to the sol when heated for 10 minutes at 100° C (212° F) and be fluid enough to be easily transferred to the impression tray. At this time the sol should be homogeneous and free of lumps. The sol also should revert to a gel at a temperature of 37° C (98.6° F) or higher up to 45° C (113° F).

The flexibility of the gel for most commercial products at the time of removal from the mouth is 4% to 15% when a stress of 14.2 psi (1000 gm/cm^2) is applied. A few hard-set materials, however, have a flexibility of 1% to 2%. Although the agar impression is flexible, it does not completely recover from being deformed during removal from undercut areas. The amount of permanent deformation depends on the amount of deformation and length of time that it is deformed during removal, in a manner described for alginate impressions. For example, the percentage of permanent deformation of a typical agar impression subjected to 10% deformation for 30 seconds would be about 1%.

The strength values of importance for agar impressions are the tear strength and the compressive strength. A variety of values are reported in the literature, since the values depend on the rate of deformation during testing. For rates of loading comparable with those used clinically, agar impression materials of the tray type have tear strengths of 4 lb/in (715 gm/cm) and compressive strengths of 116 lbs/in^2 (8000 gm/cm^2). The syringe materials have poorer mechanical properties, about one third those for tray materials.

Manipulation

The tray material, usually in a tube, is placed in one of the water baths of a hydrocolloid conditioner at 100° C (212° F) for 10 to 15 minutes. A typical hydrocolloid conditioner is pictured in Fig. 8-18. The conditioner has three temperature-controlled water baths, one for liquefying the gel, a second for storage of the sol, and a third for tempering the sol before placing it in the mouth.

After the agar gel has been converted to a sol, the tube is transferred to the second water bath, maintained at 60° to 66° C (140° to 150° F). At these temperatures the agar sol will remain fluid during the day. When an impression is to be made, the stored agar sol is squeezed into a perforated water-cooled metal impression tray. The tray, filled with the agar sol at 60° to 66° C (140° to 150° F), is tempered (further cooled) to 43° to 46° C (110° to 115° F) in the third water bath so that the impression material will not burn the oral tissues. The tray containing the tempered material is removed from the bath, and the outer skin, or surface, of the agar sol is scraped off; then the water hoses are connected, and the tray is positioned in the mouth by the dentist.

After the tray has been properly positioned, water at 13° C (55° F) is circulated through the tray. Water may also be sprayed on the tray to facilitate jelling of the sol. When the agar has jelled, the peripheral seal around the impression is broken, and the impression is removed rapidly from the mouth with a single stroke. The impression is rinsed thoroughly with water, is disinfected and rinsed

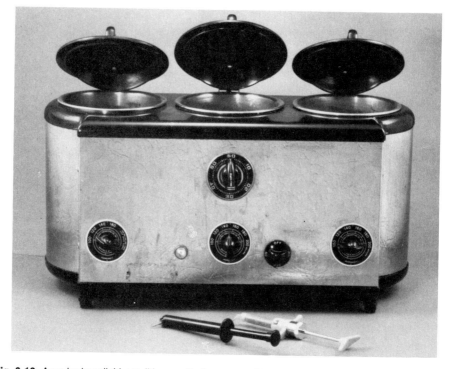

Fig. 8-18. Agar hydrocolloid conditioner with three controlled-temperature water baths for liquefying, tempering, and storing agar.

with water, and the excess is removed by shaking the impression and then gently directing a stream of air onto the impression without dehydrating the surface.

Storage of agar impressions should be avoided. Storage in air results in dehydration, and storage in water causes swelling of the impression. Storage in 100% relative humidity results in shrinkage from syneresis. **If storage is unavoidable, it should be limited to 1 hour in 100% relative humidity.**

The impression is poured in plaster or stone, and when set the agar impression should be removed promptly, since the impression will dehydrate, become stiff, and be difficult to remove without a portion of the model being fractured. In addition, prolonged contact of the agar impression with the plaster and stone will result in a rougher-than-normal surface on the model.

AGAR-ALGINATE IMPRESSION MATERIAL

Agar-alginate impressions are taken using a syringe-type agar that is injected around the preparation. Then a tray containing a thinner-than-normal alginate mix is placed over the agar before it jells. The alginate cools the agar quickly

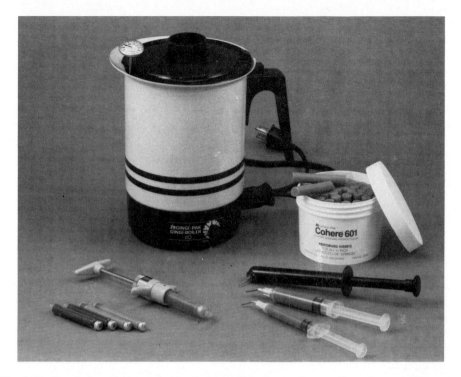

Fig. 8-19. Agar hydrocolloid supplied in glass cartridges for use in reusable syringes, in disposable syringes, and in bulk for use in reusable syringes, plus a simple heater for liquefying and storing agar for use in taking agar-alginate impressions.

enough that by the time the alginate sets, the agar has jelled, and the combination impression may be removed. When a compatible agar and alginate combination is used, no separation occurs between the two materials on removal of the impression. This technic eliminates the use of water-cooled impression trays, and simpler and less expensive heating equipment is needed.

Manipulation and properties

The agar is supplied in a glass cartridge that is used with a reusable syringe. The agar is also supplied in disposable plastic syringes and as sticks in a jar that are placed in a reusable syringe. Examples of these materials and a temperature bath are shown in Fig. 8-19. The agar is heated in boiling water, usually for 6 minutes, and can be used immediately or stored at 65° C (149° F). The alginate is a regular-set type that is mixed with 10% more water than usually recommended to increase the working time and fluidity.

The agar is syringed around the preparation; then the mixed alginate is placed in a perforated impression tray and promptly is seated on top of the agar before it jells. The alginate usually sets in about 3 minutes, at which time the agar has jelled and the impression can be removed. A cross section of an agar-alginate impression is shown in Fig. 8-20 and shows that the stiffer alginate has pushed the agar in the gingival direction during placement.

The bond strengths between compatible agars and alginates are from 800 to 1000 gm/cm². **Since some combinations are not compatible, the manufacturer's suggestions should be followed.** The accuracy of the agar-alginate system has been compared to rubber impression materials and was found to be of the same order. It is noteworthy that the use of the agar-alginate systems limits the selection of the die material to a gypsum product.

Alginate is an irreversible hydrocolloid impression material, which owes its wide usage to the simplicity of the system and technic of usage combined with adequate flexibility, strength, and clinical accuracy for study models of dentulous patients. Alginates do not yield adequate surface detail on high-strength stone models to be used to make highly precise crown and bridge restorations. Agar is a reversible hydrocolloid impression material with respect to temperature but requires considerable auxillary equipment such as three temperature-controlled water baths and water-cooled impression trays. Its properties are similar to alginates except that adequate surface detail results when high-strength stone is poured against it, and it can be used in precision crown and bridge work. Both agar and alginate impressions should be poured promptly, since they change dimensions when stored in air and

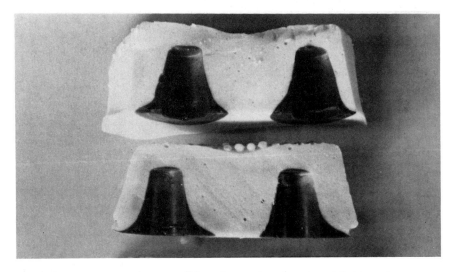

Fig. 8-20. Cross section of an agar-alginate impression after removal from a perforated tray.

water. When stored in 100% relative humidity, they can be stored for up to an hour before significant changes take place. The combined agar-alginate technic has simplified the equipment used to take agar impressions and yields suitable crown and bridge impressions.

POLYSULFIDE RUBBER IMPRESSION MATERIALS

The first rubber impression material was a polysulfide. It was flexible but did not have the major changes in dimensions during storage of agar and alginate. Furthermore, the rubber impression was much stronger and more resistant to tearing than agar or alginate. The rubber could be **electroformed** and therefore metal dies or models, as well as gypsum models, could be prepared. The metal dies were hard enough that a great deal more finishing of gold castings could be carried out on them, rather than on the patient's tooth. In addition, epoxy dies could be made in the rubber impressions.

> Electroforming is a process in which metal is deposited from solution onto the surface of a rubber by use of an electric current.

Composition

The polysulfide materials are supplied as two pastes, with one tube labeled catalyst or accelerator and the other marked base. A few examples are pictured in Fig. 8-21. Three types are classified as light-, regular-, or heavy-bodied de-

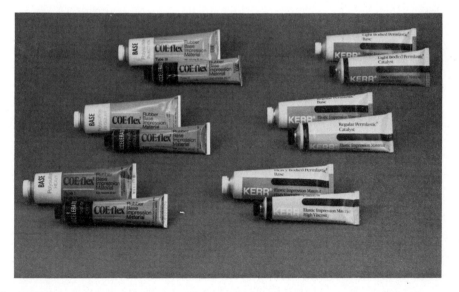

Fig. 8-21. Examples of two-paste polysulfide rubber impression materials. *Top to bottom,* Light-, regular-, and heavy-bodied materials.

pending on their viscosity and how easily they flow under load. The light-bodied class is used as a syringe material in combination with a tray material, and the regular material is used alone. The light-bodied material is also used for denture impressions in combination with a custom-made tray, as described earlier in this chapter.

The base material consists of about 80% low–molecular weight organic polymer, containing reactive mercaptan groups (—SH), and 20% reinforcing agents, such as titanium dioxide, zinc sulfate, copper carbonate, or silica. The accelerator, or catalyst, tube contains a compound that causes the mercaptan groups to react to form a polysulfide rubber. The catalyst is carried by an inert oil such as dibutyl or dioctyl phthalate. The most common catalyst is lead dioxide, with or without manganese dioxide; using it results in the paste's being dark brown to dark gray. Another catalyst system is copper hydroxide and when mixed with the white base paste a blue-green color results.

Setting reaction

The overall simplified setting reaction involves the oxidation of the mercaptan groups from two different molecules in the presence of the catalyst that joins the molecules together, forming disulfide groups. The following illustrates the setting reaction:

$$\text{Mercaptan} + \text{Lead dioxide} \rightarrow \text{Polysulfide} + H_2O$$

The following is a schematic representation of the chemical reaction for these mercaptan molecules.

$$HS\!-\!R\!-\!SH \xrightarrow{\ PbO_2 + S\ } HS\!-\!R\!-\!S\!-\!Pb\!-\!S\!-\!R\!-\!SH \rightarrow HS\!-\!R\!-\!S\!-\!S\!-\!R\!-\!SH + H_2O$$

It should be understood that many of these reactions take place, since any —SH group can react.

The molecular weight of the mercaptan is 2000 to 4000; thus each reaction with two —SH groups increases the molecular weight by about this amount. It is understandable that a limited number of these individual reactions is necessary to yield a high—molecular weight rubber.

The reaction is sensitive to moisture and temperature. Increases in either one will accelerate the setting reaction.

Properties

Properties of clinical interest are (1) toxicity, (2) color of the base and accelerator, (3) time required for mixing, (4) working time, (5) consistency, (6) permanent deformation during removal, (7) dimensional stability, (8) flow after setting, (9) flexibility, (10) reproduction of detail, (11) compatability with die and model materials, and (12) deterioration during storage of the unmixed material.

Table 8-4. Qualitative Rating of Physical and Mechanical Properties of Rubber Impression Materials

Property	Polysulfide	Condensation silicone	Addition silicone	Polyether
Working time	Moderately long	Short	Short-moderate	Short
Setting time	Moderately long	Short-moderate	Short-moderate	Short
Shrinkage on setting	Moderately high	High-moderate	Very low	Low
Permanent deformation in compression	Moderately high	Moderately high	Very low	Moderately high
Flexibility during removal	High	Moderate	Low-moderate	Low
Tear strength	Moderate-high	Low-moderate	Moderate	Low
Flow after setting under small forces	Moderately high	Low	Very low	Very low
Wettability by gypsum mixes	Moderate	Poor	Poor-good	Good
Gas evolution after setting	No	No	Yes-no	No
Detail reproduction	Excellent	Excellent	Excellent	Excellent

Although most of the accelerator pastes contain lead dioxide, they have been shown to have no toxic effects when the materials are used as directed. Manufacturers supply the base as a white paste and the accelerator paste in a contrasting color. It is easy to determine when the two pastes are mixed uniformly by the absence of streaks. A mix free of streaks can readily be made in 45 seconds, and certainly no more than 1 minute should be required.

A qualitative ranking of physical and mechanical properties for polysulfide impression materials is given in Table 8-4. For the purpose of comparison, rankings are also reported for two types of silicone and polyether rubber impression materials, which are discussed in the following two major sections.

In general, the working time for polysulfide rubber impression materials decreases as the consistency becomes stiffer (light- to heavy-bodied). The working time is an indication of the maximum time allowed before the impression material should be in the mouth, with typical values being 5 to 7 minutes. The final setting time is usually in the range of 8 to 12 minutes from the start of mixing.

The permanent deformation values of 2% to 3%, obtained when the material is held under 12% compression for 30 seconds, indicate that the polysulfides are not perfectly elastic and that compression during removal of the impression material should be kept to a minimum. The permanent deformation of polysulfide rubber is slightly higher than that for hydrocolloid impression materials, but materials having values of less than 3% are acceptable.

Polysulfide rubber impression materials shrink 0.3% to 0.4% during the first 24 hours, and thus models and dies should be prepared promptly. Studies indicate that accuracy is slightly improved if the models or dies are prepared 30 minutes after removal, but certainly no long delays should occur. Materials with a dimensional change of -0.4% or less have been clinically successful. The flow values are determined by placing a small load on cylinders of set impression material 1 hour after mixing. The test evaluates the flow of the impression material when it is placed under the compressive forces. Examples of this test would be measuring the flow of an impression that is placed on the bench top with the tray on top of the rubber or measuring the flow resulting if the impression is tightly wrapped for sending to a laboratory. Even though the material has set, flow of 0.3% to 0.9% can occur in 15 minutes, resulting in distortion of the impression.

The flexibility of the polysulfides varies considerably, with the heavy-bodied materials having generally lower values. Materials having values between 2% and 20% are believed satisfactory for clinical use, and polysulfides have values well within this range.

Polysulfide rubber provides excellent reproduction of surface detail and is readily capable of reproducing fine lines 0.025 mm wide. The materials are highly compatible with model plaster and high-strength stones, and impressions are easily metallized by electroforming (electroplating). Silverplating is usually preferred to copper-plating, although the use of silver cyanide plating solutions require special care because of their poisonous nature. The polysulfide materials have excellent shelf life but should not be stored in a warm location; the tubes should be checked to determine if the caps are on tightly before they are stored. **The shelf life can be extended by storing unused material in the refrigerator.**

The resistance of the polysulfide materials to tearing is 22 lb/in (4000 gm/cm), or about eight times the values reported for hydrocolloid impression materials. It should be emphasized that the strength and permanent deformation properties of the polysulfide materials continue to improve for a number of hours after they are set. Several minutes extra in the mouth results in noticeable improvement; however, the time in the mouth has a practical limitation. The time before preparing dies also must be balanced with the knowledge that the shrinkage, as a result of the chemical reaction, is increasing.

Manipulation

Two-paste type. Equal lengths of the base and accelerator are extruded onto a paper pad as shown in Fig. 8-22, A. Some manufacturers mark their pads at 1-inch intervals as an aid for measuring. The procedure of extruding the accelerator on top of the base is not recommended, since delays may occur before mixing, and a reaction starts at the interface and may result in a nonhomogeneous mix. A tapered, stiff-bladed spatula such as the one shown in Fig. 8-22, A, is recommended. The accelerator is mixed with the base for 5 to 10 seconds in a circular motion with the end of the spatula, as shown in Fig. 8-22, B. The blade of the spatula is wiped on the pad and then with a paper towel; this pro-

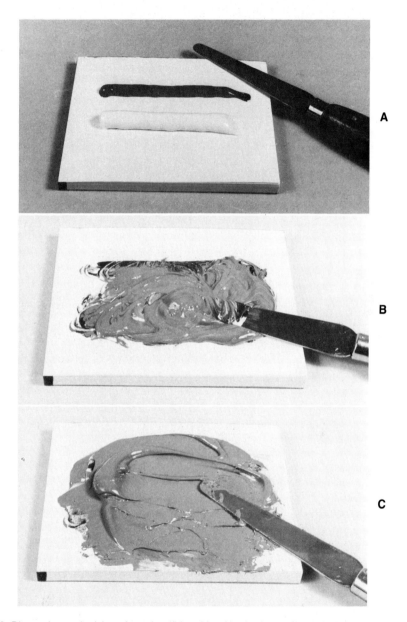

Fig. 8-22. Dispensing and mixing of a polysulfide rubber impression material. **A,** Base and accelerator extruded onto a paper mixing pad. **B,** Initial mixing of the base and accelerator. **C,** Final mixing of the base and accelerator.

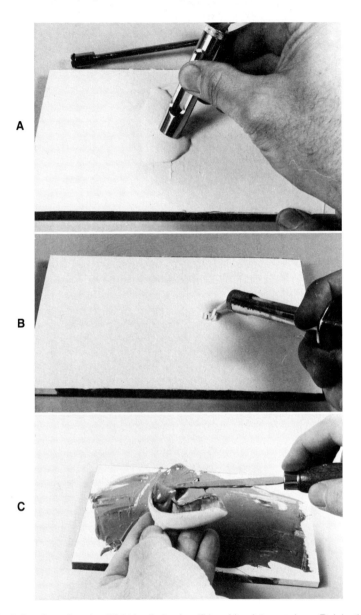

Fig. 8-23. A, Loading of a mixed light-bodied polysulfide rubber into a syringe. **B,** Injection of the rubber. **C,** Placing a regular- or heavy-bodied material into an impression tray.

cedure makes it easier to obtain a mix free from streaks later. The mixing is continued with a wide sweeping motion (Fig. 8-22, *C*) until the mix is free from streaks and uniform in color. The mixing should be accomplished in about 45 seconds.

If the material is light-bodied, it is loaded into a syringe, as shown in Fig.

8-23, *A;* it is then ready for injecting into the cavity preparation, as shown in Fig. 8-23, *B.* If the material is a regular- or heavy-bodied material, it is placed in a tray, as shown in Fig. 8-23, *C.* The tray has been constructed to provide a uniform space of about 2 mm for the impression material. Custom trays of acrylic are generally used, and the inside of the tray is painted with a rubber cement adhesive. **The solvent from the adhesive layer is then allowed to evaporate;** otherwise the polysulfide material may separate from the tray during removal from the mouth. Sometimes holes are drilled through the tray to provide mechanical retention of the impression material.

A wide variety of technics are used to make impressions. It is sufficient to point out that, if a light-bodied material is used, it is injected into the impression area and then the tray containing the heavy-bodied material is placed over the light-bodied material and the tray is seated. The light- and heavy-bodied materials set together to give a single impression, with the light-bodied material recording the surface and supported by the heavy-bodied material and the tray. Impressions may also be accomplished with a single mix of regular-bodied material.

When the material has set, the impression is removed with a steady force. A snap removal of the impression is not possible or necessary as with hydrocolloids, since the tear strength of the polysulfides is much higher. **If tearing of the rubber impression occurs, the second time the impression is taken it should be left in the mouth several minutes longer to obtain a higher tear strength.** After the removal of the impression, it is checked for completeness and detail and then is thoroughly cleaned by rinsing with tap water and then disinfected and rinsed again with water. The excess water is shaken off, and any residual moisture is removed by a gentle stream of air. The preparation of the die or model is the next step and is discussed in detail in Chapter 9. As pointed out earlier, preparation of the die or model should not be delayed, since dimensional change from continued reaction goes on for some time.

SILICONE RUBBER IMPRESSION MATERIALS

The impetus for the development of silicone impression materials resulted from several criticisms of the polysulfide materials, such as their objectionable odor, the staining of linen and uniforms by the lead dioxide, the amount of effort required to mix the base with the accelerator, the rather long setting times, the moderately high shrinkage on setting, and the fairly high permanent deformation.

Composition

Two types of silicones are used as impression materials: (1) condensation and (2) addition (sometimes called vinyl silicone) types. The names identify the type of polymerization reaction.

Condensation type. The material is supplied as a base and an accelerator, or catalyst. The base is a paste containing a moderately low–molecular weight silicone liquid, called a **dimethylsiloxane,** which has reactive—OH groups. Reinforcing agents such as silica are added to give the proper consistency to the paste and stiffness to the set rubber. The accelerator is usually supplied as a liquid but may be provided as a paste by the use of thickening agents. The accelerator consists of a tin organic ester suspension and an alkyl silicate such as ortho-ethyl silicate.

The silicone pastes are supplied in light-, regular-, and heavy-bodied consistencies, as well as a very heavy consistency called a putty. The consistency is controlled by the selection of the molecular weight of the dimethylsiloxane and the concentration of reinforcing agent. Higher molecular weights are used with the heavier-bodied materials. The concentration of the reinforcing agent increases from 35% for light-bodied consistency to 75% for the putty consistency.
Addition type. The material is supplied as a two-paste or a two-putty system, with one containing a low–molecular weight silicone having terminal vinyl groups, reinforcing filler, and a chloroplatinic acid catalyst and the other containing a low–molecular weight silicone having silane hydrogens and reinforcing filler. The two are mixed in equal lengths of paste or equal quantities of putty, and the addition reaction occurs between the vinyl and hydrogen groups with no by-product being formed.

Setting reaction

Condensation type. A simplified verbal and chemical description of the reaction that converts the mixed paste to a rubber is given as follows:

Dimethylsiloxane + Ortho-ethyl silicate + Tin octoate → Silicone rubber + Ethyl alcohol

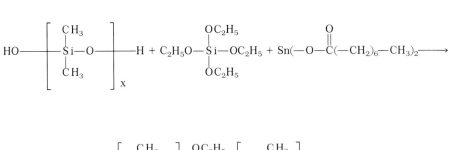

The multifunctional ethyl silicate produces a network or cross-linked structure that partly accounts for the low values of permanent deformation and flow. The ethyl alcohol produced as a by-product in the reaction gradually evaporates and contributes to the rather high shrinkage during the first 24 hours after setting. The incorporation of large amounts of filler in the putty consistency results in a reduction of the dimensional change. The setting reaction is sensitive to moisture and heat, with increases in either resulting in shorter setting and working times. These effects are more important than with polysulfide materials, since the normal setting and working times are shorter for this silicone. **Addition type.** A simplified setting reaction is as follows:

Hydrogen-containing siloxane + Vinyl-terminal siloxane + Chloroplatinic acid → Silicone rubber

$$\underset{\underset{CH_3}{|}}{\overset{\overset{CH_3}{|}}{\sim\sim Si}}-H + CH_2=CH-\underset{\underset{CH_3}{|}}{\overset{\overset{CH_3}{|}}{Si}}\sim\sim + H_2PtCl_6 \rightarrow \sim\sim\underset{\underset{CH_3}{|}}{\overset{\overset{CH_3}{|}}{Si}}-CH_2-CH_2-\underset{\underset{CH_3}{|}}{\overset{\overset{CH_3}{|}}{Si}}\sim\sim$$

The vinyl siloxane is difunctional, and the hydrogen-containing siloxane is multifunctional. No volatile by-product is formed in this reaction, and minimal dimensional change occurs during polymerization. Increases in temperature increase the rate of reaction and shorten the setting time. If hydroxyl groups are present in the addition silicone, a side reaction occurs that results in the formation of hydrogen. The hydrogen is gradually released from the set impression material and produces bubbles in gypsum dies prepared less than 1 hour, or epoxy dies less than 24 hours, after the impression is taken. **Some products permit the immediate pouring of dies by controlling the presence of hydroxyl groups or by the inclusion in the impression material of a hydrogen absorber such as palladium.** Thus manufacturer's directions for the time of preparation of dies from a particular silicone should be followed.

Silicone impression materials are not readily wetted by mixes of gypsum products, since they are hydrophobic and mixes form contact angles against silicones of about 100°. Some products contain surfactants such as detergents and become hydrophilic with contact angles of about 40°. **Hydrophilic silicones permit gypsum models and dies to be prepared with fewer air bubbles.**

A hydrophobic surface is poorly wetted by water with a contact angle of >90°. A hydrophilic surface is readily wetted by water with a low contact angle.

Consistencies

Condensation type. This type of silicone is supplied as a light-bodied material, as a putty-base material, and as a catalyst. The light-bodied base material is usually supplied in a tube and the putty is usually supplied in a jar as shown in Fig.

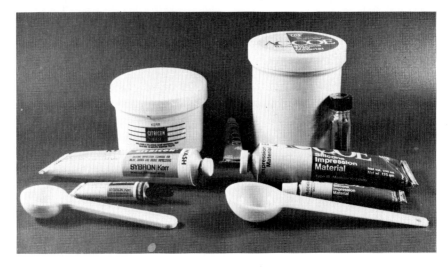

Fig. 8-24. Condensation silicone putty-wash systems.

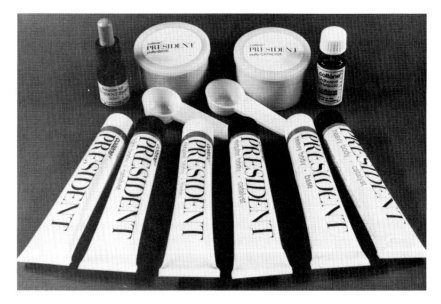

Fig. 8-25. Addition silicone system with light, regular, heavy, and putty consistencies.

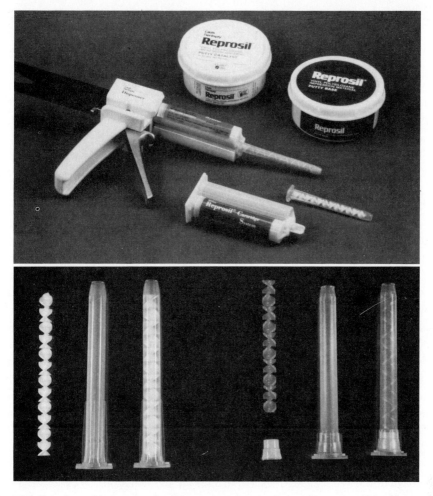

Fig. 8-26. *Top,* Automixing system for light- and medium-bodied addition silicones. *Bottom,* Disassembled and assembled static mixing tips.

8-24. The catalyst is supplied in a tube either as a liquid or a paste.

Addition type. This silicone is supplied as a light-, medium-, or heavy-bodied base, as catalyst pastes, and as a base and catalyst putty (very heavy-bodied) in jars as shown in Fig. 8-25. The light- and medium-bodied materials are also available in a dual cartridge system with the base paste in one cartridge and the catalyst paste in the other as shown in Fig. 8-26, *top.* The cartridge is placed in a mixing gun, and by a rachet device plungers extrude the pastes through a static mixing tip shown disassembled in Fig. 8-26, *bottom.* During the extrusion through the static mixing tip the two pastes are folded over each other and exit the tip in a mixed condition. The mixing tip is left on until the next mix, at which time it is replaced by a new tip. **These so-called automixing systems result in mixes with fewer bubbles than with spatulated mixes.**

Addition silicones are also available as single material that can be used as both a light- and a heavy-bodied material. These products are sometimes called monophase materials. They are formulated so that under high shear forces, such as when they are extruded from an injection syringe, they have a low viscosity, whereas when they are under low shear forces, such as when they are placed in an impression tray with a spatula, they have a high viscosity. Thus a single mix can be used as both a syringe and a tray material. These products are available as a two-paste system either in two tubes or in a cartridge system.

Properties

Condensation type. The qualitative ratings of the physical and mechanical properties of condensation silicones are presented in Table 8-4. The working time is shorter for the silicones compared with the polysulfides, and the setting times likewise are shorter, in the range of 6 to 8 minutes. The viscosity of the silicones is less than for comparable polysulfides, and as a result they are easier to mix. The dimensional change during 24 hours after setting is larger for the condensation type of silicones than the polysulfides; however, a large decrease in dimensional change occurs when the filler content is increased, as with the putty materials. It should be emphasized that **most of the dimensional change occurs during the first hour after setting** and that the percentage of the 24-hour values for both silicones and polysulfides as a function of time follows the curve shown in Fig. 8-27.

The permanent deformation of the condensation silicones is lower than that of the polysulfides and is related to the higher cross-linking in silicones. Although the putty has higher values for permanent deformation than the light-bodied material, in practice little permanent deformation takes place in the putty, since it is so stiff that most of the deformation occurs in the light-bodied material during removal of the putty-wash impression. The flow values 1 hour after setting are also much lower for the silicones than the polysulfides, and the flexibility of the silicones is lower. These differences again reflect the higher cross-linking of the silicones and the more rapid setting reaction and reinforcing agent concentration.

The materials are nontoxic, although direct contact of the skin with the catalyst is to be avoided, since allergic reactions have been noted. The base material is white, and dyes are added to the colorless catalyst to indicate the completion of mixing. The materials therefore may be any color desired.

The silicones readily reproduce fine details of the surface and easily reproduce a V-shaped groove with a width of 0.025 mm. They are compatible with model plaster and high-strength stone, but care must be taken when models or

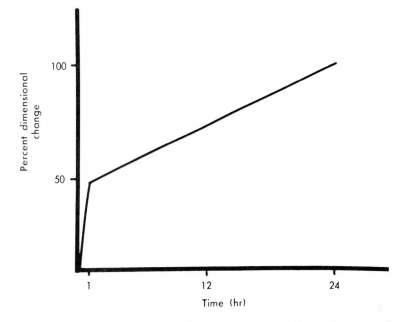

Fig. 8-27. Percent of dimensional change of silicone and polysulfide rubber impression materials with time.

dies are poured, since the wettability is poor. They can be metallized with silver or copper by electroplating; however, copperplating is generally not used. Because of the large dimensional change after setting, stone dies are more frequently made than metal dies. The silicones have reasonable shelf life, but it is usually shorter than for polysulfides; thus large quantities should not be purchased or stored.

The tear strength of the silicones is about 17 lb/in (3000 gm/cm), which is lower than that for polysulfide impressions but still substantially higher than the tear strength for hydrocolloids, and it causes no clinical problems.

Addition type. The properties for the addition type of silicone impression materials are listed in Table 8-4. The dimensional change and permanent deformation are noteworthy improvements of the addition silicones over the condensation silicones. The dimensional change in 24 hours of about −0.1% is very low. The permanent deformation at the time of removal from the mouth of about 0.2% is the lowest of all the impression materials. The percent flow values of the addition silicones are likewise very low.

These properties indicate the superior accuracy of the addition silicones. It should be pointed out that the working time is shorter for the addition silicones than for the polysulfides and that the flexibility is lower than for other rubber impression materials except the polyether material. Removal of the addition silicone impressions from undercut areas may present difficulties because of this stiffness, and extra space should be provided for the impression material when a custom tray is used.

Tissue culture tests on both the base and catalyst pastes have been negative and indicate that addition silicones cause less tissue reaction than the condensation silicones.

The addition silicones have been successfully silverplated or copperplated and easily reproduce lines smaller than 0.025 mm.

Manipulation

Condensation type. The larger dimensional change of condensation silicone materials compared with polysulfides encouraged manufacturers to supply the silicones in a putty-wash (very light-bodied) combination. The putty is so stiff that it must be dispensed with a scoop, as shown in Fig. 8-24. Depressions are made in the surface of the putty, and the appropriate number of drops or the appropriate length of catalyst is added. A stiff spatula is used to mix the putty and liquid or paste catalyst. Once the catalyst is well incorporated, mixing may be continued by hand for 30 seconds or until free from streaks. Initial mixing by hand is inadvisable, since high concentrations of the catalyst would contact the skin and possibly cause an allergic response. It is recommended that the hands be moist during the 30-second mixing to prevent sticking. Mixing can also be done while wearing rubber gloves. The putty is placed in a perforated stock tray or an adhesive-treated nonperforated tray, and a preliminary impression is made before preparing the teeth. The impression tray is rocked to provide 1 to 2 mm of space for the wash material, and the putty is allowed to set. After cavity preparation the wash material is mixed as is any syringe material, and the material is injected into the impression area and sometimes into the putty-impression. The tray, plus the putty impression, is inserted and held firmly until the wash material sets. The putty-wash system increases the accuracy of the impressions, since the putty has a lower dimensional change than the wash material. Also, the dimensional change of the putty affects accuracy very little, since it occurs before the final impression is taken, and the dimensional change of the thin layer of wash material is small.

Addition type. The four consistencies of one manufacturer's addition silicone are shown in Fig. 8-25. Scoops are supplied for dispensing the putty base and catalyst. A retarder liquid *(top left)* is supplied that, when added, extends the working time. A tray adhesive is also shown in Fig. 8-25 *(top right)*.

The two pastes of the light-, regular- and heavy-bodied materials are dispensed onto a mixing pad in equal lengths and spatulated in the same manner as described for the polysulfide materials. The base and catalyst are formulated to have contrasting colors. The addition silicones are less viscous than polysulfides and can be readily mixed in 30 to 45 seconds to a streak-free mix.

The base and catalyst putties are dispensed in equal quantities and are mixed by hand until free from streaks. **The two putties should not be mixed when latex rubber gloves are worn,** since components in the rubber will retard or prevent the setting by poisoning the platinum catalyst. Vinyl gloves or bare hands are acceptable. If latex gloves must be worn they should be washed thoroughly using a detergent and dried just before mixing the putties.

These four consistencies can be used in a variety of impression technics to take a light-bodied-heavy-bodied impression, a light-bodied putty impression, or a regular-bodied impression. In addition, a monophase two-paste system can be used to take a syringe-tray impression.

The automix system shown in Fig. 8-26 supplies light- and regular-bodied, as well as monophase, silicones in cartridges and the putty consistency in jars. These allow the same impression technics to be used as with the previous four consistencies. The cartridge is inserted into the gun and the cap on the end removed. The plungers are advanced by the trigger until base and catalyst paste is extruding uniformly. The tip is wiped off, and a static mixing tip is placed on the end of the cartridge. The trigger is used to extrude and mix the base and catalyst through the mixing tip. The material is thoroughly mixed as it exits the tip. The light- and regular-bodied materials together with the putty can be used as described to take a variety of impressions.

POLYETHER RUBBER IMPRESSION MATERIALS

Polyether systems offer the possible combination of better mechanical properties than those of polysulfides along with less dimensional change than those of condensation silicone impression materials. They appear to have other limiting features, however, such as short working time and high stiffness.

Composition and setting reaction

Polyether rubber impression materials are supplied as a base and catalyst system. The base is a moderately low–molecular weight polyether, containing ethylene imine terminal groups. These terminal groups are reacted together by the action of an aromatic sulfonic acid ester catalyst to form a cross-linked high–molecular weight rubber as illustrated by the following, in which R is a series of organic groups:

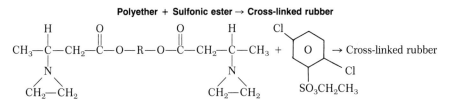

Polyether + Sulfonic ester → Cross-linked rubber

Properties

The properties of polyether impression materials are listed in Table 8-4. The working time is the shortest of any of the three rubber impression materials, and the consistency is listed as regular-bodied but is heavy compared with that of other regular-bodied materials. It is also available as a light- and heavy-bodied polyether system. **The working time is short enough that the viscosity noticeably increases during the mixing of the material.**

The permanent deformation of the polyethers is less than that of the polysulfides but is not as low as that of the silicones, whereas the polyethers exhibit less flow under small loads 1 hour after setting than do either the polysulfide or the condensation silicone impression materials. The low flow is caused by the rubber being cross-linked and by its high stiffness. The high stiffness is indicated by the low flexibility of 3% compared with 5% and 7% for condensation silicone and polysulfide regular-bodied types. The low flexibility may cause problems in the removal of the impression from the mouth, and a 4-mm rather than 2-mm thickness of rubber between the tray and teeth is recommended.

The dimensional change of polyethers is lower than that of any other rubber impression material except the addition silicones. The polyether absorbs water and changes dimensions if stored in contact with water until equilibrium is reached. The times involved in normal electroplating do not cause any problems with accuracy. **However, polyether impressions should not be stored in water and should be washed, disinfected, and dried after removal from the mouth.**

The viscosity of the mixes can be reduced by using a thinner. An equal length of thinner mixed with the base and catalyst results in an increase of the working time to 4 minutes and the flexibility to 6% without any significant loss of other physical or mechanical properties. These impressions also can be readily silverplated to produce accurate dies.

The aromatic sulfonic acid ester catalyst can cause skin irritation, and direct contact with the catalyst should be avoided. Thorough mixing of the catalyst with the base should be accomplished to prevent any irritation of the oral tissues.

Manipulation

The polyether materials are supplied in two tubes, one containing the base and the other the catalyst, as shown in Fig. 8-28 (*left* and *center*). Equal lengths are extruded onto a paper mixing pad. Mixing is accomplished as with the other rubber impression materials, and a uniform mix free of streaks should be obtained in 30 to 45 seconds. A decrease or increase of 25% in the amount of catalyst can be used to lengthen or shorten the working or setting time. Increases in the temperature of the room will shorten the working and setting times. A

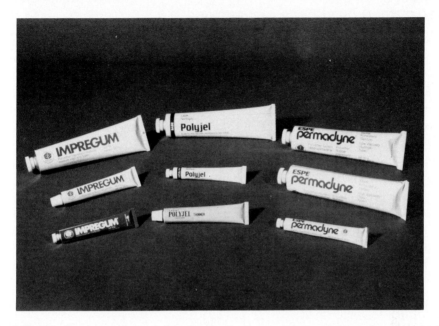

Fig. 8-28. Polyether impression materials showing the base, catalyst, and thinner for regular-bodied materials *(left* and *center)* and a light- and heavy-bodied polyether and the catalyst *(right).*

thinner supplied in a third tube may be used in amounts up to equal lengths of the base paste to increase the working time and flexibility. Polyethers are also supplied as a light- and heavy-bodied base paste (Fig. 8-28, *right*) and as a catalyst that is used with either consistency.

The use of a tray that allows for a thickness of at least 4 mm of impression material helps in the removal of the fairly stiff impression. A stock or individual tray may be used, but in either instance an adhesive should be used. The material is generally used in a single-mix technic, but a syringe-tray technic may be used. If a syringe-tray technic is desired, it is better to use the light and heavy consistency product.

The impression should be pulled slowly to break the seal and then removed in a single stroke; it should be rinsed with cold water, disinfected, and blown dry. The impression should not be stored in water or in direct sunlight, and the dies or models should be prepared promptly.

Unreacted polyether may be removed with organic solvents such as acetone or chloroform or with soap and water. The set rubber may be removed with chloroform or other chlorinated solvents, such as trichloroethylene.

Polyether materials have good shelf life and should be usable after 2 years of storage at room temperature.

DISINFECTION OF RUBBER IMPRESSIONS

A variety of disinfectants including (1) neutral glutaraldehyde, (2) acidified glutaraldehyde, (3) neutral phenolated glutaraldehyde, (4) phenol, (5) iodophor, and (6) chlorine dioxide were used to disinfect polysulfide, addition silicone, and polyether impressions. The impressions were immersed in appropriately diluted solutions for 10 minutes, except for chlorine dioxide, in which they were immersed for only 3 minutes. The accuracy of high-strength stone dies poured into these impressions was excellent for addition silicones and acceptable for the polysulfides, whereas it was unacceptable for polyethers. As a result, disinfection of polyether impressions by immersion is not recommended except for very short (2 to 3 minutes) times in chlorine compound disinfectants. Also, the surface quality of high-strength stone dies poured against the impressions is acceptable. **Overall, the selection of the impression material is of greater importance than the selection of the disinfectant. Since times for disinfection vary, product data should be used to determine the appropriate immersion time.**

Rubber impression materials are distinguished from hydrocolloid impression materials by their stability in air after setting, their excellent reproduction of surface detail, their higher tear strengths, and their ability to allow the preparation of dies other than of the gypsum type. Polysulfides are characterized by rather long working and setting times, moderately high permanent deformation and flow, and high flexibility. Condensation and addition silicones have fairly short working and setting times and moderate flexibility and tear strength; however, the addition silicones have very low shrinking on setting, flow, and permanent deformation, making them the most accurate impression material. Polyether impression materials, although accurate, have short working and setting times, low tear strength, and are very stiff. The wettability of the polyethers and the hydrophilic addition silicones by mixes of gypsum are good. Polysulfides and silicones can be disinfected by immersion, with the least effect on accuracy being with the addition silicone.

Self-test questions

In the following multiple choice questions, one or more responses may be correct.
1 Which of the following statements are true?
   a. An impression gives a negative reproduction of a tooth.
   b. An impression gives a positive reproduction of the soft tissue.
   c. The die of a mandibular molar is a positive duplication of the tooth.
   d. The die of a maxillary molar is a negative duplication of the tooth.
   e. When an impression rests on its tray, the lowest area of the impression is the cuspal surface.

2 Indicate whether the following impression materials are classified as rigid or flexible:
___ **a.** Agar hydrocolloid
___ **b.** Polyether rubber
___ **c.** Zinc oxide–eugenol
___ **d.** Alginate hydrocolloid
___ **e.** Polysulfide rubber
___ **f.** Silicone rubber
___ **g.** Impression plaster
___ **h.** Dental impression compound

3 Which of the following statements are true?
a. Impression compound is hard at mouth temperature but flows at 45° C to record detail.
b. Time must be allowed during heating or cooling of impression compound to obtain a uniform temperature.
c. Softening of impression compound by kneading in warm water increases the flow when it hardens at mouth temperature.
d. Impression compound is used as a check impression to determine if undesirable undercuts are present in the cavity preparation.
e. Water spray of 16° to 18° C should be used to cool impression compound because colder water is uncomfortable for the patient and can cause increased internal stress in the impression.

4 Zinc oxide–eugenol impression material:
a. Is used as a wash impression in a thin layer in a tray
b. Is rigid and used to record impressions of completely or partially edentulous arches
c. Is supplied as a two-paste system
d. Sets by forming a matrix of zinc eugenolate around unreacted zinc oxide particles
e. Sets faster in the presence of water
f. Shrinks 0.5% during setting
g. Can be removed from a patient's lips by wiping with oil of orange

5 Indicate which of the functions listed in the right-hand column correspond to the components of alginate impression material listed in the left-hand column:
___ **a.** Calcium sulfate   1. Soluble alginate
___ **b.** Sodium alginate   2. Retarder, reacts first with $CaSO_4$
___ **c.** Water   3. Insoluble alginate
___ **d.** Sodium phosphate   4. Gel formation
___ **e.** Calcium alginate   5. Provides soluble calcium ions
___ **f.** Diatomaceous earth   6. Controls consistency of mix and flexibility of impression

6 The alginate hydrocolloid:
a. Consists of calcium alginate that has precipitated into a fibrous network with water occupying the intervening capillary spaces
b. Is a reversible hydrogel
c. Sets by a double decomposition-precipitation reaction
d. Usually contains salts to counteract the inhibiting effect of alginate on the setting of gypsum model material

7 Regular-setting alginate should:

a. Develop a smooth, creamy consistency free of graininess in less than 30 seconds

b. Set within 2 to 4½ minutes

c. Set more slowly if mixed with cold water

d. Set more slowly if mixed to a thin consistency

8 The permanent deformation of alginate can be minimized clinically by:

a. Increasing the time in the mouth before removal of the impression

b. Using a mix of thinner consistency

c. Decreasing the percent deformation during removal of the impression

d. Using more material between the tray and teeth

9 Which of the following statements are true?

a. Alginate impressions should be stored for as short a period as possible.

b. Alginate gels expand when stored in water.

c. Alginate gels shrink when stored in air or 100% relative humidity.

d. Alginate gels can be stored in 100% relative humidity without serious dimensional changes for about an hour.

10 Which of the following statements are true for alginate?

a. The can of alginate should be aerated, or fluffed up, before each opening.

b. The powder-dispensing cup should be slightly overfilled to allow the powder to fill the cup after compaction.

c. The powder should be added to the water and initially stirred to wet the particles.

d. Graininess in the mix and poor detail in the impression can result from inadequate mixing.

e. Alginate should be mixed with a vigorous stropping or wiping action.

11 Which of the following statements are true with respect to alginates?

a. Mixed alginate is generally added to the anterior portion of the tray and pushed toward the posterior part.

b. Patient gagging can be minimized by reducing the amount of alginate in the posterior palatal area.

c. The posterior portion of the tray is usually seated first.

d. Sufficient alginate should be present in the anterior part of the tray to record the soft tissues.

e. Setting is completed when the surface is no longer tacky.

12 Which of the following statements are true for alginate impressions?

a. The impression should be rinsed with water to remove any saliva or blood.

b. Excess water that collects in cuspal areas of the impression causes the gypsum model to be weak in these areas.

c. The impression should be placed face down on the bench to allow excess water to drain.

d. The impression can be stored for a short period if tightly wrapped in a damp towel.

e. Alginate not supported by the tray need not be cut away, since it is away from the area of interest.

13 Indicate the correspondence of the functions listed in the right-hand column to the components of agar hydrocolloid listed in the left-hand column:

___ **a.** Agar   1. Gel formation
___ **b.** Borax   2. Preservative
___ **c.** Potassium sulfate   3. Strength improver
___ **d.** Benzoates   4. Ensures proper setting of gypsum die materials
___ **e.** Water

14 Agar hydrocolloid:
  a. Converts to a sol when heated to 65° C
  b. Exhibits syneresis, since it solidifies at a lower temperature than that at which it liquefies
  c. Is permanently deformed about 1% when compressed 10% for 30 seconds
  d. Has a tear strength of about 30 lb/in

15 Agar impressions:
  a. Should be rinsed free of saliva or blood before pouring a gypsum model
  b. Can be electroplated with silver
  c. Should be stored for only a limited time before a model is prepared
  d. If stored for up to 1 hour, should be kept at 100% relative humidity

16 Indicate which of the rubber impression materials listed in the right-hand column contain the components listed in the left-hand column, and indicate the function of each component in the left-hand column by selecting the matching item in the right-hand column:
  ___ **a.** Polymer containing ethylene imine terminal groups   1. Polysulfide
  ___ **b.** Dimethylsiloxane with terminal hydroxy groups   2. Condensation silicone
  ___ **c.** Polymer-containing mercaptan groups   3. Polyether
  ___ **d.** Tin octoate and alkyl silicate   4. Addition silicone
  ___ **e.** Lead dioxide   5. Catalyst
  ___ **f.** Sulfonic acid ester   6. Base
  ___ **g.** Silica   7. Filler
  ___ **h.** Chloroplatinic acid

17 A comparison of the properties of rubber impression materials would indicate that:
  a. Condensation silicones show less dimensional change than polysulfides or polyethers.
  b. Polyethers are stiffer than silicones or polysulfides.
  c. Polyethers show less flow than condensation silicones or polysulfides.
  d. Addition silicones show less permanent deformation than polysulfides or polyethers.
  e. Condensation silicones show less working time than polysulfides but more than polyethers.

18 Which of the following statements about the manipulation of rubber impression materials are true?
  a. A flexible spatula should be used for mixing.
  b. The accelerator (or catalyst) initially is mixed with the base for 5 to 10 seconds in a circular motion with the tip of the spatula.
  c. Mixing by a wide sweeping motion should be accomplished within 1½ minutes.
  d. Increasing the temperature of the room will lengthen the working and setting time.

19 Tearing of a polysulfide rubber impression material when removing it from the mouth can be minimized by:
  a. Use of an alginate material instead
  b. Allowing the impression to remain in the mouth an additional 2 minutes
  c. Removal with a rapid, uniform motion

20 Which of the following properties apply to a regular-bodied addition silicone impression material?
  a. Working time of 2 to 4 minutes
  b. Dimensional change of −0.1%
  c. Permanent deformation of 0.05%
  d. Flow of 0.5%
  e. Flexibility of 10%
  f. Positive tissue culture tests on the mixed material
  g. Silverplating not possible

21 Which of the following statements apply to polyether impression materials?
  a. Polyether impressions are inaccurate because they absorb water and change dimensions.
  b. An equal length of thinner mixed with the base and catalyst doubles the working time and flexibility.
  c. These impressions cannot be readily silverplated.
  d. Their higher stiffness can be compensated for by increasing the thickness of rubber between the impression area and the tray.

22 The impression material that shows the least dimensional change as a result of disinfection by immersion is:
  a. Alginate
  b. Agar
  c. Polysulfide
  d. Addition silicones
  e. Polyether

23 Which of the statements are true for addition silicones?
  a. They release hydrogen after setting, and high-strength stone models should not be poured until 1 hour after setting.
  b. They are hydrophilic, whereas condensation silicones are hydrophobic.
  c. They are supplied as monophase systems.
  d. They are supplied as automix systems.
  e. The putties should be mixed while wearing latex gloves to protect the operator from the catalyst.

24 Which statements are true for immersion disinfection of impression materials?
  a. The accuracy of polyether impressions is the least affected.
  b. Selection of the type of disinfectant is more important than selection of the impression material.
  c. Addition silicones are the least affected by disinfection.
  d. None of the above.

Suggested supplementary readings

Council on Dental Materials, Instruments and Equipment, Council on Dental Practice, and Council on Dental Therapeutics: Infection control recommendations for the dental office and the dental laboratory, *J Am Dent Assoc* 116:241, 1988.

Craig RG: On making good impressions, *Dent Advis* 1:1, 1984.

Craig RG: Review of dental impression materials, *Adv in Dent Res* 2:51, 1988.

Craig RG, Urquiola NJ, Liu CC: Comparison of commercial elastomeric impression materials, *Oper Dent* 15:94, 1990.

Drennon DG, Johnson GH: The effect of immersion disinfection of elastomeric impressions on the surface detail and reproduction of improved gypsum casts, *J Prosthet Dent* 63:233, 1990.

Farah JM, Powers JM, eds: Crown and bridge impression materials, *Dent Adv* 6(2):1, 1989.

Johnson GH, Drennon DG, Powell GL: Accuracy of elastomeric impression materials disinfected by immersion, *J Am Dent Assoc* 116:525, 1988.

Look JO, Clay DJ, Gong K, Messer HH: Preliminary results from disinfection of irreversible hydrocolloid impressions, *J Prosthet Dent* 63:701, 1990.

Vermilyea SG, Powers JM, Craig RG: Polyether, polysulfide and silicone impression materials. II. Accuracy of silverplated dies, *J Mich State Dent Assoc* 57:405, 1975.

chapter
nine

Model and Die Materials

A model, cast, or die used in dentistry is a replica of the hard or soft oral tissues or both. Specifically, a model is a replica that is used primarily for observation. A study model is used in orthodontics, for example, to observe the progress of treatment. A cast is a working model; it is a replica on which is fabricated an appliance or a restoration. A cast must be made of a material that is strong and resistant to abrasion because it is subjected to the stresses of carving and finishing procedures. By definition a cast is a replica of more than one tooth; for example, a quadrant or a full arch. A cast may be partially or completely edentulous. A die is a working replica of a single tooth or several teeth.

Relationship between replica and impression. The relationship between a replica and an impression is illustrated for a full-arch, partially edentulous impression in Fig. 9-1. When the replica and impression are viewed as shown, two observations can be made. One is that low points of the impression (in this case, the cusp tips) are high points of the replica. A second observation is that the right side of the impression becomes the left side of the replica. Because of the close relationship between replica and impression, **flaws that exist in the impression will be reproduced in the replica.** Care must be taken not to perpetuate flaws in successive procedures because they may interfere with the fit of the finished appliance or restoration.

TYPES AND SELECTION

The materials used to make models, casts, or dies from dental impressions may be classified in groups as follows:

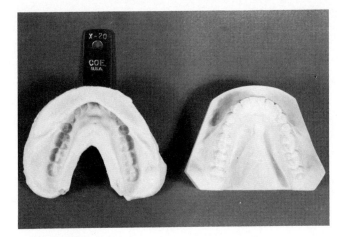

Fig. 9-1. Relationship between an impression and a replica for a full arch. (Courtesy Dr. Lon T. Smith, University of Texas Health Science Center at Houston, Dental Branch, Houston, Texas.)

Gypsum Products	Metal	Resin
Model plaster	Electroplated copper	Epoxy
Dental stone	Electroplated silver	
Dental stone, high-strength	Low-fusing alloy	

The selection of one of these materials is determined by the particular impression material in use and the purpose for which the replica is to be used. Often a system consisting of an impression material and model or die material is chosen because of the requirements of a particular clinical situation.

The types of models or dies that can be made in certain impression materials are limited because of their incompatibility or other technical problems. For example, only gypsum materials and investments can be used to make models or dies from the hydrocolloid impression materials. On the other hand, dies made from gypsum products, electroplated silver, and epoxy can be fabricated in polysulfide rubber base impressions. In the latter example, selection of the die material depends to a large extent on the purpose for which the cast or die is intended. If a master cast is desired from a polysulfide impression as a replica for use in complete denture prosthetics, dental stone should be used. If, however, a polysulfide impression of a tooth preparation is being used to fabricate an inlay, electroplated silver may be chosen as the die material. Impression materials that are compatible with the model and die materials commonly used are listed in Table 9-1.

Table 9-1. Compatibility of Cast or Die Materials with Impression Materials

Cast or die material	Impression material
Gypsum product	Compound
	Zinc oxide–eugenol
	Agar or alginate
	Plaster, if coated with separator
	Polysulfide rubber base
	Silicone (all types) rubber base
	Polyether rubber base
Electroplated copper	Compound
	Silicone (all types) rubber base
Electroplated silver	Polysulfide rubber base
	Silicone (addition hydrophobic) rubber base
	Polyether rubber base
Epoxy resin	Silicone (all types) rubber base (some require separator)
	Polysulfide rubber base, if coated with separator
	Polyether rubber base

DESIRABLE QUALITIES

A number of qualities are required of a material to be used for making casts or dies. These qualities, some of which may not be exhibited by every material, are accuracy, dimensional stability, ability to reproduce fine detail, strength and resistance to abrasion, ease of adaptation to impression, color, safety (noninjurious to health), and economy of time.

Accuracy and dimensional stability are properties of primary concern because casts and dies are used to fabricate appliances and restorations that must fit the prepared hard or soft oral tissues. Cast and die materials must reproduce an impression accurately and remain dimensionally stable under normal conditions of use and storage. Expansion or contraction that may occur during setting and dimensional changes in response to variations in temperature are required to be at a minimum. Strength and abrasion resistance are necessary for the cast or die material to be durable and to be able to withstand the manipulative procedures required for forming and finishing the chosen restorative metal.

Some of the qualities just cited are described in more detail in conjunction with the properties of several cast and die materials to be examined subsequently.

GYPSUM PRODUCTS

Gypsum materials are used extensively to make models, casts, and dies in dentistry. Examination of Table 9-1 indicates the variety of impression materials that are compatible with gypsum. Model plaster is used for study models, which are for record purposes only. Dental stone is stronger and more resistant to abrasion than is plaster and is used primarily for casts of full-arch impressions. Casts made of dental stone are durable enough to be used for forming mouth protectors. Dies that are used for fabricating gold restorations such as inlays, crowns, and bridges require strength and resistance to abrasion that exceed the properties of dental stone. A third gypsum material, high-strength dental stone, is able to withstand most of the manipulative procedures involved in the production of appliances and restorations. In addition, this material is dimensionally stable over long periods of time.

Chemical and physical nature

Setting reaction. Three forms of gypsum materials are commonly used as model and die materials—model plaster, dental stone, and high-strength dental stone. All forms of gypsum materials are obtained from the mineral gypsum, which is the dihydrate form of calcium sulfate. Gypsum has the chemical formula $CaSO_4 \cdot 2H_2O$. On heating during the manufacturing process, gypsum loses $1\frac{1}{2}$ moles of its 2 moles of water of crystallization and is converted to the hemihydrate form of calcium sulfate. Calcium sulfate hemihydrate has the chemical formula $CaSO_4 \cdot \frac{1}{2} H_2O$, which is sometimes written $(CaSO_4)_2 \cdot H_2O$.

When calcium sulfate hemihydrate in the form of plaster, stone, or high-strength stone is mixed with water, a chemical reaction takes place, and the **hemihydrate is converted back to the dihydrate form of calcium sulfate.** This chemical reaction, which is exothermic, is written as follows:

$$CaSO_4 \cdot \tfrac{1}{2} H_2O + 1\tfrac{1}{2} H_2O \rightarrow CaSO_4 \cdot 2H_2O + Heat$$

| **Plaster** | **Water** | **Gypsum** |

The amount of water necessary to react completely with 100 gm of calcium sulfate hemihydrate to form calcium sulfate dihydrate is 18.61 gm. The actual mechanism of setting or hardening is the result of a difference in solubility between the hemihydrate and dihydrate forms of calcium sulfate. During setting, growth and subsequent interlocking of gypsum crystals occur, as shown in Fig. 9-2. The interlocking contributes to the strength and dimensional change of the gypsum. Manipulative procedures that influence the difference in solubility and the growth of the dihydrate crystals can influence the physical and mechanical properties of the gypsum mass.

Physical form. Although plaster, stone, and high-strength stone have the same chemical formula, the method of removing part of the water of crystallization is different for each form.

Plaster is produced by heating gypsum in an open kettle at a temperature of approximately 115° C. The hemihydrate powder that results is a porous, irregularly shaped material called **β-calcium sulfate hemihydrate.** The plaster re-

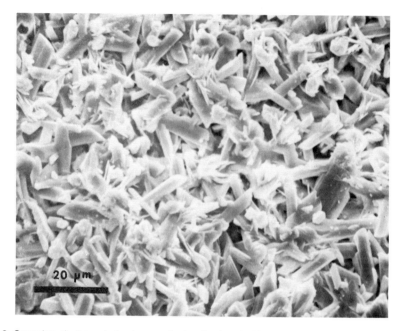

Fig. 9-2. Scanning electron photomicrograph showing interlocking crystals of set high-strength dental stone on the surface of a die.

ferred to in this chapter is commonly known as model plaster. Orthodontic plaster is a mixture of model plaster and dental stone and is used for models in orthodontics. Neither of these should be confused with a third type of plaster, called **impression plaster,** the properties and usage of which are different from those of the model plasters.

Dental stone is manufactured by removing part of the water of crystallization of gypsum under pressure and in the presence of water vapor at 125° C. The hemihydrate particles of this material are uniform in shape, as shown in Fig. 9-3, and less porous than the particles of plaster. Dental stone is designated as **α-calcium sulfate hemihydrate.**

High-strength dental stone is produced by boiling gypsum in a 30% solution of calcium chloride. The hemihydrate particles obtained in this fashion are the least porous of the three types of hemihydrate particles.

Plaster, stone, and high-strength stone are made up of hemihydrate particles whose size, shape, and porosity differ for each material. These physical differences in the hemihydrate particles are the basic factors that determine the manipulative conditions for mixing the particles and the properties and usage of the hardened gypsum product.

Excess water. Plaster, stone, and high-strength stone, when mixed with water,

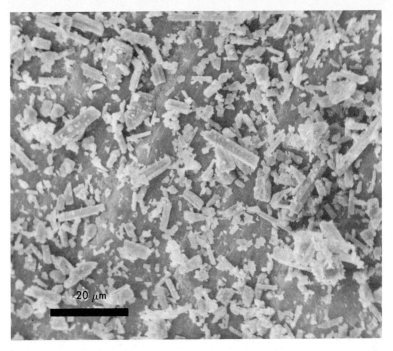

Fig. 9-3. Powder particles of a dental stone (α-calcium sulfate hemihydrate).

Table 9-2. Amount of Water Needed to Mix Gypsum Materials*

Gypsum	Mixing water (ml per 100 gm of powder)	Excess water (ml per 100 gm of powder)
Model plaster	45-50	26.4-31.4
Dental stone	30-32	11.4-13.4
High-strength dental stone	19-24	0.4-5.4

*Recommended water-powder ratio varies with each product.

set to form a hard mass. The actual amount of water necessary to mix the calcium sulfate hemihydrate is greater than the amount required for the chemical reaction (18.61 gm of water per 100 gm of hemihydrate) as shown in Table 9-2. The water required, in addition to that necessary for the chemical reaction, is called excess water and serves to wet the hemihydrate powder particles in such a way that they can react to form dihydrate crystals. The excess water itself does not react with the hemihydrate crystals, however, and is eventually lost by evaporation once the gypsum is set. **The excess water serves only to aid in mixing the powder particles and is replaced by voids during evaporation.**

The amount of excess water necessary to mix the hemihydrate powder depends on the size, shape, and porosity of the particles. Porous, irregularly shaped hemihydrate crystals require more water to facilitate wetting and mixing than do less porous, more regularly shaped crystals. Thus **plaster requires more water to mix than do stone and high-strength stone.** High-strength stone requires the least amount of excess water because its hemihydrate crystals are regularly shaped and dense. Therefore, once setting has occurred, the gypsum mass made from high-strength stone will be denser than either plaster or stone masses.

The amount of water necessary to mix plaster, stone, and high-strength stone is recommended by the manufacturer and is different for each product (Table 9-2). Model plasters require the largest amount of water to mix, whereas the high-strength stones require the least. Deviation from the amount of water recommended by the manufacturer will change both the consistency of the material and the properties of the set mass.

Properties

Initial and final setting times. The initial setting time is also called the working time. During the working time the material can be mixed and poured into the impression. Although the chemical reaction is initiated at the moment the powder is mixed with water, only a small portion of the hemihydrate is converted to gypsum at this early stage. The freshly mixed mass has a semifluid consistency and can be poured into a mold of any shape. As the reaction proceeds, however, more hemihydrate crystals react to form dihydrate crystals. The viscosity of the reacting mass begins to increase rapidly, and at some point the mass can no longer flow into the fine detail of the impression. At this point the material has reached the initial setting time and should no longer be manipulated.

The initial setting time can be detected clinically by a phenomenon known as loss of gloss. At some stage in the chemical reaction, the excess water on the surface is absorbed into the hardening mass of gypsum crystals. At this time the surface of the gypsum no longer reflects light and appears dull. When loss of gloss occurs, further manipulation of the gypsum mass should be avoided. For gypsum materials that meet the requirements of the ANSI–ADA Specification No. 25, the initial setting time must occur within 8 to 16 minutes from the start of the mix.

The final setting time is defined as the time at which the material can be separated from the impression without distortion or fracture, the time at which the chemical reaction is practically completed. The final setting time is usually measured arbitrarily by some form of penetration test, such as that using the Gillmore needle. Although the final setting time of many gypsum materials used in model and die applications occurs within 20 minutes from the start of the mix,

Table 9-3. Knoop Hardness and Surface Roughness of Several Die Materials

Die material	Knoop hardness (kg/mm²)	Surface roughness (microinches)
Epoxy	25	2.0
High-strength stone without hardener	77	16.0
High-strength stone with hardener	79	11.0
Electroplated silver	128	2.4
Electroplated copper	134	1.2

Modified from Fan PL, Powers JM, Reid BC: *J Am Dent Assoc* 103:408, 1981.

Table 9-4. Relationship Between Contact Angle of High-Strength Stone on Various Impression Materials and Number of Bubbles on Cast

Material	Contact angle of high-strength stone (degrees)	Number of bubbles on cast
Agar	40	—
Alginate	44	—
Polyether	49-51	9-28
Polysulfide	67-77	39-43
Silicone (hydrophilic)	50	—
Silicone (hydrophobic)	92-98	56-69

Modified from Lorren RA, Salter DJ, Fairhurst CW: *J Prosthet Dent* 36:176, 1976.

common practice allows the gypsum mass to harden for 45 to 60 minutes before removing it from the impression.

Reproduction of detail. Gypsum dies do not reproduce surface detail as well as electroplated or epoxy dies because the surface of the set gypsum is porous on a microscopic level (see Fig. 9-2). The porosity of the set gypsum causes the surface to be rough compared with other die materials (Table 9-3). The use of a hardener solution instead of water during mixing may reduce surface roughness for some high-strength stones. Air bubbles frequently are formed at the interface of the impression and gypsum cast because the freshly mixed gypsum does not wet some impression materials well. As shown in Table 9-4, the number of bubbles formed on a cast is related to the wettability of the impression material as described by the contact angle of freshly mixed gypsum on the impression. **The frequency of bubbles can be reduced dramatically by use of vibration during pouring of the cast.**

Compressive strength. The strength of gypsum materials is directly related to the density of the set mass. Because high-strength dental stone is mixed with the least amount of excess water, it is the densest of the gypsum materials and the strongest. Model plaster, being the least dense, is the weakest of the group.

The minimum values of 1-hour compressive strength required of materials to pass the ANSI–ADA Specification No. 25 are 1280 psi (9 MN/m^2) for model plaster, 2980 psi (21 MN/m^2) for dental stone, and 4980 psi (35 MN/m^2) for high-strength dental stone. The 1-hour compressive strength is actually a measure of the wet strength of the gypsum because the excess water has not yet been lost. Once the gypsum has dried, which may take as long as 7 days for a large model, the strength is increased. This so-called **dry strength is approximately twice the value of the wet strength (1-hour).**

Tensile strength. The tensile strength of gypsum materials is important in structures in which bending forces tend to occur, as in the removal of casts from flexible impression materials. Because of the brittle nature of gypsum materials, the teeth on a cast will fracture rather than bend.

The 1-hour tensile strength of model plaster is approximately 330 psi (2.3 MN/m^2). When dry, the tensile strength of model plaster doubles. The tensile strength of high-strength dental stone is twice that of plaster in the wet or dry condition. **Plaster, stone, and high-strength stone are all considerably weaker in tension than in compression.**

Hardness and abrasion resistance. The surface hardness of gypsum materials is related to their compressive strength. The higher the compressive strength of the hardened mass, the higher the surface hardness. The hardness of high-strength stone is three times that of an epoxy die but about half that of an electroplated die (Table 9-3). Resistance to abrasion also increases with increasing compressive strength. **Maximum hardness and resistance to abrasion are reached once the dry strength has been attained.** High-strength dental stone is the most resistant of the gypsum materials to abrasion, but in practical use the abrasion resistance of even high-strength stone is not as high as is desirable. The lack of a smooth, uniform surface, as shown in Fig. 9-2, may explain the moderate abrasion resistance of high-strength stone. Attempts to improve the abrasion resistance of gypsum by impregnating the die with methyl methacrylate monomer that then is allowed to polymerize have not been successful. The idea of drying models, casts, or dies in an oven to obtain dry compressive strength and dry surface hardness of the gypsum quickly is not practical because the water of crystallization might be attacked, which would reduce the strength instead of increasing it. The use of a hardening solution in place of water may increase hardness substantially and improve abrasion resistance of some high-strength stones as a result of a smoother surface (see Table 9-3).

Dimensional accuracy. All gypsum materials show a measurable linear expansion on setting. The expansion results from the growth of the calcium sulfate dihydrate crystals and their impingement on one another. The magnitude of ex-

Table 9-5. Marginal Openings of Castings Made on Undersized Dies

Taper of preparation degrees	Die error (%)		
	0.1	0.2	0.3
2	135 μm	270 μm	405 μm
5	57 μm	115 μm	172 μm
15	23 μm	46 μm	68 μm

Modified from Price WR Jr, Chai L, Eames WB, and Wallace SW: *J Dent Res* 55:B235, 1976.

pansion, however, varies from one type of gypsum material to another. Normally model plaster develops a setting expansion of 0.2% to 0.3%, dental stone about 0.08% to 0.1%, and high-strength stone about 0.01% to 0.08%. ANSI–ADA Specification No. 25 lists maximum permissible values of setting expansion of 0.3%, 0.2%, and 0.1% for model plaster, stone, and high-strength stone, respectively. **Dies made from high-strength stone generally are undersize but are more accurate than dies made by silverplating or from epoxy materials** (which are also undersize). Accuracy is affected also by the dimensional change associated with the impression material during setting and by the taper of the preparation. A more highly tapered full-crown preparation will show less marginal discrepancy in the casting made on an undersized die than will a preparation that has nearly parallel axial walls (Table 9-5).

The setting expansion may be controlled by different manipulative conditions, as well as by the addition of some chemicals. These factors are discussed in the section on manipulation.

If during the setting process the gypsum materials are immersed in water, the setting expansion will increase. The **hygroscopic** expansion of plaster, stone, and high-strength stone is approximately twice the normal setting expansion of these materials.

> Setting expansion of gypsum under water is termed hygroscopic expansion.

Manipulation

Selection of product. The selection of a particular type of gypsum material should be based on the clinical usage of the material and the properties required. Dental model plaster (Type II) is the least expensive of the gypsum materials but has low strength and high setting expansion. Model plaster should be chosen for applications in which strength is not required and dimensional accuracy is not critical. The ease of trimming models made of model plaster is a definite advantage of selecting plaster for study models. High-strength dental stone (Type IV) is the most expensive of the gypsum materials. Its hardness, strength, and dimensional accuracy make high-strength stone desirable for use in fabri-

Table 9-6. Examples of Commercial Gypsum Model and Die Materials*

Manufacturer	Model plaster (Type II)	Dental stone (Type III)	High-strength dental stone (Type IV)
Dentsply	Model Plaster	Castone	Glastone
Miles Dental	Lab Plaster	Denstone	Die Stone
	Model Plaster	TruStone	
Sybron/Kerr	Kerr Snow White Plaster No. 1	Rapid Stone	Vel Mix Stone
Whip-Mix	Laboratory Plaster	Microstone	Die-Rock
	Model Plaster, Grade A	Quickstone	Silky-Rock

*Certified products according to ANSI–ADA Specification No. 25.

Table 9-7. Effect of Water-Powder Ratio on Setting Time and Compressive Strength of Model Plaster with Normal Spatulation

W-P ratio (ml/gm)	Initial setting time (min)	1-hour compressive strength (psi [MN/m^2])
0.45	8	1800(12.6)
0.50	11	1600(11.2)
0.55	14	1300(9.1)

Modified from Craig RG, editor: Restorative dental materials, ed 8, St. Louis, 1989, Mosby–Year Book.

cating gold restorations. Dental stone (Type III) has properties that are intermediate to those of plaster and high-strength stone. It may be chosen when a more durable study model is required or for use as a working model in complete denture technics. A list of current gypsum products is given in Table 9-6.

Water-powder ratio. Model plaster is mixed with a water-powder ratio of 45:100, in which the water is measured volumetrically in milliliters and the powder is measured in grams. In comparison, dental stone requires about 30 ml of water and high-strength stone 19 to 24 ml of water for each 100 gm of powder to produce a workable consistency.

Deviation from the water-powder ratio recommended by the manufacturer affects setting time, strength, and setting expansion. The effect of water-powder ratio on setting time and compressive strength of model plaster is shown in Table 9-7. Increasing the water-powder ratio produces a thinner mix that takes longer to set. As mentioned previously, a mix with a thinner consistency is weaker because more excess water is used. When a gypsum product is mixed with a lower water-powder ratio, the mixed mass is thicker and more difficult to manipulate, but the set gypsum is usually stronger. Setting expansion is also influenced by the water-powder ratio with thicker mixes showing increased expansion.

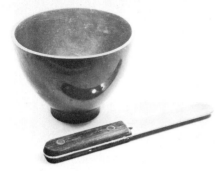

Fig. 9-4. Flexible rubber mixing bowl and metal spatula with a stiff blade.

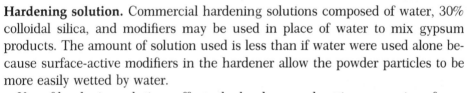

Fig. 9-5. Mechanical spatulator for use with small gypsum mixes.

Hardening solution. Commercial hardening solutions composed of water, 30% colloidal silica, and modifiers may be used in place of water to mix gypsum products. The amount of solution used is less than if water were used alone because surface-active modifiers in the hardener allow the powder particles to be more easily wetted by water.

Use of hardening solutions affects the hardness and setting expansion of gypsum dies. Increases in hardness of high-strength stone dies poured against impressions are 2% for silicones, 20% for polysulfide, 70% for agar, and 110% for polyether. High-strength stones mixed with hardener show a slightly higher setting expansion of 0.07% as compared with 0.05% for mixes with water alone. Scraping resistance is also improved for high-strength stones mixed with hardener.

Spatulation. In a typical mixing sequence, measured amounts of water and powder are added to a flexible rubber mixing bowl (Fig. 9-4) of an appropriate size and design. **The water is dispensed in the bowl first; the powder is then added and allowed to settle into the water for approximately 30 seconds.** This technic minimizes the amount of air incorporated into the mix during the initial spatulation. To obtain a smooth mix, the powder and water should be mixed slightly with a spatula having a stiff blade. Further spatulation can be continued by hand or with the aid of a mechanical spatulator (Fig. 9-5).

By hand, the spatulation is carried on by stirring the mixture vigorously and at the same time wiping the inside surfaces of the bowl with the spatula to be

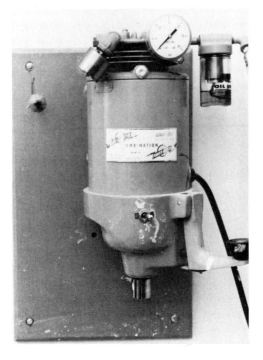

Fig. 9-6. Power-driven mechanical spatulator with a vacuum attachment.

sure that all the powder is wet and mixed uniformly with water. The average time of hand spatulation is typically 1 minute, with the rate of spatulation being approximately two revolutions per second.

The use of a hand-mechanical spatulator or a power-driven mechanical spatulator (Fig. 9-6) for mixing gypsum materials is a convenient method for providing a smooth mix. Vacuuming the mix during or after spatulation usually yields a product with reduced porosity because most of the air incorporated in the mix during spatulation is eliminated. An automatic vibrator is also of considerable aid in removing air bubbles during mixing.

The time and rate of spatulation have a definite effect on the setting time and expansion of gypsum materials. Within practical limits **an increase in the amount of spatulation will shorten the setting time. The setting expansion is also increased by increasing the time or rate of spatulation.** Both setting time and setting expansion are decreased by vacuum mixing.

Accelerators and retarders. The setting time of gypsum materials can be altered by methods more practical than varying the water-powder ratio or the time and rate of spatulation. By the addition of suitable chemicals, the rate of the chemical reaction can be changed to a few minutes or several hours. **Accelerators** are chemicals that increase the rate of reaction so that the setting time is reduced to several minutes. **Retarders** are chemicals that have the opposite effect.

Many accelerators and retarders work on the principle of changing the solubilities of the hemihydrate and dihydrate crystals so that the conversion of hemihydrate to dihydrate is increased or decreased. An accelerator causes the hemihydrate to be much more soluble than the dihydrate, thus accelerating the chemical reaction. Examples of accelerators are potassium sulfate (K_2SO_4) and calcium sulfate ($CaSO_4$) dihydrate crystals.* A 2% solution of K_2SO_4 in water is an excellent accelerator. Addition of this salt solution to plaster reduces the setting time from approximately 10 to about 4 minutes. If a small amount of set ($CaSO_4$) dihydrate is ground and mixed with plaster, for example, the dihydrate crystals will act as an effective accelerator. The set gypsum used in this manner is called terra alba and, in concentrations of 0.5% to 1%, is very effective. A practical way of shortening the setting time of gypsum materials in the dental office is to use the slurry water from the model trimmer to mix the gypsum product.

A retarder causes the hemihydrate to have only slightly higher solubility than the dihydrate, causing the chemical reaction to slow. Borax with the formula $Na_2B_4O_7 \cdot 10H_2O$ is a dependable retarder that may prolong the setting time of some gypsum products for several hours when added to the powder in a concentration of 2%. **Colloidal systems such as blood, saliva, agar, or alginate also retard the setting reaction of gypsum products,** although they do not function by altering the solubilities of the hemihydrate and dihydrate. If these colloids are in contact with the gypsum mass during setting, a soft, easily abraded surface of gypsum is obtained. To avoid this problem, impressions should be thoroughly rinsed in cold water to remove traces of blood and saliva before the impression is poured.

Temperature and humidity. The temperature of the water used for mixing, as well as the temperature of the environment, has an effect on the setting time of gypsum materials. It has been found by experience that by increasing from a room temperature of 20° C to a body temperature of 37° C, the rate of the reaction increases slightly, and the setting time is shortened. As the temperature is raised above 37° C, however, the rate of reaction decreases, and the setting time is lengthened. At 100° C the solubilities of hemihydrate and dihydrate are equal, in which case no reaction can occur and the gypsum will not set.

Gypsum materials are hydroscopic to some extent and can absorb water vapor from the humid atmosphere to form $CaSO_4$ dihydrate. Although it was stated earlier that the presence of $CaSO_4$ dihydrate crystals in plaster can shorten the setting time, experience has shown that exposure of plaster, stone, or high-strength stone to high humidity lengthens the setting time. **For best results all**

---

*Calcium sulfate ($CaSO_4$) dihydrate crystals accelerate the chemical reaction by serving as sites where new dihydrate crystals can form as the reaction progresses.

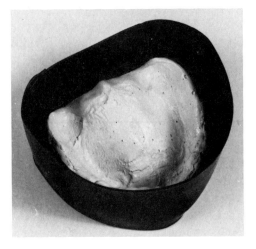

Fig. 9-7. Use of boxing wax to form a mold around an impression.

gypsum products should be kept in a closed container when not in use to protect them from the atmospheric humidity.

Construction of a model or cast. There are several common methods for the construction of a model or cast. In one method, strips of a soft wax called boxing wax are wrapped around the impression to form a mold for the gypsum (Fig. 9-7). Generally, the wax is extended approximately ½ inch beyond the tissue side of the impression to provide a base for the model. In manipulating the soft wax, care must be taken not to deform the impression material. The mixture of plaster or stone and water is then allowed to run into the impression under vibration in such a manner that the mixture pushes air ahead of itself as it fills the impressions of the teeth and other irregularities. It is common practice to pour the teeth of a cast or model in dental stone and then to pour the remainder of the impression in model plaster. This dual technic allows for strong teeth in the model and for easy trimming of the base and is referred to in the explanation of the following methods.

A second method for the construction of a model or cast begins with filling the impression with stone as already described. The filled impression can then be inverted and placed on a pile of freshly mixed plaster that has been placed on a glass plate. The consistency of the stone is thick enough that the mass will remain in the impression when it is inverted. The plaster mass on the plate should not be allowed to extend over the impression tray, since this would make removal of the impression from the set gypsum difficult. Before the gypsum sets, it is practical to shape the base with a spatula to reduce the time required at the model trimmer when the gypsum has set.

In a third method, the impression filled with stone is inverted and placed in a rubber mold called a model former (Fig. 9-8) in which freshly mixed plaster has

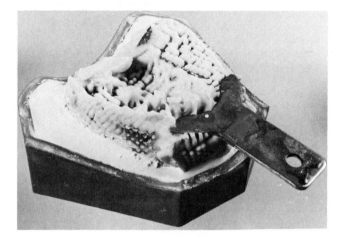

Fig. 9-8. Model former made of flexible rubber, with dental stone and plaster poured and the impression in the correct position.

been vibrated. Before setting occurs, the surfaces of the plaster can be smoothed with a wet finger. Regardless of the method used to construct the model or cast, the gypsum should not be separated from the impression until it has thoroughly hardened. Gypsum materials are usually allowed to harden for 45 to 60 minutes before the impression is removed and the model or cast trimmed. Careful attention paid to constructing the base of the model can save valuable time at the model trimmer.

When a gypsum material has been poured into an alginate impression and the initial set of the gypsum has occurred, the poured impression should be placed in an atmosphere of high relative humidity. This is best achieved by the use of a humidor, but when one is not available, the impression can be carefully wrapped in a wet towel for a short time. If an alginate impression is left uncovered on the bench for a period of time, the alginate will lose moisture to the air and subsequently may absorb moisture from the surface of the gypsum during setting with a detrimental effect on the surface quality of the cast. If the alginate is allowed to become dry, it loses its flexibility and becomes hard; it may be difficult to remove the model or cast from the dried impression.

Models can be disinfected with a spray of iodophor used according to manufacturer's instructions. In a hospital dental clinic, a model poured from a nondisinfected impression can be aseptically wrapped and sterilized in ethylene oxide.

METAL-PLATED DIES

Metal dies can be made by copperplating compound impressions or by silver-plating rubber-base impressions. When a cast or die is made in this manner, the process is referred to as **electroplating.** With other die materials, such as the gypsum products, the possibility of a dimensional change occurring as the die material sets is always present. No such expansion or contraction occurs in the electrodeposition of a metal.* This type of die reproduces the impression less accurately than high-strength stone but is tougher and more abrasion resistant and allows satisfactory finishing and polishing of metal restorations on the die. Plating usually requires 12 to 15 hours to produce a suitable thickness of metal.

Copperplating

Copperplated dies are most commonly made from compound or addition silicone rubber impressions. A copperplating apparatus suitable for dental use consists of a transformer and rectifier to reduce the voltage of the domestic supply and convert the AC to DC current. The low-voltage direct current passes through a variable resistor that is used to regulate the rate at which metal is deposited. A milliammeter indicates the current passing through the plating bath. An electrolytically pure copper plate is attached at the anode, whereas the impression to be plated is attached at the cathode. Both anode and cathode are immersed in an electrolytic solution, containing an acidic solution of copper sulfate. The surface of the impression is coated with a conductor of electricity before it is attached to the cathode by wires embedded in the impression.

Silverplating

Silverplated dies are restricted to the polysulfide, polyether, and some hydrophobic silicone rubber impression materials. The process of silverplating is similar to that of copperplating but a smaller current is required in silverplating. An apparatus used for silverplating is shown in Fig. 9-9. A pure silver anode is used with a silver cyanide plating solution.

The silverplating solution is poisonous; extreme care should be taken that the hands, workbench area, and clothing do not become contaminated. The addition of acid to the solution will produce hydrogen cyanide gas, an extremely poisonous one. **Silverplating solution therefore must be kept as a basic solution (pH > 7).** Copperplating should not be done in the same area in which silverplating is done because the risk of contaminating the basic silverplating solution with acidic copperplating solution is too high. **The silverplating bath should be kept covered at all times to control evaporation and dissipation of fumes.**

The surface of the impression is made conductive by brushing the areas to be plated with powdered silver, which adheres well to rubber-base impressions, allowing a uniform layer of silver to be electrodeposited (Fig. 9-10). Dispersions of silver powder in a volatile liquid are also available.

---

*Although the plating process itself does not cause a dimensional change, the rubber impression material can shrink before the initial plating is deposited.

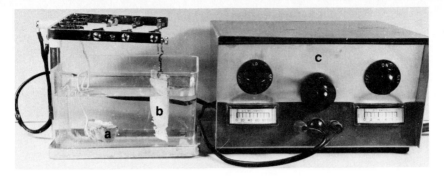

Fig. 9-9. Silverplating apparatus. *a,* Impression (cathode); *b,* silver bar (anode); *c,* DC power supply.

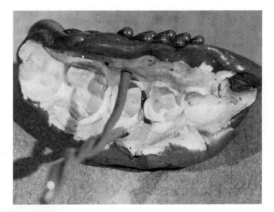

Fig. 9-10. Polysulfide impression showing electrical connecting wires and a layer of silver deposited by electroplating. (From Craig RG, editor: *Restorative dental materials,* ed 8, St. Louis, 1989, Mosby–Year Book.)

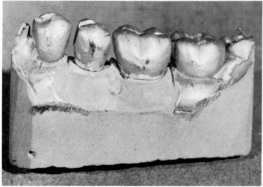

Fig. 9-11. Silverplated cast with a stone base made from the impression shown in Fig. 9-10. (From Craig RG, editor: *Restorative dental materials,* ed 8, St. Louis, 1989, Mosby–Year Book.)

When electroplating is completed, acrylic resin, dental stone, or a low-fusing metal is added to the inside of the electroplated shell. The impression is boxed with wax, and dental stone is poured to complete the cast (Fig. 9-11). Typically the electroplated dies are removable to allow more convenient fabrication of the restoration.

Table 9-8. Examples of Commercial Epoxy Die Materials

Product	Manufacturer
Epoxydent	Oxy Dental
Epoxy Die Material	Dentsply
Epoxy Die Resin	George Taub
Pri-Die	J.F. Jelenko

EPOXY DIES

Dies of epoxy for use in fabricating crowns, bridges, and inlays can be made in polyether, polysulfide, or silicone rubber impression materials, although a silicone separator must be used with polysulfide impressions. **Epoxy dies are tougher and more abrasion resistant than high-strength stone dies but are not as accurate or as stable dimensionally.** Four commercial epoxy die materials are listed in Table 9-8.

Composition

Epoxy die materials are two-component systems that include a resin and a hardener. The viscous resin may be a difunctional epoxy to which filler may be added.

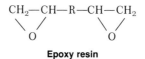

Epoxy resin

The hardener is a polyamine that, when mixed with the resin for about a minute, causes polymerization. The hardener is toxic and should not come into contact with the skin during mixing and manipulation of the unset material.

Properties

Epoxy die materials have a working time of about 15 minutes and set within 1 to 12 hours, depending on the product. Although the Knoop hardness number of the epoxy die (25 KHN) is less than that of high-strength stone (77 KHN), the compressive strength of 16,000 psi (110 MN/m^2) after 7 days and the abrasion resistance of the epoxy die are superior. The dimensional change (shrinkage) during polymerization is between 0.03% and 0.3% and continues to occur for up to 3 days. Because the epoxy materials are so viscous when poured, porosity can occur. One manufacturer minimizes porosity by centrifuging the impression after the epoxy has been poured. Most epoxy dies should not be used until 16 hours after pouring, since they harden slowly; however, a few epoxy materials set rapidly enough to be used in 30 minutes.

Gypsum products—model plaster, dental stone, and high-strength dental stone—are used extensively in dentistry to make models, casts, and dies. Although chemically similar, plaster, stone, and high-strength stone require different amounts of water for mixing and exhibit different values of strength, abrasion resistance, and setting expansion. These properties are affected by manipulative variables, such as water-powder ratio and conditions of spatulation, and by the evaporation of the excess water. Metal-plated and epoxy dies are alternatives to high-strength stone dies. Epoxy dies are more abrasion resistant than gypsum dies but not as accurate or as dimensionally stable.

Self-test questions

In the following multiple choice questions, one or more responses may be correct.

1 Match the model and die materials listed in the right-hand column with their compatible impression materials listed in the left-hand column:

   ___ **a.** Polyether rubber base   1. Gypsum
   ___ **b.** Zinc oxide–eugenol   2. Electroplated silver
   ___ **c.** Agar   3. Epoxy resin (without separator)
   ___ **d.** Silicone rubber base   4. Electroplated copper
   ___ **e.** Alginate
   ___ **f.** Impression compound
   ___ **g.** Polysulfide rubber base

2 The amount of water that reacts chemically with 100 gm of a dental gypsum product is:
  a. Dependent on the water-powder ratio of the product
  b. 50 gm
  c. 30 gm
  d. 18.6 gm

3 Excess water mixed with model plaster:
  a. Serves to wet the hemihydrate particles so they can react
  b. Is bonded to the precipitated dihydrate crystals
  c. Is eventually lost by evaporation once the gypsum is set
  d. Improves the ease of mixing the powder particles

4 Which of the following statements are true with respect to gypsum products?
  a. The amount of excess water necessary to mix the hemihydrate powder depends on the size, shape, and porosity of the particles.
  b. Dental stone requires more excess water to mix than does model plaster.
  c. The set mass will be denser and stronger if the excess water for a particular product is increased.
  d. The rate of growth of the dihydrate crystals will be reduced if the hemihydrate crystals are mixed in more excess water than recommended.

5 Which of the following statements are true?
   a. The initial setting time characterizes the start of the chemical reaction of model plaster.
   b. The initial setting time of model plaster can be detected clinically by the phenomenon known as loss of gloss.
   c. Common practice allows the model plaster to harden for 45 to 60 minutes before removing it from the impression.
   d. The setting time of gypsum can be altered easily by the operator with the use of accelerators or retarders.

6 Which of the following statements are true?
   a. The strength of gypsum materials is indirectly related to the density of the set mass.
   b. Because high-strength stone is mixed with the least amount of excess water, it is the strongest of the gypsum materials.
   c. The wet strength of gypsum is about twice the dry strength.
   d. The wet strength is a measure of strength of gypsum before all the water has reacted.

7 Which of the following statements are true?
   a. All gypsum materials show a measurable linear expansion during setting that results from the growth of calcium sulfate dihydrate crystals.
   b. Model plaster develops a setting expansion of 0.2% to 0.3%.
   c. Dental stone develops a setting expansion of 0.08% to 0.1%.
   d. High-strength stone develops a setting expansion of 0.01% to 0.08%.

8 Increasing the water-powder ratio of high-strength stone would:
   a. Lengthen the initial setting time
   b. Increase the 1-hour compressive strength
   c. Increase the setting expansion
   d. Increase the amount of excess water used to mix the material

9 Which of the following statements are true for manipulation of model plaster?
   a. The powder is added to the water in the mixing bowl.
   b. Spatulation can be described best as a whipping action.
   c. Hand mixing should be done in a stiff plastic bowl with a spatula that has a flexible blade.
   d. The average time of hand spatulation is 1 minute.

10 Increasing the amount of spatulation of model plaster, dental stone, or high-strength stone causes:
   a. A shorter setting time
   b. Dihydrate crystals to form faster
   c. A decrease in the setting expansion

11 Indicate which of the following are retarders and which are accelerators for the setting of model plaster, dental stone, or high-strength stone:

a. 2% solution of K_2SO_4	**e.** Saliva
b. Blood	**f.** Agar
c. Slurry water from model trimmer	**g.** Alginate
d. $CaSO_4$ dihydrate crystals	**h.** Borax

12 Which of the following statements are true?
    a. It is common practice to pour the teeth of an impression in model plaster and the base in dental stone.
    b. In manipulating boxing wax to form a mold around an impression, care must be taken not to deform the impression.
    c. To minimize the difficulty of removing the impression from the set gypsum, model plaster should not be allowed to extend over the impression tray.
    d. Before the model plaster sets, it is practical to shape and smooth the base with a spatula to reduce time at the model trimmer.
    e. An alginate impression poured with gypsum should be stored in an atmosphere of high relative humidity for short periods.

13 Which of the following statements about copperplating are true?
    a. The copperplating solution contains copper sulfate and is basic in pH.
    b. The copperplating solution contains cyanide salts and is acidic in pH.
    c. The impression compound is coated with a colloidal dispersion of graphite to make the surface conductive.
    d. The silverplating solution is poisonous and must be kept as a basic solution (pH > 7).
    e. After electroplating, the inside of the electroplated shell is filled with high-strength stone, acrylic plastic, or low-fusing metal.

14 Which of the following statements are true?
    a. Epoxy dies are less resistant to abrasion than stone dies.
    b. Epoxy dies expand about 0.1% during hardening.
    c. Polysulfide impression materials require a separator with epoxy die materials.
    d. Epoxy dies are stronger than stone dies.

Suggested supplementary readings

Fan PL, Powers JM, Reid BC: Surface mechanical properties of stone, resin, and metal dies, *J Am Dent Assoc* 103:408, 1981.

Garber DK, Powers JM, Brandau HE: Effect of spatulation on the properties of high-strength stones, *J Mich Dent Assoc* 67:133, 1985.

chapter
ten

Waxes

Waxes are composed of high–molecular weight organic molecules. The principal component in beeswax, for example, is an ester, myricyl palmitate:

$$C_{15}\,H_{31}-C\overset{O}{\overset{\|}{-}}O-C_{30}\,H_{61}$$

Dental waxes are composed of natural and synthetic waxes, gums, fats, fatty acids, oil, natural and synthetic resins, and pigments.

More than 200 years ago beeswax was first employed to produce impressions of areas of the mouth; since then waxes have continued to be used in dentistry. Currently few procedures in restorative dentistry can be carried to completion without the use of wax.

Wax products can be broadly classified as pattern, processing, or impression waxes. Pattern waxes include inlay, casting, and baseplate waxes and are used to form models of a restoration or appliance. Processing waxes include boxing, utility, and sticky waxes. They are used as auxiliary materials, for example, to aid in the production of casts, in the extension of impression trays, or in soldering. Corrective and bite waxes are used as impression materials to record detail in the oral cavity.

PATTERN WAX

Inlays, crowns, and bridge units are formed by a metal-casting process that employs the lost wax pattern technic. A pattern of wax that duplicates the shape and contour of the desired metal casting is constructed (Fig. 10-1). The carved wax pattern is embedded in a gypsum-silica investment material to form a mold with a sprue leading from the outer surface of the mold to the pattern (see Fig. 12-4). The wax is subsequently eliminated by heating, and the mold is further

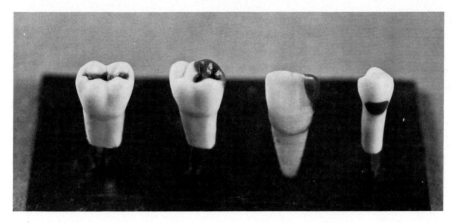

Fig. 10-1. Different wax patterns on dies. *Left to right,* Classes 1, 2, 4, and 5.

conditioned to receive the molten alloy. The lost-wax process is described in more detail in Chapter 12.

Composition

The principal waxes used to formulate inlay, crown, and bridge waxes are paraffin, microcrystalline wax, ceresin, carnauba, candelilla, and beeswax. For example, a wax may contain 60% paraffin, 25% carnauba, 10% ceresin, and 5% beeswax. Hydrocarbon waxes constitute the major portion of this formulation. The formula for hydrocarbon wax is as follows:

$$CH_3—(CH_2)_{15\text{-}42}—CH_3$$

By the use of higher melting hydrocarbon waxes or by the addition of an ester wax such as carnauba wax, inlay waxes of various hardness can be formulated. The description of hardness is an indication of the resistance of the wax to flow. Types I and II dental inlay casting waxes are recognized by ANSI–ADA Specification No. 4 revised in 1984. Type I is a medium wax that is prescribed for forming direct patterns in the mouth. Type II is a softer wax that is used as an indirect technic wax in the production of inlays and crowns. Inlay waxes are generally produced in blue, green, or purple rods or sticks about 7.5 cm long and 6 mm in diameter. Some manufacturers supply the wax in the form of small pellets or cones or in small metal ointment jars.

Properties

The accuracy and ultimate usefulness of the resulting metal casting is dependent to a large degree on the accuracy and fine detail of the wax pattern. The specification has been developed for dental inlay casting waxes to define certain physical properties that are extremely critical in their limitations. Among these properties are excess residue on burnout, flow, and linear thermal expansion.

Excess residue. Since wax patterns are to be melted and vaporized from the investment mold, **it is essential that no excess residue remain in the mold form to cause incomplete casting of the margins of restorations.** The specification therefore limits the nonvolatile residue of inlay waxes to a maximum of 0.10%.

Flow is the slippage of wax molecules over each other

Flow. This property is highly dependent on the temperature, composition of the wax, force causing the deformation, and length of time that the force is applied. **Flow greatly increases as the melting range of the wax is approached or as the load and its length of application are increased.**

The amount of flow required from a wax depends on its use. The Type I wax is prescribed for forming direct patterns in the mouth. **Low flow values are required at mouth temperature to minimize any tendency to distortion of the pattern on removal from the cavity preparation.** At 37° C a maximum of 1% flow is allowable for a Type I wax. When forming a wax pattern directly in the mouth, one must heat the wax to a temperature at which it will have sufficient flow under compression to reproduce the prepared cavity walls in great detail. However, this temperature must not be so high as to cause damage to the vital tooth structure or to be uncomfortable to the patient. Thus at 46° C a Type I wax must have a flow within the range of 70% to 90%.

A Type II wax is used to prepare patterns on a die and is therefore a softer wax. The Type II waxes show greater flow than Type I waxes both below and above mouth temperature. The required low flow of the direct wax and greater ease of carving of the softer indirect wax are desirable working characteristics for each of their respective technics.

Thermal expansion. Waxes expand when subjected to a rise in temperature (Fig. 10-2) and contract as the temperature is decreased. In general, dental waxes have the largest values of coefficient of thermal expansion of any material used in restorative dentistry. For example, the linear coefficient of thermal expansion of one Type I wax between 22° and 37.5° C is $323 \times 10^{-6}/°$ C. **The coefficients of thermal expansion of inlay waxes are high enough that temperature changes in wax patterns after the establishment of critical dimensional relationships may serve as a major contributing factor in inaccuracy of the finished restoration.**

The manufacturer is required to provide thermal expansion data for the Type I wax so that compensation may be determined for the shrinkage that occurs when the wax pattern is cooled from mouth temperature, at which it was formed, to room temperature, at which it will be invested. The maximum allowable expansion (or shrinkage when the wax cools) between 25° and 30° C and between 25° and 37° C is 0.20% and 0.60%, respectively.

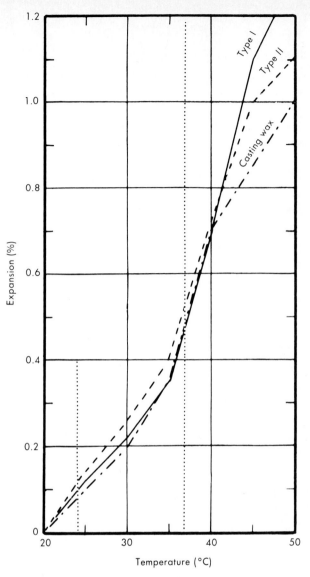

Fig. 10-2. Expansion of inlay and casting waxes from 20° to 50° C, showing percentage dimensional change from mouth temperature to room temperature. (From Craig RG, editor: *Restorative dental materials,* ed 8, St. Louis, 1989, Mosby–Year Book.)

Mechanical properties. The elastic modulus, proportional limit, and compressive strength of waxes are low compared with other materials, and these properties are strongly dependent on the temperature. For example, an inlay wax shows a change in modulus from 110,000 to 7000 psi (759 to 48 MN/m²) between 23° and 40° C. The modulus of inlay wax is important in the hygroscopic casting procedure in which nonuniform deformation can occur in wax patterns of crowns as the wax is subjected to stresses during setting of the investment.

The proportional limits and compressive strengths of waxes exhibit the same trends as their elastic moduli. The compressive strength of an inlay wax, for example, decreases from 12,000 to 70 psi (83 to 0.5 MN/m^2) between 23° and 40° C. Over this temperature range, inlay wax is considered a brittle material, although it does possess some flow at stresses below its proportional limit, which changes from 700 to 30 psi (4.8 to 0.2 MN/m^2) between 23° and 40° C.

Residual stress. Regardless of the method used to prepare a wax pattern, residual stress exists in the completed pattern. When released by the action of time and temperature, residual or internal stress can result in a nonuniform dimensional change, or distortion. In addition, the coefficient of thermal expansion can be dramatically affected by the presence of residual stress. When a wax is cooled under tensile forces, for example, the wax may actually contract when it is subsequently reheated. Any change in a pattern from any cause may be reflected in the lack of fit of the final casting.

Stress remaining in a wax as a result of manipulation is residual stress.

The manipulation of wax must be directed toward both minimizing the development of residual stress and keeping that which is developed from being released. Residual stress is developed in wax when the solid is subjected to stress well below its melting range, such as the stress that occurs during a carving procedure or during cooling under pressure. Residual stress can be minimized by manipulating the wax at temperatures as high as practical. In general, the higher the temperature of the wax at the time that the pattern is adapted and shaped, the less the tendency for distortion in the prepared pattern.

Wax can be softened uniformly by heating at about 50° C for at least 15 minutes before use. Because waxes are composed of molecules with a range of molecular weights, they have melting ranges rather than specific melting points. If the wax is used in the molten state, it should be added to the die in small increments to minimize the dimensional changes caused by solidification and thermal contraction. Carving instruments and the die can be warmed to about 37° C on a heating pad or under an incandescent lamp to minimize the introduction of residual stresses in the wax. It is most important to have the temperature of the wax at the moment of contact with the cavity or die well above the annealing temperature (50° C) if detail is to be recorded.

Since the release of residual stress and subsequent warpage are associated with storage time and temperature, **greater warpage naturally results at higher storage temperatures and during longer storage times. Warpage can be minimized by investing a wax pattern immediately or within 30 minutes.** If storage cannot be avoided, the pattern can be stored in a refrigerator but should be allowed to warm to room temperature before investing. It may be necessary to readapt the margins if the pattern has been stored.

CASTING WAX

The pattern for the metallic framework of removable partial dentures and other similar structures is fabricated from casting waxes (Fig. 10-3). These

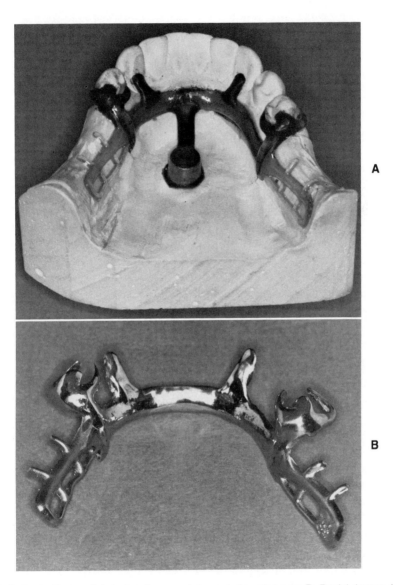

Fig. 10-3. A, Cast with a partial denture framework formed of casting wax. **B,** Partial denture framework after being cast in metal.

waxes are available in sheets, ready-made shapes, and in bulk. Little is known of the exact composition of the casting waxes, but it is reasonable to assume that they contain ingredients found in some inlay waxes.

Casting wax sheets are used to establish minimum thickness in certain areas of the partial denture framework, such as the palatal and lingual bar, and to produce the desired contour of the lingual bar. Clasps and retention meshes in various sizes are supplied as preformed shapes.

Casting wax sheets and ready-made shapes generally possess a slight degree of tackiness to help maintain their position on the cast until they are sealed in final position to the cast with a hot spatula. Since these waxes are casting pattern waxes for partial denture cast restorations, they must vaporize with minimum residue. Currently no ANSI–ADA specification for casting waxes exists.

BASEPLATE WAX

Baseplate wax derives its name from its use on the baseplate tray to establish the vertical dimension, the plane of occlusion, and the initial arch form in the technic for complete denture restoration. The normally pink color provides some esthetic quality for the initial stage of construction of the denture before processing. Baseplate wax serves as the material to produce the desired contour of the denture after the teeth are set in position (Fig. 10-4, *lower left*). As a result the contoured wax establishes the pattern for the final plastic denture.

Baseplate waxes may contain 70% to 80% paraffin-based waxes or commercial ceresin with small quantities of other waxes, resins, and additives. A typical composition might include 80% ceresin, 12% beeswax, 2.5% carnauba, 3% natural or synthetic resins, and 2.5% microcrystalline or synthetic waxes. The baseplate waxes are normally supplied in sheets 7.5 cm wide, 15 cm long, and 0.13 cm thick in pink or red.

Three types of waxes are included in the ANSI–ADA Specification No. 24 for baseplate wax. Type I is a soft wax for building contours and veneers. Type II is a medium wax to be used for patterns to be tried in the mouth in temperate climates, and Type III is a hard wax for patterns to be tried in the mouth in tropical weather. Flow requirements for these waxes are listed in Table 10-1. The maximum flow allowed at any given temperature decreases rapidly from Type I to III. The flow requirements of Type III baseplate wax are comparable to those of the Type I inlay wax. **Flow is important for the waxes used in patterns to be tried in the mouth** because excessive flow could cause changes in vertical dimensions and occlusion. The linear coefficient of thermal expansion for baseplate waxes has been reported to be between $200 \times 10^{-6}/°$ C and $390 \times 10^{-6}/°$ C from 25° to 37° C. The specification limits the expansion of the wax to 0.8% between 25° and 40° C

There is residual stress within the baseplate wax holding and surrounding

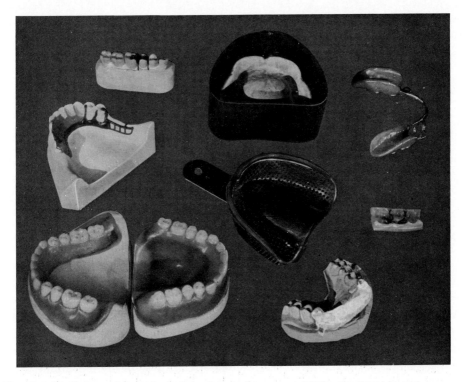

Fig. 10-4. Applications of waxes in dentistry. Inlay pattern, *upper left;* boxing of an impression, *upper center;* baseplate, *lower left;* casting wax, *left center;* utility wax, *center;* sticky wax, *lower right;* corrective impression, *upper right;* and bite, *right center.* (From Craig RG, editor: *Restorative dental materials,* ed 8, St. Louis, 1989, Mosby–Year Book.)

Table 10-1. Flow Requirements for Dental Baseplate Wax

| Wax | Temperature (°C) | Flow (%) | |
		Minimum	Maximum
Type I	23	—	1.0
	37	5.0	80.0
	45	—	—
Type II	23	—	0.6
	37	—	2.5
	45	50.0	90.0
Type III	23	—	0.2
	37	—	1.2
	45	5.0	50.0

Modified from ANSI–ADA Specification No. 24 for baseplate wax, 1971; addendum, 1986.

Table 10-2. Summary of Requirements of Working Properties for Dental Boxing, Utility, and Sticky Waxes

Type of wax	Color	Working properties
Boxing	Green or black	Smooth, glossy surface on flaming; pliable at 21° C but retains shape at 35° C; seals easily to plaster with hot spatula
Utility	Orange or dark red	Pliable and tacky at 21° to 24° C; sufficient adhesion to stick to itself
Sticky	Dark or vivid	Sticky when melted; adheres closely; not more than 0.2% residue on burnout

Modified from Federal Specification U-W-138, May, 1947, for boxing wax; Federal Specification U-W-156, August, 1948, for utility wax; Federal Specification U-W-00149a (DSA-DM), September, 1966, for sticky wax.

the teeth of a wax denture pattern, which results from differential cooling, "pooling" the wax with a hot spatula, and physical manipulation of the wax below its most desirable working temperature. Allowing the finished denture pattern to stand for long periods can result in distortion of the wax and movement of the teeth. **The waxed denture should be flasked soon after completion to maintain the greatest accuracy of tooth relations.**

BOXING WAX

One method that was discussed in Chapter 9 for forming a plaster or stone cast from an impression of the edentulous arch requires that a wax box first be formed around the impression (Fig. 10-4, *upper center*). Freshly mixed plaster or stone is then poured and is vibrated into the boxed impression. The boxing technic usually consists of first adapting a long narrow stick or strip of wax to fit around the impression below its peripheral height, then following it with a wide strip of wax, thus producing a form around the entire impression. Since the impression may be made partially or totally from a material that is easily distorted, such as a hydrocolloid, it is desirable to have a boxing wax that is readily adaptable to the impression at room temperature as indicated in Table 10-2.

UTILITY WAX

In numerous instances an easily workable, adhesive wax is desired. A standard perforated tray for use with alginate impression materials, for example, may easily be brought to a more customized contour by a utility wax (Fig. 10-4, *center*). This is done to prevent sag and distortion of the impression material. A soft and pliable adhesive wax may also be used on the lingual portion of a bridge pontic to stabilize it while a labial plaster splint is poured.

Utility wax probably consists largely of beeswax, petrolatum, and other soft waxes. It is usually supplied in stick and sheet form in a dark red or orange color. In orthodontics it is called periphery wax and is supplied in white sticks.

STICKY WAX

A suitable sticky wax for prosthetic dentistry is formulated from a mixture of waxes and resins. Such a material is sticky when melted and adheres closely to the surfaces on which it is applied. However, at room temperature the wax is firm and free from tackiness and possesses a quality of brittleness. Sticky wax is used to assemble metallic or resin pieces in a fixed temporary position and to seal a plaster splint to a stone cast in the process of forming porcelain facings (Fig. 10-4, *lower right*). Because **sticky wax is brittle at room temperature,** any unwanted movement of the pieces held together by the wax will cause it to fracture rather than distort. The pieces can then be easily rejoined in the proper relationship.

CORRECTIVE IMPRESSION WAX

Corrective impression wax is used as a wax veneer over an original impression to contact and register the detail of soft tissues in a functional state (Fig. 10-4, *upper right*). Corrective waxes appear to be formulated from hydrocarbon waxes such as paraffin and ceresin and may also contain metallic particles. **The flow of these waxes at 37° C is 100%; thus they are subject to distortion on removal from the mouth.**

BITE REGISTRATION WAX

Bite registration wax is used to articulate accurately certain models of opposing quadrants (Fig. 10-4, *right center*). Bite registrations are frequently made from 28-gauge casting wax or from baseplate wax. Specially formulated bite waxes appear to be formulated from beeswax or hydrocarbon waxes such as paraffin or ceresin. Certain products contain aluminum or copper particles. The flow of several bite registration waxes at 37° C ranges from 2.5% to 22%, indicating that **these waxes are susceptible to distortion on removal from the mouth.**

Dental waxes are formulated from high–molecular weight organic molecules to function as pattern, processing, or impression waxes. Time and temperature affect the flow, thermal expansion, mechanical properties, and development and release of residual stresses of waxes. Distortion of waxes can be minimized by manipulation at proper temperatures, careful handling, and prompt investment of patterns.

Self-test questions

In the following multiple choice questions, one or more responses may be correct.

1 Which of the following statements are true?
   a. Paraffin waxes are saturated hydrocarbons, melt in the range of 40° to 71° C, and are soft.
   b. Beeswax contains esters and hydrocarbons and is characterized by its brittleness at mouth temperature.
   c. Carnauba wax is hard and brittle and melts at higher temperatures than paraffin.
   d. Synthetic waxes have dependable properties and are used frequently in dental formulations to replace natural waxes.

2 The coefficient of thermal expansion of a dental inlay wax is about:
   a. -50×10^{-6}/° C
   b. 20×10^{-6}/° C
   c. 80×10^{-6}/° C
   d. 200×10^{-6}/° C

3 Residual stress:
   a. Is developed in wax when it is cooled under stress
   b. Results in a uniform dimensional change that can be compensated for in the casting process
   c. Can be minimized by the manipulation of a wax at a temperature as high as is practical
   d. Can cause warpage that increases at higher storage temperatures and during longer storage times

4 A pattern wax might be used to:
   a. Make a corrective impression
   b. Form a mold around an impression
   c. Form the general size and contour of a restoration

5 Casting waxes possess useful properties such as:
   a. Tackiness
   b. No residue other than carbon
   c. Minimum values of flow at mouth temperature
   d. Specified values of coefficient of thermal expansion

6 At 37° C the flow values of certified Types I, II, and III dental baseplate waxes are respectively:
   a. <1.2%, <2.5%, 5% to 80%
   b. <2.5%, <1.2%, 5% to 80%
   c. <1.2%, 5% to 80%, <2.5%
   d. 5% to 80%, <2.5%, <1.2%

7 Which of the following statements are true?
   a. Boxing wax is used for forming a mold around an impression before a gypsum cast is poured.
   b. Utility wax must stick to itself.
   c. Sticky wax must have less than 0.2% residue on burnout.

d. Utility wax is used to prevent sag and distortion of an alginate impression in a tray.

e. Sticky wax is used to assemble metallic or resin pieces in a fixed temporary position and is brittle at room temperature.

8 Which of the following statements apply to bite registration waxes?

a. They are used to articulate models of opposing quadrants accurately.

b. Formulations are made from carnauba wax.

c. The flow of these waxes at 37° C is from 5% to 80%.

d. These waxes can be distorted when removed from the mouth.

Suggested supplementary readings

Craig RG, Eick JD, Peyton FA: Properties of natural waxes used in dentistry, *J Dent Res* 44:1308, 1965.

Craig RG, Eick JD, Peyton FA: Strength properties of waxes at various temperatures and their practical applications, *J Dent Res* 46:300, 1967.

Craig RG, Powers JM, Peyton FA: Differential thermal analysis of commercial and dental waxes, *J Dent Res* 46:1090, 1967.

Craig RG, Powers JM, Peyton FA: Thermogravimetric analysis of waxes, *J Dent Res* 50:450, 1971.

Powers JM, Craig RG: Penetration of commercial and dental waxes, *J Dent Res* 53:402, 1974.

Powers JM, Craig RG: Thermal analysis of dental impression waxes, *J Dent Res* 57:37, 1978.

chapter eleven

Gold and Nonprecious Alloys

Gold foil was the original metallic restorative dental material. Because of the difficulty and time it takes to compact gold foil, it has been largely replaced by silver amalgam and cast gold inlays. High-gold-content alloys have until recently been the main materials for cast crown and bridgework. Since 1973, because of the escalation in the price of gold, these high-cost alloys are steadily being replaced by lower-gold-content alloys, palladium-silver alloys, and nickel alloys. Partial denture frameworks are usually cast with cobalt-chromium alloys, less frequently with nickel-chromium alloys, and only occasionally with gold alloys. In this chapter **noble metal content includes only gold, platinum, and palladium.** Although silver is often considered as "precious," it is not noble, since it tarnishes readily and is relatively inexpensive. The total noble metal content of dental alloys is required by regulation to be listed on the package.

> Noble metals include gold, platinum, palladium, and iridium.

GOLD CONTENT

The **karat** (also spelled **carat**) is the traditional unit expressing gold content in an alloy. Pure gold is 24 karat. Therefore a 12-karat alloy contains half as much gold, or is 50% gold. The following formula illustrates this system:

> Karat is a measure of gold content.

$$\frac{\text{Karat} \times 100}{24} = \% \text{ Gold}$$

Gold content may also be expressed in terms of **fineness.** The fineness is obtained by multiplying the percent of gold content by 10. Therefore a 24-karat alloy would have a fineness of 100×10, or 1000, and a 12-karat alloy would be 500 fine. Articles of jewelry containing 50% gold would be marked 12 K, since K is the symbol for karat. The symbol for fineness is F.

Fineness is the percentage of gold multiplied by 10.

DIRECT GOLD FILLING MATERIALS

The pure element gold contributes tarnish resistance and high ductility to a restoration. Pure gold (24 K) is so ductile and malleable that it may be drawn out into extremely fine wires and rolled down to extremely thin foils. Still thinner sheets may be made by beating between parchment paper to form gold foil, which may be used to form a restoration directly in a prepared cavity by compacting layer on layer. This fabrication process is carried out with instruments called **condensers.** Force is applied by striking the condenser with a mallet or by using an automatic mechanical condenser. Each condensed layer of foil is **welded** to form an atomic bond. In the process of mechanical working, the gold is also strengthened and hardened. The properties of condensed gold are comparable to those of a 22-K gold alloy.

Direct gold filling materials are forms of gold that are compacted in the patient's tooth to form restorations.

In addition to gold foil, other forms of pure gold are available for fabricating direct restorations (Fig. 11-1). Gold formed by rapid electrolysis forms "sponge gold." Thin strips of compressed electrodeposited gold powder are known as mat gold. Other forms of gold are **fibrous foil** and a **powdered gold-calcium alloy.** Powdered gold also is available enclosed in a foil envelope.

For the gold to weld easily with another piece of gold, it must have a clean or uncontaminated surface. Gold with such a surface is known as **cohesive gold.** It has been found that **annealing** gold foil immediately before use makes it more cohesive. This process involves a **degassing** of the surface by heat applied in the **annealing furnace** or alcohol flame. In the tray method, the material is heated for 10 minutes at 454° C. The alcohol annealing technic is the method of choice for powdered gold, which contains an indicator. The powdered gold is heated directly over the alcohol flame until an organic indicator produces a yellow flame and the pellet appears a dull red color. Annealing is a process of heating gold foil to remove surface impurities to make it cohesive.

Although gold foil restorations have been found to serve well over many years, **the technic of condensing the foil to a satisfactory condition is largely dependent on the skill of the operator.**

Gold foil can be condensed directly to form a restoration by a process of mechanical condensation. The process is highly technic selective and time consuming but can produce long-lasting small fillings.

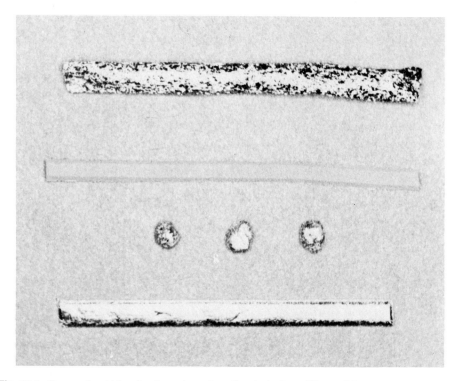

Fig. 11-1. Forms of gold for direct condensation. *Top to bottom,* Fibrous foil, mat gold, powdered gold, and powdered gold-calcium alloy (Electraloy). (From Dennison JB: Restorative materials for direct application. In Craig RG, editor: *Dental materials: a problem-oriented approach,* St. Louis, 1978, Mosby–Year Book.)

GOLD ALLOYS FOR CASTING

A wide variety of gold alloys may be made by the addition of copper, silver, metals of the platinum group, and other metals for casting. In dentistry, gold alloys are classified by ANSI–ADA specifications as Type I, II, III, or IV. Noble metal contents and hardnesses are given in Table 11-1. The softer Type I alloys are used for simple inlays. Type II alloys are indicated for larger two- or three-surface inlays (Fig. 11-2), and Type III alloys are designed for crown and bridge applications. Type IV alloys are used for partial dentures.

Casting is a process of pouring a molten alloy into a mold to form restorations.

In addition to the four ANSI–ADA types of alloys, gold alloys are available for **porcelain-fused-to-metal** restorations and low-karat yellow and white alloys. The escalation in the price of gold (Fig. 11-3) has given rise to the wider use of

Table 11-1. Noble Metal Content and Hardness of ANSI–ADA Types I to IV Gold Alloys

Type	Gold plus platinum group metals (minimum %)	Vickers hardness number (softened condition)
I (soft)	83	50-90
II (medium)	78	90-120
III (hard)	78	120-150
IV (extra hard)	75	150+

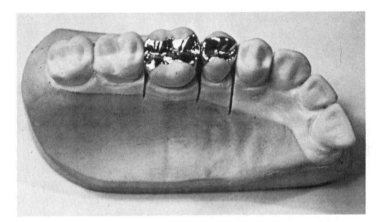

Fig. 11-2. Highly polished cast gold inlays

lower karat alloys. These low-karat alloys retain a light gold color with gold content as low as 40% if the palladium content is not higher than 6%. They also contain about 54% of copper and silver combined. **A higher incidence of short-term tarnish is reported with these alloys in clinical studies;** however, there is less tarnish than expected if sufficient palladium is present. It is too early to fully assess the long-term tarnish resistance of these alloys. The gold contents of several low-karat commercial alloys are given in Table 11-2.

Porcelain-fused-to-metal restorations have an outer coating of porcelain for a natural appearance.

White gold alloys, which have been used since the 1930s, contain lower percentages of gold (around 30%) and greater amounts of palladium (10% to 35%), silver (35% to 66%), and copper (6% to 25%). Palladium acts as a potent whitener but absorbs gases during melting that can produce porous castings.

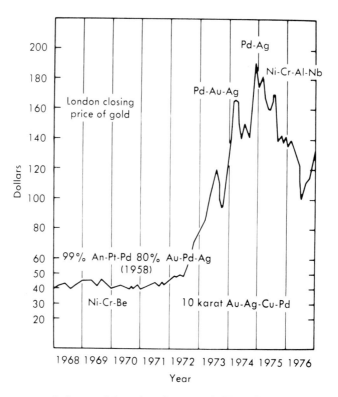

Fig. 11-3. Appearance of alloys and the price of pure gold. (From O'Brien WJ: Evolution of dental casting. In Valega TM, editor: *Alternatives to gold alloys in dentistry,* Conf. Proc. DHEW Pub. No. [NIH]77-1227, Jan, 1977, Washington, DC, U.S. Government Printing Office.)

Table 11-2. Low-Gold-Content Casting Alloys

Alloy	Gold content
Maxigold*	60
Midigold*	50
Midas†	46
Forticast†	42
Minigold*	40

*Williams Gold, Inc, Buffalo, NY 14214.
†Jelenko, Armonk, NY 10504.

INGREDIENTS OF GOLD ALLOYS

The most important elements in dental gold alloys are gold, copper, silver, platinum group metals, and zinc. A few alloys for use with porcelain contain iron, indium, and tin. The role of these ingredients is discussed briefly. **Gold contributes strongly to the color, tarnish resistance, and ductility.** Alloys for dental use should be at least 16 K for reliable tarnish resistance. **Copper contributes hardness and strength to pure gold,** which is too soft alone; gives the alloy a reddish appearance; and lowers the fusion temperature and tarnish resistance. Silver serves to balance the red color given by copper. **Silver also contributes to the hardness and strength of the alloy but lowers tarnish resistance.** The platinum group metals added to dental alloys are platinum, palladium, and iridium. **Platinum may be added to strengthen the alloy and raise the fusion point. Palladium,** which is much less expensive than platinum, **serves the same function but whitens the alloy.** Alloys with more than 6% palladium take on a whiter color. Higher percentages of palladium result in **white gold alloys.** Since palladium is less expensive than gold, these alloys have lower costs. Palladium absorbs hydrogen and other gases, and white gold alloys may be more porous when cast.

White gold alloys are gold-based alloys that have a silver color.

Gold alloys seen under the microscope show the crystal or **grain structure** and any porosity present. The microstructure shown in Fig. 11-4 shows porosity within and along the grain boundaries. The average diameter of a grain is the **grain size.** Fine-grained alloys have many small grains, whereas coarse-grained alloys have relatively large grains. Fine-grained alloys are generally stronger and more ductile than coarse-grained alloys of the same general composition. The average grain size in a gold casting is about 300 μm as compared with only 60 μm for a fine-grained alloy. **Iridium is frequently added as a grain refiner.**

Grains are tiny crystals of a metal.

Grain refiners produce smaller grains.

Porosity is the presence of a Swiss cheese structure seen under the microscope.

Zinc is usually present in dental gold alloys in low percentages, around 0.5%. Since zinc is chemically active, it acts as a **deoxidizing** element and reduces the oxygen content. Oxygen released during solidification results in porosity. Alloys for bonding with porcelain use small quantities of **iron, tin, and indium as hardening and bonding agents.** These alloys must also have high fusion temperatures to resist melting during the porcelain-firing procedure. Conventional gold alloys should never be mixed with alloys used with porcelain.

Hardening agents increase hardness and strength.

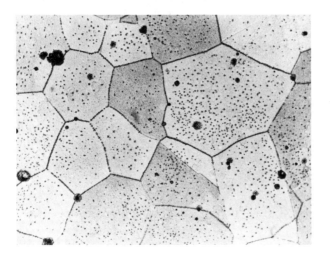

Fig. 11-4. Grain structure of a cast gold inlay showing porosity and a range of grain sizes.

BIOCOMPATIBILITY OF ALLOYS

Of the pure metals, gold and palladium are the least toxic, followed by silver, nickel, then copper. Lower gold content alloys with high copper contents showed greater cell toxicity, as well as a greater incidence of tarnish. Palladium additions reduce the toxicity of copper more effectively than gold. Nickel alloys have the special problem of being a common allergen, with as many as 6% of the female population and 2% of the male population being sensitive to them.

SOLDERS

Soldering is a method of joining metal components together by fusion with a lower melting alloy. **Brazing** is the preferred term, when the joining alloy melts above 500° C, and soldering generally refers to the lower melting lead-tin solders. Dental gold soldering alloys are used to join individual units to form a bridge. The crowns and other units to be joined are embedded in a soldering investment. The brazing alloy is torch melted and is drawn into the spaces by capillary action. It is essential that the units to be joined are thoroughly cleaned and oxidation is prevented by using the reducing portion of the torch flame and fluxing.

Brazing is the joining of two metals with a low melting alloy.

The composition of the solder depends on the alloys being joined. For the ANSI–ADA types of alloys, gold solders with a lower gold content containing additional zinc and tin are used. The solder must be completely molten at a temperature at least 80° C (150° F) below that of the cast gold alloy. **Dental gold solders are often stamped with two numbers that relate to the karat of the cast**

gold and to the solder's fineness. For example, a 16-650 solder is designed for use with a 16-K cast gold, and the solder fineness is 650.

Solders for gold alloys used to fabricate porcelain-fused-to-metal restorations must not soften during firing of the porcelain on the completed bridge. Therefore **solders designed specifically for these alloys must be used.**

Silver solders are used to join wires and other components together in fabricating orthodontic appliances. They are used with stainless steel, as well as precious metals.

The fluxes used to prevent oxidation of parts being soldered contain borates or fluorides in paste or liquid form.

The brazing of nickel alloys used for porcelain-fused-to-metal restorations requires a highly skilled technician. In most cases, these bridges are cast in one piece to avoid the brazing process.

Fluxes are low melting compounds that remove and prevent oxidation.

HEAT TREATMENT OF GOLD ALLOYS

Conventional cast gold alloys that contain sufficient copper may be easily **heat treated** to produce a softer or harder alloy. They are softened by heating for 15 minutes at 705° C (1300° F) and then cooling rapidly to room temperature in water. A heat hardening treatment takes place when the alloys are heated at 370° C (700° F) for 15 minutes and then cooled in air. Heat hardening produces an increase in strength but also a reduction in ductility.

Heat treatment is a process of heating a metal to improve its properties.

In practice, dental gold castings are heat treated by either quenching or slowly cooling the casting in the mold. To produce a softer casting, the entire mold is quenched in water when the metal appears dull red in shaded areas of the room. A harder and stronger but less ductile casting is produced by allowing it to cool to room temperature in the mold. Gold alloys to be used with porcelain do not harden by the same mechanism as conventional cast golds. They harden as the result of the formation of a **platinum-iron compound** during slow cooling from the porcelain-fusing temperature. The presence of copper in conventional gold alloys has been found to discolor the porcelain.

ALLOYS FOR BONDING TO PORCELAIN

Several types of alloys are used to cast substructures for porcelain-fused-to-metal crowns and bridges. All have coefficient of thermal expansion values matched to porcelain enamels (i.e., $13\text{-}14 \times 10^{-6}/°$ C). A layer of porcelain enamel is fused to the alloy to give natural esthetics (Fig. 11-5). The nature and properties of these alloys are discussed and compared.

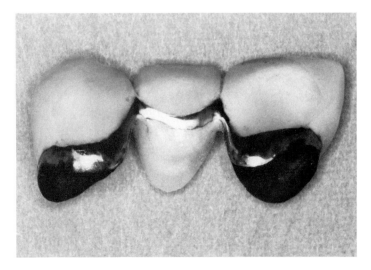

Fig. 11-5. Porcelain-fused-to-gold-alloy bridge. The alloy is visible only on the lingual surface.

Table 11-3. Comparison of Properties of Alloys for Bonding to Porcelain

Properties	High gold	Palladium-silver	Palladium-copper	Nickel-chromium
Strength	Adequate	Adequate	Adequate	Adequate
Density (gm/cm³)	15	11	10.6	8
Hardness	Softer than tooth enamel	Softer than tooth enamel	Softer than tooth enamel	Ranges between softer and harder than tooth enamel for different alloys
Stiffness	Flexible	Flexible	Flexible	Stiffer
Tarnish resistance	Adequate	Adequate	Adequate	Adequate
Thermal expansion coefficient ($\times 10^{-6}/°$ C)	14.8	14.6	14.1	14.0
Fabrication problems	Minor	Greening of porcelain	Sagging during firing of long-span bridges	Casting, soldering, bonding to porcelain
Cost	High	Moderate	Moderate	Low

High-gold alloys

The first group consists of alloys with a noble metal content (e.g., gold plus platinum and palladium) of around 98%. The content balance consists of **iron, tin, and indium,** which produce hardening and form an oxide layer that bonds with porcelain. These alloys have higher melting temperatures than traditional crown and bridge alloys, but are otherwise similar in properties. They were used extensively from 1958 until the price of gold escalated in 1972 (Fig. 11-3). The properties of these alloys are described in Table 11-3.

Gold alloys with a total noble metal content of 80% have largely replaced the original higher karat alloys. These alloys are slightly less expensive and found to be generally satisfactory. The properties of these alloys differ only slightly from alloys of higher noble metal content. They are stronger, slightly harder, more ductile, and less dense.

Palladium-silver alloys

Palladium-silver alloys form a second group of precious metal alloys for use with porcelain. These alloys contain 50% to 60% palladium, 30% to 40% silver, and a lower percentage of base metals for hardening. A lower density is the main difference in physical properties that distinguishes them from gold alloys, as indicated in Table 11-3. Their significantly lower cost has made them widely used among precious metal alloys. **The main problem with their use is a green discoloration of porcelain by silver contamination.** This discoloration may be prevented by rigid adherence to technics designed to reduce the vaporization and diffusion of silver during porcelain baking.

Palladium-copper alloys

Palladium-copper alloys offer an alternative to the palladium-silver alloys. These alloys contain 70% to 80% palladium, 10% to 15% copper, and 5% to 10% gallium. They are similar to the palladium-silver alloys in properties with two differences: they **do not produce greening, which is caused by silver, and they tend to sag more at porcelain firing temperatures.** Therefore they are not recommended for long-span bridgework. (See Table 11-3 for a comparison of their properties.)

Nickel-chromium alloys

Nickel-chromium alloys have become widely used substitutes for the higher-cost precious metal alloys. They are commonly referred to as **nonprecious alloys** and contain 70% to 80% nickel, approximately 15% chromium for corrosion resistance, and metals including aluminum, beryllium, and manganese.

The nickel-chromium alloys have coefficient of ther-

Nonprecious alloys for crowns and bridges are referred to as nickel alloys, but the preferred term is nickel-chromium.

mal expansion values in the same range as the gold alloys they replace. As Table 11-3 indicates, a wide range of mechanical properties exists for these alloys, depending on their formulation. The early nickel alloys were too hard, with a Vickers hardness of around 400 that made polishing and finishing difficult. More recently, softer alloys have become available. Generally, nickel alloys are more difficult to cast and solder than gold or palladium-silver alloys. Also, around 6% of the female population and 2% of the male are allergic to nickel. However, **nickel alloys are stiffer than the noble and precious metal alloys,** which is an advantage, since porcelain needs rigid support to prevent fracture.

Other nonprecious metal alloys such as cobalt-chromium and stainless steel have been developed for porcelain-fused-to-metal crowns and bridges, but they are still in the experimental stage.

Another application of nickel-chromium alloys is the use of resin-bonded bridges. These bridges, often referred to as "Maryland bridges," have a porcelain-fused-to-metal pontic bonded to adjacent teeth by metal extensions. The metal extensions are electrolytically etched and bonded to the etched lingual surfaces of the abutment teeth with resin cements. The strength of the bond depends upon the proper etching of the nickel-chromium alloy and the tooth enamel. **The main advantage of these bridges is that little or no cavity preparation of the abutment teeth is necessary. The main disadvantage is the possibility of short-term failure of the bond.**

COBALT-CHROMIUM ALLOYS

Most partial denture frameworks (Fig. 11-6) are fabricated with alloys that are basically 60% cobalt and 25% chromium, with small additions of nickel, carbon, molybdenum, and other substances. Their density is about half that of the Type IV gold alloys, resulting in lighter prostheses.

These alloys have replaced gold-base alloys mainly on the basis of their lower cost and adequate mechanical properties. An alloy with the brand name of Vitallium was first introduced in 1930 and is a cobalt-chromium alloy. Since then other nickel-chromium and cobalt-chromium-nickel alloys have been introduced. Chromium is added for tarnish resistance, since chromium oxide forms an adherent and resistant surface layer; cobalt contributes rigidity to the alloy; and nickel increases the ductility of the alloy.

Several ingredients in minor amounts in cobalt-chromium alloys have an important influence on their properties. Molybdenum strengthens the alloys. Carbon is usually present in small amounts up to 0.4%. Carbon compounds (carbides) are found finely dispersed along the grain boundaries (Fig. 11-7). Introducing too much carbon embrittles the alloys. **Beryllium** is added in a few alloys

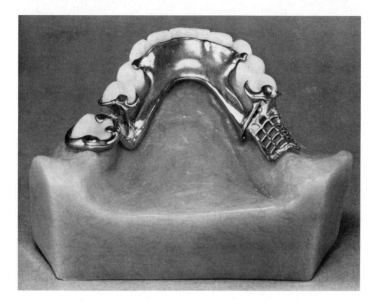

Fig. 11-6. Cobalt-chromium-nickel partial denture.

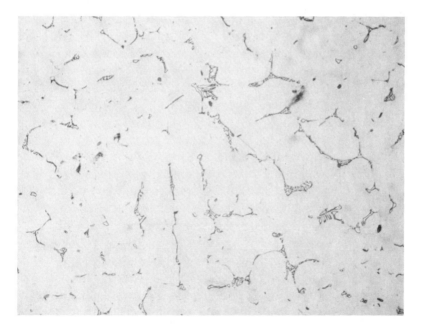

Fig. 11-7. Microstructure of cobalt-chromium alloy showing carbides finely dispersed along the grain boundaries. (×400.)

Table 11-4. Comparison of Properties of Cobalt-Chromium Alloys with Gold Alloys

Properties	Cobalt-chromium	Gold Type IV
Strength	Adequate	Adequate
Density (gm/cm³)	8	15
Hardness	Harder than tooth enamel	Softer than tooth enamel
Stiffness	Stiff	More flexible
Melting temperature (° C)	~1300	~900
Casting shrinkage (%)	2.25	1.25-1.65
Heat treatment	Complicated	Simple
Price	Reasonable	High for large castings
Tarnish resistance	Adequate	Adequate

to reduce the melting temperature so that similar calcium sulfate investments used with gold alloy may be employed. Silicon and manganese are added in small amounts to increase castability.

Beryllium is a toxic element present in small amounts in nonprecious alloys.

The strengths of most cobalt-chromium dental casting alloys are comparable to those of hard gold alloys (Type IV) as shown in Table 11-4, but the cobalt-chromium alloys are about 50% harder, which makes polishing more difficult than with gold alloys. The density of the gold alloys is about two times greater than that of the cobalt-chromium alloys. Therefore a partial denture of cobalt-chromium alloy would weigh twice as much if fabricated in gold. With the exception of the nickel-chromium (Ticonium) alloys with beryllium, the cobalt-chromium alloys must be cast at much higher temperatures than are gold alloys. Induction casting machines using high frequency are especially equipped for casting these alloys. Since it is difficult to judge temperatures in the white heat range, electro-optical pyrometers are used. High-heat investments, such as the phosphate and silicate types, must be used for casting all but the lower fusing nickel-chromium alloys. **The casting shrinkage of cobalt-chromium alloys is much greater than that of gold alloys. Obtaining sufficient accuracy for crowns and bridges is more difficult,** but nickel-base alloys are available for these applications.

Cobalt-chromium dental alloys are about twice as stiff as gold ones, as indicated by their higher moduli of elasticity. Gold alloys have greater ductility than the average cobalt-chromium–base dental alloys. This ductility is an advantage of gold alloys, since it means less brittleness. However cobalt-chromium-nickel and cobalt-chromium-tantalum alloys have been developed with elongation values around 10%.

The cobalt-chromium-nickel alloys are much lower in cost than gold alloys.

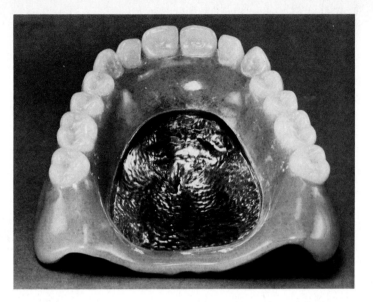

Fig. 11-8. Complete denture with the palatal area composed of a cobalt-chromium alloy.

They are lighter and stiffer, which are advantages in many applications. However, gold alloys are easier to cast, polish, and adjust without breakage. **The cobalt-chromium-nickel alloys have almost completely replaced gold alloys for partial dentures** and are also used for the palatal areas of complete dentures (Fig. 11-8).

Gold foil was the first type of metallic restoration used in dentistry. Several types of direct gold restorative materials are available, including sponge gold, mat gold, and powdered gold, as well as the traditional foil. Cast gold restorations have largely replaced direct gold restorations and are available in Types I, II, III, and IV. The main elements present in these alloys are gold, palladium, copper, and silver. Zinc is added as a deoxidizer and iridium as a grain refiner. In recent years, low-karat alloys have been introduced as an economy measure. These alloys show a higher incidence of tarnish than the higher karat ANSI–ADA alloys. Today, most cast alloy restorations are bonded with an outer veneer of porcelain. Several special alloys are available for these porcelain-fused-to-metal restorations, including gold, palladium-silver, palladium-copper, and nickel-chromium. Although the nickel-chromium alloys are less expensive, they are more difficult to fabricate, and they can provoke allergic reactions in sensitive patients. Most partial denture frameworks are cast from cobalt-chromium alloys, which are tarnish resistant and stiffer than gold alloys.

Self-test questions

In the following multiple choice questions, one or more responses may be correct.

1 The noble metals used in dentistry include:
  a. Gold
  b. Platinum
  c. Palladium
  d. Silver

2 Precious metals include:
  a. Gold
  b. Platinum
  c. Palladium
  d. Silver

3 The gold content of an 18-K alloy is:
  a. 50%
  b. 75%
  c. 100%
  d. 30%

4 Gold foil has the following number of karats:
  a. 12
  b. 16
  c. 18
  d. 24

5 Which of these statements apply to the use of gold foil?
  a. Fabrication of foil is accomplished with instruments called condensers.
  b. Force is applied to the foil by striking the condenser with a mallet or by using an automatic mechanical condenser.
  c. Each layer of foil is welded to form a covalent bond.
  d. The mechanical working or condensation decreases the strength of the gold and increases the hardness and brittleness.
  e. The properties of well-condensed gold foil are comparable to those of a 22-K cast gold alloy.

6 Which statements apply to the handling of cohesive gold?
  a. For the gold increments to weld easily, the surface must be free from contamination.
  b. Annealing gold foil immediately before use is not important as long as it is annealed within an hour before condensation.
  c. Annealing involves degassing the surface by heat to remove contaminants.
  d. In the tray method the gold is heated for 10 minutes at 545° C.
  e. Annealing hardens the gold.
  f. An alcohol flame is used when heating the gold in a flame.

7 The use and content of noble metals in gold alloys classified by the ANSI–ADA are described in which of the following ways?
  a. Type I contains a maximum of 83% noble metal and is used for simple inlays not subject to occlusal forces.
  b. Type II contains a minimum of 78% noble metal and is used for inlays requiring higher strength.

   c. Type III contains a minimum of 70% noble metal and is used for crowns, bridge abutments, and inlays subject to high occlusal forces.

   d. Type IV contains a minimum of 75% noble metal and is used in partial dentures.

8 The minimum gold content of low-karat casting alloys used for dental restorations is around:

   a. 60%

   b. 40%

   c. 75%

   d. 25%

9 White gold alloys contain:

   a. About 50% gold

   b. 10% to 35% palladium as a whitener

   c. 10% to 20% silver

   d. 6% to 25% copper

10 Which of these statements apply to low-karat gold-colored alloys?

   a. They contain as little as 40% gold.

   b. They contain 26% palladium.

   c. They contain about 54% copper and silver combined.

   d. They are as equally resistant to tarnish as are Type III alloys.

11 Indicate the function of the components listed in the left-hand column by selecting the correct answer listed in the right-hand column:

___ **a.** Gold	1. Increases hardness
___ **b.** Copper	2. Increases ductility
___ **c.** Silver	3. Produces fine-grained alloys
___ **d.** Zinc	4. Improves tarnish resistance
___ **e.** Platinum	5. Increases the melting point
___ **f.** Palladium	6. Serves as a scavenger for oxygen
___ **g.** Iridium	7. Reduces the melting point
	8. Reduces tarnish resistance
	9. Whitens the alloy

12 With respect to the grain structure of gold alloys:

   a. Fine-grained alloys generally are stronger than coarse-grained alloys.

   b. Coarse-grained alloys are more ductile than fine-grained alloys.

   c. The average grain size of a fine-grained alloy is 300 μm.

13 Which of the following statements apply to gold soldering?

   a. The units to be joined must be thoroughly cleaned.

   b. The units should be heated in the reducing portion of the flame.

   c. A flux should be used.

   d. The solder should be completely molten 10° C (50° F) below the melting temperature of the units.

14 The purpose of adding small amounts of iron, tin, and indium to high-karat gold alloys for bonding to porcelain include:

   a. To provide corrosion resistance

   b. To cause hardening

   c. To lower the fusing temperature of the porcelain

   d. To form oxides that bond with porcelain

15 Which of these statements apply to porcelain-fused-to-metal alloys?
  a. Palladium-silver alloys present special problems, since the silver may produce a green color in the porcelain.
  b. Nickel-chromium alloys have coefficients of expansion near those of available porcelains.
  c. Nickel-chromium alloys have caused problems with high hardness.
  d. No concern exists with nickel sensitivity of patients.

16 Which of the following statements about alloys for bonding to porcelain are true?
  a. The strengths of the high-karat gold alloys are comparable to those of the palladium-silver alloys.
  b. The nickel-chromium alloys contribute to a green discoloration of porcelain.
  c. The main advantages of the nickel alloys are low cost and higher stiffness.
  d. Some patients may be allergic to nickel alloys.

17 Compared with Type IV gold alloys, cobalt-chromium alloys:
  a. Are about half as dense
  b. Have higher casting shrinkage
  c. Are easier to finish and polish
  d. Use the same type of melting and casting equipment

18 Indicate the function of the components listed in the left-hand column in cobalt-chromium-nickel alloys by selecting the correct answer listed in the right-hand column:
  ___ **a.** Chromium   1. Forms carbides
  ___ **b.** Cobalt   2. Increases strength
  ___ **c.** Nickel   3. Increases modulus
  ___ **d.** Carbon   4. Increases tarnish resistance
  ___ **e.** Beryllium   5. Increases ductility
  ___ **f.** Molybdenum   6. Decreases melting temperature
  ___ **g.** Aluminum

19 Compared with Type IV gold alloys, cobalt-chromium alloys:
  a. Are stronger
  b. Have a modulus of elasticity about twice that of gold alloys
  c. Are about 50% harder
  d. Shrink less during cooling from the casting temperature

20 Which of the following comparisons between nickel-chromium, cobalt-chromium, and gold alloys are true?
  a. Nickel-chromium and cobalt-chromium alloys are both lower in density than high-karat gold alloys.
  b. Nickel-chromium and cobalt-chromium alloys are stiffer than gold alloys.
  c. Nickel-chromium and cobalt-chromium alloys are tarnish resistant in the mouth.
  d. Nickel-chromium and cobalt-chromium alloys are heat treated in the same way as are gold alloys.

Suggested supplementary readings

Bertolotti RL: Alloys for porcelain fused to metal restorations. In O'Brien WJ, editor, *Dental materials: properties and selection,* Chicago, 1987, Quintessence.

Craig RG, Hanks CT: Cytotoxicity of experimental casting alloys evaluated by cell culture tests, *J Dent Res* 69:1539, 1990.

Valega TM, editor: Alternatives to gold alloys in dentistry, HEW Pub. No. (NIH)77-1227, Washington, DC, 1977, U.S. Government Printing Office.

chapter twelve

Dental Casting of Metals

The purpose of this chapter is to describe and to discuss the general process of preparing a dental casting. Many variations in technics exist that are outside the scope of this textbook. However, an overall understanding of the process is needed for the purpose of educating patients.

Several **casting** methods are used by dental laboratories, including the so-called thermal expansion technic and the hygroscopic technic. The purpose of this chapter is to convey only the general features of casting inlays; the various methods are not described in detail. Emphasis is placed on the thermal expansion technic.

Casting is a process of forming an object by pouring a molten metal into a mold.

The **lost wax process** is used for casting inlays, crowns, and partial dentures. **Accuracies of ±0.05% in dimensions are possible** if all the steps in the process are carefully controlled. The sequence used to cast a gold inlay is as follows:

1. A wax pattern in the shape of the final inlay is prepared in the mouth on the prepared tooth (direct technic) or on a die (indirect technic).
2. The wax pattern is attached to a sprue pin and mounted on a base.
3. The wax pattern is invested by pouring a slurry of gypsum investment around the pattern, which is surrounded by a cylinder.
4. After hardening of the investment, the wax pattern is burned out in a furnace, leaving a mold with a hollow cavity in the shape of the wax pattern.
5. Next the casting alloy is melted and forced under pressure to fill the mold.
6. Finally, the casting is removed from the mold, cleaned in acid, and polished. Each of these steps is discussed with reference to critical factors.

WAX PATTERN

The wax **pattern** of an inlay may be formed in the patient's mouth on the prepared tooth **(direct method)** or on a die replica of the prepared tooth **(indirect method)** (Fig. 12-1).

A pattern is a model of the restoration to be cast.

Type I **dental inlay wax** is specified by the American Dental Association for use in the direct technic. A Type II wax with greater flow properties is designed for use with the indirect method. In the direct method, a piece of wax is heated above a flame until it is soft and then it is pressed firmly into the cavity preparation. When the indirect technic is employed, melted wax is applied to the die with a small spatula until the pattern is built up. A lubricant is used to coat the die in the indirect method to facilitate separation from the die material.

Wax is a potential source of inaccuracy because of its high coefficient of thermal expansion and its tendency to distort after being formed. A wax pattern formed in the mouth at 37° C will shrink about 0.4% when cooled to room temperature. Therefore an additional compensation must be used in the direct method. Inlay patterns prepared by either method have a tendency to distort with time when stored at room temperature. Therefore they should be invested soon after formation. If this cannot be done, storage in a refrigerator will reduce the rate of distortion. Before investing, the pattern on the die should be allowed to warm to room temperature. Care must be taken not to damage the thin margins of the pattern after removal from the die, especially when the pattern is cold.

Waxes that are used for patterns have the advantage of being plastic when heated, which allows shaping. Their main disadvantage is that they are thermally unstable and will expand and contract with temperature changes and distort if left standing.

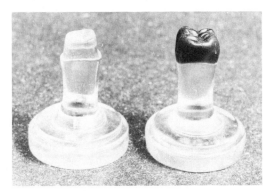

Fig. 12-1. *Left,* Die replica made from the prepared tooth for the indirect method; *right,* wax pattern for restoration.

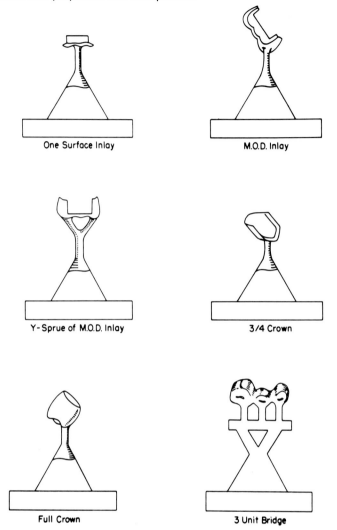

One Surface Inlay

M.O.D. Inlay

Y-Sprue of M.O.D. Inlay

3/4 Crown

Full Crown

3 Unit Bridge

Fig. 12-2. Sprue designs for inlay, crown, and bridge castings. (From O'Brien WJ, Ryge G, editors: *Outline of dental materials and their selection,* Philadelphia, 1978, WB Saunders.)

SPRUING

The wax pattern is attached to a short pin called a **sprue.** After investing, the sprue is removed to leave a channel for molten metal to enter the mold cavity. The sprued pattern is then mounted on a sprue base and is surrounded with a casting ring, as shown in Figs. 12-2 to 12-4. **The sprue pin should be attached to the pattern at its thickest portion.**

A sprue forms a channel for the molten alloy to enter the mold cavity.

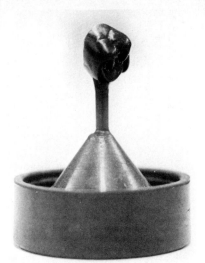

Fig. 12-3. Wax pattern and the attached sprue on a sprue base.

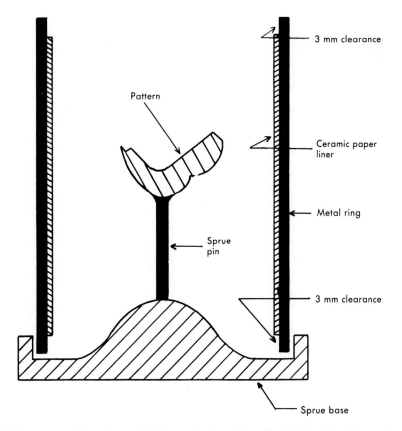

Fig. 12-4. Arrangement of pattern within the casting ring. (From Craig RG, editor: *Restorative dental materials,* ed 8, St. Louis, 1989, Mosby–Year Book.)

Sprues for inlays and crowns should be short and 10 to 12 gauge (0.1 to 0.08 inch [2.6 to 2.1 mm]) in diameter to prevent solidification of the gold alloy before the casting. The casting ring is lined with a layer of moistened ceramic paper to provide a cushion against which the mold can expand during setting and heating.

INVESTING

The material used to form a mold for dental gold casting consists of a binder and a refractory. The **binder** is calcium sulfate hemihydrate ($CaSO_4 \cdot \frac{1}{2} H_2O$), and the **refractory** is either quartz or cristobalite, which are both forms of silica (SiO_2). When this material is mixed with water, the following setting reaction takes place:

A **binder** is a material that holds the material together.

A **refractory** is a material that resists heat.

$$CaSO_4 \cdot \frac{1}{2} H_2O + 1 \frac{1}{2} H_2O \rightarrow CaSO_4 \cdot 2 H_2O$$

(Hemihydrate + Water → Gypsum)

Phosphate-bonded investments are used instead of gypsum investments for high-fusing gold and nonprecious alloys. **The powder consists of a mixture of silica, magnesium oxide, and ammonium phosphate.** During mixing with water, the following setting reaction takes place:

$$NH_4H_2PO_4 + MgO \rightarrow NH_4MgPO_4 + H_2O$$

During heating of the mold, additional reactions take place between silica and the phosphate compounds to produce a mold resistant to high temperatures. Phosphate-bonded investments are much stronger than gypsum investments and are more difficult to break up after casting.

It is important to weigh out the investment powder and to measure the mixing water in a graduated cylinder to obtain an accurate casting. The powder is added to the water in a rubber bowl and is mixed by hand to a smooth consistency. To reduce porosity when set, the investment may then be placed under a vacuum to draw out air bubbles from the slurry. Equipment is also available for mechanically mixing the investment under reduced pressure.

The wax pattern may be prepared for investment contact by treatment with a wax pattern detergent solution and by painting with the investment slurry. The detergent solution makes the wax more wettable by the investment. However, **any excess solution must be blown off before investing.** Painting the pattern with some of the mixed investment using an artist's paintbrush is often done instead of vacuum investing to reduce the possibility of porosity in the set investment. After being coated with the mixed investment, the pattern is immediately invested. A vibrator can also be used during investing to reduce porosity of the investment.

Careful handling of the investing procedure is necessary for a well-fitting, smooth, and bubble-free casting.

INVESTMENT EXPANSION

Several means are used to compensate for the shrinkage accompanying the casting process. First of all, patterns made by the **direct technic** at mouth temperature shrink when cooled to room temperature. To compensate for this shrinkage, the investment mix water should be around 37° C to expand the pattern to its original size.

In the direct technic, the wax pattern is formed in the cavity preparation at mouth temperature.

Expansion of the investment is used to compensate for the **shrinkage of the gold casting** as it cools during the casting procedure. A total of 1.5% to 2% mold expansion is the aim in most gold casting. During the setting of the investment, an expansion of 0.25% takes place because of the gypsum crystallization process.

The thermal expansion technic depends on normal setting expansion and on heating to a temperature of 482° to 650° C (900° to 1200° F), depending on the investment and the pattern material to obtain full thermal expansion. **The investment is allowed to set in air for at least 45 minutes.** After removal of the base former and sprue former, the mold is heated to burn out the wax pattern and to obtain thermal expansion.

Additional expansion, called **hygroscopic expansion,** is obtained if the investment is allowed to set in contact with water. This may be accomplished by immersing the invested ring in a temperature-controlled water bath or by adding a measured amount of water to the surface of the investment mold before the initial set. A hygroscopic expansion of 1.5% may be obtained with a hygroscopic investment and a water bath immersion. A hygroscopic expansion technic reduces the need for thermal expansion, and a burnout temperature of 468° C (875° F) is used. Hygroscopic technics require the use of special investments and equipment.

In summary the balance of shrinkage and expansion is as follows:

Wax shrinkage + Gold shrinkage = Wax expansion + Setting expansion + Hygroscopic expansion + Thermal expansion

WAX ELIMINATION

Heating the mold to eliminate the wax pattern and to expand the mold is called the **burnout procedure.** The wax pattern must be eliminated completely to obtain full castings. The mold is placed in a burnout oven with the sprue hole facing downward to facilitate the outward flow of the molten wax. After 30 minutes the mold is turned over with the sprue hole up. The furnace pyrometer

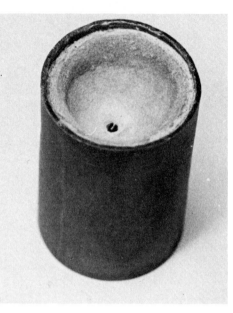

Fig. 12-5. Investment mold after wax burn out.

should be calibrated periodically to ensure accurate temperature control. Molds should be kept away from the walls of the furnace to promote their uniform heating. Molds for the thermal expansion technic should be heated gradually to the burnout temperature of 482° to 650° C (900° to 1200° F) to prevent cracking of the mold material. For the same reason, it is safest to place the molds in a cold or warm furnace rather than directly into a red-hot furnace. If the mold is for the **hygroscopic technic,** it is heated to 482° C, and may be placed directly into a preheated furnace. It is also important to heat soak the mold at the final burnout temperature for at least 30 minutes to allow the inner core of the mold to reach the furnace temperature. More complete wax elimination and thermal expansion are obtained in this way.

Heating gypsum molds above 650° C may result in the formation of sulfur dioxide gases that will contaminate the gold castings. This "sulfur contamination" makes castings harder to clean and may lead to brittleness.

The mold should be removed from the furnace and should be placed on the casting machine just before casting. The metal should be ready to cast at this time to prevent cooling of the mold while waiting (Fig. 12-5).

CASTING THE ALLOY

Gold alloys may be melted for casting by the use of a gas-air blowtorch (Fig. 12-6) or in an electric casting machine (Fig. 12-7). It is essential to maintain a reducing atmosphere during melting of the alloy to prevent oxygen absorption.

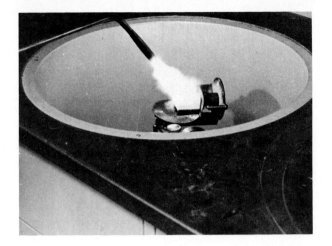

Fig. 12-6. Gold alloy that has been melted with a gas-air blowtorch; the investment ring is in position for casting.

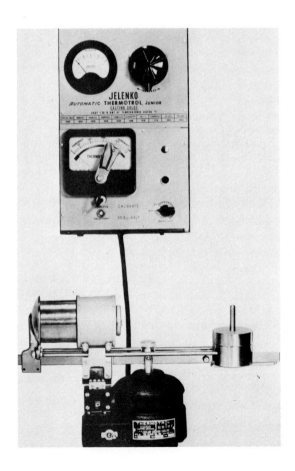

Fig. 12-7. Electric casting machine. (Courtesy Jelenko, Armonk, NY.)

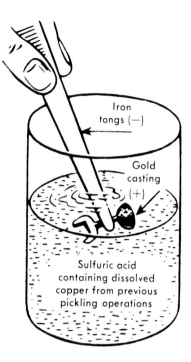

Fig. 12-8. Electric cell with gold casting and iron tongs.

This may be accomplished by keeping the reducing portion of the torch flame in contact with the alloy or by using a graphite crucible with the electric casting machine. The addition of a small amount of reducing **flux** capable of dissolving metal oxides also reduces the oxygen absorption. Oxygen absorption may result in porosity in the casting.

Flux is a low melting salt (e.g., Borax) that removes oxides.

The alloy should be cast when fully fluid, which occurs at around 70° C (150° F) above the melting point. Centrifugal casting machines are most often used for casting. When the machine is rotating, the outward centrifugal force drives the molten alloy through the sprue channel to fill the mold. After the casting machine stops rotating, the mold is removed and quenched in water, and the casting is recovered by breaking away the investment mold. The casting is **pickled** in acid after casting to remove surface oxidation that gives it a dark appearance. The surface can be contaminated during this step if the gold casting comes in contact with base metals while in the acid. Creation of an electrolytic cell is possible, which would lead to the plating of metals on the casting. Tweezers with plastic-coated ends should be used to handle the casting in the acid (Fig. 12-8).

After pickling, the casting is rinsed off with water and polished with abrasive wheels, rubber wheels, pumice, tripoli, and finally, rouge (Figs. 12-9 and 12-10). The final gold casting is then ready for cementation (Fig. 12-11).

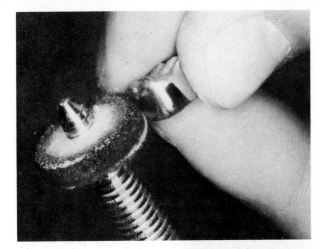

Fig. 12-9. Polishing of gold casting with felt wheel and tripoli. (Courtesy Dr. JR Savignac, Milwaukee, Wisc.)

Fig. 12-10. Final polishing of a gold crown with a cloth wheel and rouge. (Courtesy Dr. JR Savignac, Milwaukee, Wisc.)

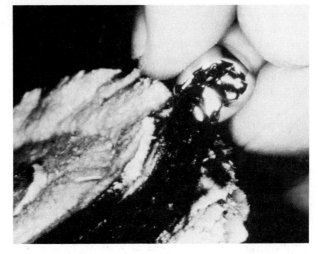

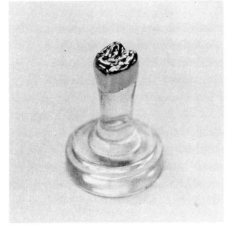

Fig. 12-11. Polished gold crown on a die.

REMINDERS FOR CORRECT MANIPULATION

1. Make the wax pattern as smooth as possible.
2. Clean the pattern and coat it with a wetting agent.
3. Invest the wax pattern as soon as possible after removal from the mouth or die.
4. Weigh out the investment powder and measure the correct amount of water with a graduated cylinder.
5. Paint the pattern with investment mix immediately before filling the ring with investment.
6. Line the casting ring with a layer of moistened ceramic paper liner to allow for mold expansion.
7. Use vacuum equipment to remove air from the investment mix.
8. Allow the investment to set for at least 1 hour before heating.
9. Do not place the mold in an oven that is hotter than 250° C to avoid cracking the investment (thermal technic). Hold the mold at the desired casting temperature for at least 30 minutes to allow it to arrive at the furnace temperature.
10. Do not heat the mold above 700° C to avoid decomposition of the investment.
11. Use new or thoroughly cleaned gold alloy scrap for casting. All investment must be removed from old castings with a brush.
12. Melt the gold in a reducing atmosphere by using an electric casting machine and graphite crucibles or the reducing zone of a torch. Line and crucible of a casting machine with a fresh piece of ceramic paper liner. Use a small amount of reducing flux during melting.
13. Wind the casting machine at least three times to provide sufficient pressure during casting of the metal.
14. Allow the mold to cool for 1 or 2 minutes before quenching in water. Quenching too quickly can result in cracked castings.
15. Pickle the casting in dilute sulfuric, hydrochloric, or phosphoric acid. Be careful to protect eyes, skin, and clothing from the acid. Do not allow the gold casting to contact base metals in the acid, and prevent accidental plating by using plastic-coated tongs.

Dental castings are made by the lost wax process. A pattern of the restoration is made in wax and used to form a mold with gypsum- or phosphate-bonded investments. The accuracy of the final casting depends on careful attention to the expansion of the mold by hygroscopic and thermal expansions to compensate for the shrinkage of the wax pattern and metal casting.

Self-test questions

In the following multiple choice questions, one or more responses may be correct.

1 For acceptable results, once the wax pattern has been formed it can be:
   a. Stored at room temperature for 24 hours to allow any distortion to occur before investing
   b. Stored in a refrigerator but warmed to room temperature before investing
   c. Stored in a refrigerator and invested when cold
   d. Invested immediately

2 Which of the following statements about gypsum investments are true?
   a. The binder is calcium sulfate hemihydrate, and the refractory is a form of silica.
   b. The investment powder is mixed with a special liquid supplied by the manufacturer.
   c. The components of the investment must be proportioned accurately to obtain a suitable casting.
   d. The investment may be mixed mechanically under a vacuum to reduce porosity in the set mold.

3 Differences in technic between hygroscopic and thermal expansion methods include:
   a. A special investment is required for the hygroscopic method.
   b. Special investment rings are used with the hygroscopic method.
   c. Heating the mold to 482° C produces sufficient thermal expansion in a hygroscopic investment, but not necessarily enough expansion in a thermal investment.

4 The purposes of heating the investment are:
   a. To increase the hygroscopic expansion of the investment
   b. To expand the mold thermally
   c. To eliminate the wax pattern from the mold

5 Which of the following statements about the wax elimination procedure are true?
   a. The mold is burned out for 30 minutes with the sprue hole down and then for 30 minutes with the sprue hole up.
   b. Thermal investments heated to 650° C must be heated gradually, whereas hygroscopic investments heated to 482° C can be placed in a preheated oven.
   c. Heating gypsum investment to about 650° C may cause sulfur dioxide gas to form that will contaminate the gold casting.
   d. The mold should be allowed to cool for 15 minutes before the metal is cast into it.

6 Which of the following describe phosphate-bonded investments?
   a. The powder contains only ammonium phosphate and magnesium oxide.
   b. Phosphate investments are weaker than gypsum investments.
   c. Phosphate-bonded investments are used with high-fusing gold alloys and nonprecious metal alloys.

7 Steps recommended in the handling of the investment are:
   a. Weigh out the investment powder and measure the water volume with a graduated cylinder.
   b. Paint the pattern with investment mix just before filling the ring with investment.
   c. Line the casting ring with a layer of dry ceramic paper.
   d. Use vacuum equipment to remove air from investment mix.

8 Rules for correct spruing include:
  a. The sprue should be attached to the thickest portion of the pattern.
  b. A Y sprue should be used for spruing a wax MOD inlay pattern, with bulky cusps separated by a thin section.
  c. The sprue should solidify at the same time as the casting.
  d. Sprues should be short and 10 to 12 gauge in diameter.
9 Which of the following are recommended procedures for casting gold alloys:
  a. Melt the gold in a reducing atmosphere.
  b. Wind a centrifugal casting machine at least three times.
  c. Quench the mold immediately after casting to prevent cracking.
10 Precautions to consider when pickling include:
  a. Avoid contact between the casting and metal tweezers in pickling acid.
  b. Protect eyes, skin, and clothing from pickling acids.
  c. After pickling, carefully rinse acid from the casting with water.

Suggested supplementary readings

Asgar K: Casting restorations. In Clark JW, editor: *Clinical dentistry*, vol 4, New York, 1976, Harper & Row.

O'Brien WJ: Evolution of dental casting. In Valega TM, editor: *Alternatives to gold alloys in dentistry*, HEW Pub. No. (NIH)77-1227, Washington, DC, 1977, U.S. Government Printing Office.

O'Brien WJ, editor: *Dental materials: properties and selection*, Chicago, 1989, Quintessence.

chapter
thirteen

Plastics in Prosthetics

The greatest volume of plastics, frequently termed polymers, is used in prosthetic dentistry. Examples of plastics used in dentistry are acrylic and rubber-reinforced acrylic polymers. Of these materials, the acrylic plastics have been the most widely used and accepted, and it is estimated that they represent 95% of the plastics used in prosthetics.

Acrylic plastics may be soft and flexible or rigid and brittle, and therefore they can be used for a wide variety of applications. Their principal use is as a complete or partial denture base to support artificial teeth. For this application a rigid plastic is desired. However, the soft acrylic plastics are used as a soft liner on the tissue-bearing surface of complete and partial dentures. Acrylic plastics have been used extensively in the manufacture of artificial denture teeth and in some applications have competed favorably with porcelain denture teeth. Esthetic facings on fixed metal bridges can be constructed from acrylic plastics and are substantially cheaper to construct than porcelain-bonded-to-metal restorations. Plastics of the acrylic type also have been used in the fabrication of individual impression trays. A variety of plastics have been used to construct athletic mouth protectors, as described earlier in Chapter 3.

POLYMERIZATION PROCESS

To understand the use, application, and care of plastics, an elementary knowledge of the **polymerization** process is necessary. In the office or laboratory use of plastics, it is convenient if the material can be mixed as a dough, molded into the desired shape, and then allowed to set in the desired shape. This objective is accomplished by polymerization as indicated in the simplified reaction shown at the top of p. 268.

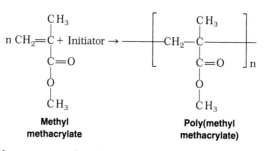

Methyl methacrylate   **Poly(methyl methacrylate)**

It is apparent that, except for the arrangement of the chemical bonds, the atoms in the units in the **polymer** are the same as those in the **monomer.** The molecular weight of this monomer is about 100; therefore if 100 of these monomers react, a polymer molecule with a molecular weight of 10,000 results. The monomer is a volatile liquid (boiling point 100° C [212° F]) with a characteristic sweetish odor that is toxic if inhaled for a prolonged period. The polymerization process converts the material to a solid having essentially no vapor pressure.

Polymerization is the conversion of low–molecular weight compounds, called monomers, to high–molecular weight compounds, called polymers.

The initiator for the reaction is an organic peroxide (usually benzoyl peroxide) that is decomposed into active **free radicals** either by heating or by the addition of an organic accelerator (usually an organic amine). In the first instance, a temperature of about 74° C (165° F) is needed to obtain reasonable rates of decomposition, and in the second instance, the organic amine causes the decomposition of the peroxide at room temperature. The products using heat for decomposition of the initiator are called **heat-curing plastics,** and those using amines are termed **chemically or cold-curing plastics.**

Monomer means one unit; polymer means many units.

A free radical is a molecular fragment with an unpaired electron.

The active free radicals react with the double bond of the methyl methacrylate monomer molecules. Once the monomer molecules are activated, they can react with additional monomer units, and a growing polymer chain results. The reaction continues until the activated molecule becomes deactivated. In typical dental processing, molecular weights of 50,000 are common, which means that 500 monomer units have reacted to form the final polymer. **Different numbers of monomer units react, and thus the final polymer molecules have various molecular weights, resulting in a material with a molecular weight distribution** rather than a material in which all the molecules have the same molecular weight.

Heat is liberated during the polymerization reaction. Thus processing conditions must be controlled to limit the heat to an acceptable level, since the monomer has a high vapor pressure. Excessively high temperatures cause vaporization of the monomer, which produces undesirable bubbles (porosity) in the final set material. The density (or weight per unit volume) of the polymer is about 25% greater than that of the monomer, and volumetric contraction occurs during polymerization. **This dimensional change must be minimized to produce appliances that fit;** methods are described in the section on processing.

Cross-linked polymers

In general, the reaction of acrylic monomer molecules occurs in such a manner that linear polymer molecules result. It has been found that it is frequently desirable to have the polymer molecules linked (or reacted) together to form a **cross-linked polymer.** These cross-linked polymers may be produced by the presence of small amounts of different monomer units with reactive double bonds on each end of the molecule, such as glycol dimethacrylates:

> **A cross-linked polymer is a high–molecular weight network polymer.**

$$CH_2=C-\overset{\displaystyle O}{\overset{\|}{C}}-O(CH_2CH_2O)_x-\overset{\displaystyle O}{\overset{\|}{C}}-C=CH_2$$
$$\underset{CH_3}{|}\qquad\qquad\qquad\underset{CH_3}{|}$$

A growing chain can react first with one end, and another growing chain can later react with the other end. Repetition of the process with other monomers results in a cross-linked polymer. **The advantage of cross-linked polymers is that they are more resistant to surface cracking, or crazing, in the mouth.** Manufacturers label these materials as cross-linking plastics.

In plastics used for esthetic facings for fixed bridges, monomers with reactive groups on each end (dimethacrylates) are used exclusively. Triethylene or tetraethylene glycol dimethacrylates are used because they have low vapor pressures (low volatility) even at temperatures of 100° to 150° C (212° to 302° F). The lower vapor pressure allows processing at elevated temperatures without danger of porosity from a high-vapor pressure monomer. The large amount of cross-linking yields a polymer that is easier to grind and finish.

Copolymers

Other modifications of methyl methacrylate polymers may be accomplished by the addition of other monomers to methyl methacrylate. For example,

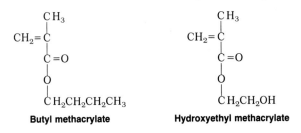

Butyl methacrylate   **Hydroxyethyl methacrylate**

Monomers such as these will react with methyl methacrylate to yield copolymers containing both units spaced randomly along the chain. Copolymerization of methyl methacrylate with butyl methacrylate results in a copolymer that is more resistant to fracture by impact forces. Addition of sufficient amounts of higher acrylic esters such as octyl methacrylate results in a copolymer that is soft and flexible at mouth temperatures and that has been used as a soft liner, which will be described later.

Copolymers consist of two or more different monomers.

Hydroxy-substituted acrylics, such as hydroxyethyl methacrylate, increase the water sorption and wettability of the copolymer by saliva. When large portions of the polymer are made from the hydroxy-substituted acrylics, the material becomes soft and flexible if placed in water or saliva; these materials have found applications as soft contact lenses and as soft liners for dentures.

Modified polymers

Acrylic polymers have been modified by the addition of compounds that do not enter into the polymerization reaction, such as oily organic esters without reactive groups, rubbers, and inorganic fillers. The addition of oils such as dibutyl phthalate plasticize the polymer, and, if enough is added, the polymer becomes rubbery. These plasticized acrylics are used as temporary soft liners for dentures. They gradually become hard as the oily plasticizer is leached out by the saliva.

Plasticize means to soften.

Butadiene-styrene rubber has been added to acrylic plastics to improve their resistance to fracture caused by impact forces. Denture base materials of this type are available with impact strengths as much as two times those of the usual acrylic polymers used for denture construction. These materials are particularly useful for patients who have a history of breaking dentures during cleaning as a result of careless handling.

Individual impression trays are frequently constructed from acrylic polymers by mixing a monomer with polymerized powder containing large quantities of inert inorganic fillers. The mixture becomes doughlike and is rolled out into a patty in the same manner as bread or piecrust dough. This patty is then adapted to a gypsum cast of the patient's mouth prepared from a preliminary alginate impression and allowed to harden. Blockout, or space, between the tray and cast is provided to allow space for the final impression material. It is then used as a tray to make a final impression. If the inorganic filler were not present, the patty would not hold its shape. The presence of the filler minimizes the change in shape of the patty and permits the preparation of an accurately adapted tray to be accomplished with ease.

VINYL PLASTICS

Copolymers of vinyl acetate and ethylene have been used for athletic mouth protectors. The structures of the monomers are as follows:

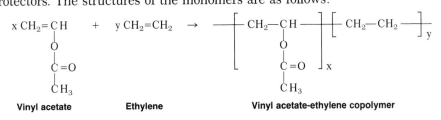

| Vinyl acetate | Ethylene | Vinyl acetate-ethylene copolymer |

The vinyl acetate-ethylene copolymers have important applications in preventive dentistry in which they are used as athletic mouth protectors, as trays in the application of fluorides, and as appliances for individuals with bruxism. These materials are described in Chapter 3.

ACRYLIC PLASTICS AS DENTURE BASES

Acrylic plastics have been supplied in a variety of forms, such as powder-liquid, gels, and sheets or blanks. Currently the powder-liquid type is the most popular. The use of the powder-liquid system simplifies the processing procedures, and, although not commonly done, a denture base can readily be processed in a dental office laboratory. Several products of the powder-liquid type are shown in Fig. 13-1. These products represent only a few of the available

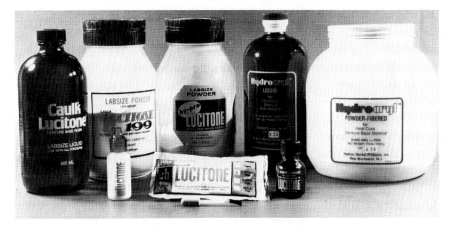

Fig. 13-1. Powder-liquid type of denture base materials. *Left to right, background,* Methyl methacrylate monomer, rubber-reinforced acrylic polymer, regular acrylic polymer, monomer for vinyl acrylic powder, and vinyl acrylic polymer; *foreground,* methyl methacrylate polymer colored for gingival shading, a foil packet of poly(methyl methacrylate), and a bottle of methyl methacrylate monomer.

denture base materials; a recent American Dental Association list of certified denture base materials includes more than fifty heat-accelerated and four chemically accelerated products. In many instances the product from one manufacturer may include clear, pigmented, and characterized (containing colored plastic fibers) variations. These materials have found wide application as denture bases for both complete and partial denture construction.

Composition

The components that may be present in the powder and liquid of an acrylic denture base material are listed in Table 13-1. The polymer is the principal component of the powder and is present as small spheres called beads or pearls, as shown in Fig. 13-2. The peroxide is present in amounts of about 1%, and, when decomposed by heat or chemicals, it initiates the polymerization reaction. Titanium dioxide is added in small amounts to increase the opacity until the material has the approximate translucency of the oral mucosa, since the pure processed polymer would be transparent. Inorganic pigments, commonly mercuric sulfide (red), cadmium sulfide (yellow), or ferric oxide (brown), are added in small amounts to match the shade of the denture base to the soft tissues. A wide range of shades is available, since considerable variation is present in the color of soft tissues of patients. A variety of stains is also available that can be applied during processing to alter further the shades commercially supplied. More and more denture base materials are being supplied that contain dyed synthetic fibers to simulate the minute blood vessels underlying the oral mucosa (characterized products).

The liquid is principally monomer, which is highly volatile. An organic inhibitor hydroquinone, is present in amounts of less than 0.1% and has the important function of preventing the monomer from polymerizing during several years of storage. The polymerization reaction can be initiated by ultraviolet

Table 13-1. Components of the Powder and Liquid of an Acrylic Denture Base Material

Powder	Liquid
Poly(methyl methacrylate) or polymer	Methyl methacrylate or monomer
Organic peroxide initiator	Hydroquinone inhibitor
Titanium dioxide to control translucency	Dimethacrylate or cross-linking agent*
Inorganic pigments for color	Organic amine accelerator†
Dyed synthetic fibers for esthetics	

*A cross-linking agent is present if the manufacturer indicates that the material is a cross-linked acrylic.

†The amine is present only if the material is labeled as a product to be processed at room temperature. Some manufacturers list them as cold-curing or self-curing materials.

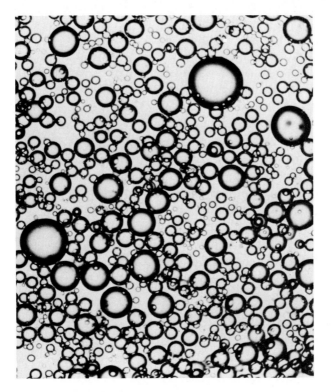

Fig. 13-2. Polymer powder of an acrylic denture base material. (From Craig RG, editor: *Restorative dental materials,* ed 8, St. Louis, 1989, Mosby–Year Book.)

light; therefore the liquid is always supplied in dark brown glass bottles that filter out this undesirable light. A dimethacrylate or other appropriate difunctional organic molecules will be present in the liquid if the manufacturer is supplying a cross-linked material. As pointed out earlier, the presence of small amounts of cross-linking agents increases the resistance of the final denture base to surface cracks, or crazing. If the acrylic denture base material is designed to be processed at room temperature, an organic amine or other organic accelerator is included to decompose the organic peroxide at room temperature so that the polymerization can be carried out without applying heat to the material.

Plasticizers, such as oily organic liquids or other high–molecular weight acrylic ester monomers, may be added to the liquid if the material is to be used as a soft liner for a denture base. Also, as described earlier in this chapter, the acrylic polymer may be a copolymer to control the impact strength of the denture base.

Properties

A summary of the more important properties of heat-processed acrylic denture base materials is given in Table 13-2. The strength properties can be summarized by the statement that **acrylic denture base materials are generally low in strength, fairly flexible, brittle, and soft and have reasonably high resistance to failure in fatigue** (1.5 million flexures before failure at a maximum stress of 2500 psi [17 MN/m^2]).

The acrylic denture bases have low thermal conductivity, and **patients will notice a substantial decrease in thermal stimulation of the oral tissues under an acrylic denture base.** The heat distortion temperature is relatively low (94° C [170° F]), and **patients should be cautioned not to clean dentures in excessively hot water,** since it may result in distortion of the base and a poorer fit of the appliance.

The volumetric polymerization shrinkage of a 3:1 polymer-monomer mix is high (6%), which represents a possible linear shrinkage of 2% during processing. Through the application of proper processing technics, the actual linear dimensional shrinkage is about 0.5%.

Water sorption of acrylic denture base materials is fairly high (0.6 mg/cm^2).

Table 13-2. Properties of Heat-Processed Acrylic Denture Base Materials

Tensile strength	8000 psi (55 MN/m^2)
Compressive strength	11,000 psi (76 MN/m^2)
Proportional limit	3800 psi (26 MN/m^2)
Elastic modulus	550,000 psi (3800 MN/m^2)
Impact strength	0.2 ft lb/in
Elongation	2%
Transverse deflection	
@3500 gm	2 mm
@5000 gm	4 mm
Fatigue strength	
@2500 psi (17MN/m^2)	1,500,000 cycles
Knoop hardness	15 kg/mm^2
Thermal conductivity	0.0006 cal/sec/cm^2(° C/cm)
Heat distortion temperature	94° C (170° F)
Polymerization shrinkage (volumetric)*	6%
Water sorption (24 hours)	0.6 mg/cm^2
Water solubility (24 hours)	0.02 mg/cm^2
Adhesion to metal	None
Adhesion to acrylic (tensile)	6000 psi (41 MN/m^2)
Color stability	Good
Taste or odor	None
Tissue compatibility	Good

*Based on a polymer-monomer mixture of 3:1.

After they are soaked in water until equilibrium, a sorption of about 2% occurs. This sorption of water causes the base to expand slightly and results in a better fit by partly compensating for the dimensional shrinkage during processing. The solubility is low, and the little that does take place is a result of the leaching out of traces of unreacted monomer into the oral fluids.

The adhesion of acrylic polymers to metal and porcelain is poor, and bonding to these materials is accomplished by mechanical retention. However, the adhesion to plastic denture teeth is good. Color stability is good, and, when properly processed, no taste or odor occurs. In addition, the compatibility of denture base polymers is good. **Instances of toxicity or allergic reactions have been shown to be related to excessive residual monomer resulting from improper processing. Room temperature-processed acrylic dentures.** The principal difference between room temperature-processed and heat-processed dentures is that more residual monomer is present in the room temperature-processed denture. The residual monomer functions as a plasticizer, and, initially, lower values for the properties usually result. As the unreacted monomer is leached out, the properties gradually improve and approach those of heat-processed acrylic dentures. Documented cases have been reported of irritation of the tissue as a result of this unreacted monomer. Nevertheless, room temperature-processed dentures have been shown to be more accurate than heat-processed ones, with a dimensional change of less than 0.1% for the former during processing.

MODIFIED ACRYLIC DENTURE BASE PLASTICS

Acrylic denture base materials have been modified by the incorporation of butadiene-styrene rubber and by the use of copolymers prepared from hydroxyethyl methacrylate monomers with methyl methacrylate. Properties of the modified acrylic materials plus those of a typical methyl methacrylate material are presented in Table 13-3.

The rubber-reinforced acrylic contains butadiene-styrene rubber grafted with methyl methacrylate, which is dispersed in a poly(methyl methacrylate) matrix. This modification increases the impact strength, which is accompanied by some increase in transverse deflection and by decrease in stiffness as indicated by the modulus in bending. A small decrease in water sorption also occurs as a result of the incorporation of the rubber.

The hydroxyethyl methacrylate-modified acrylic is the most flexible of the four types and fractures at a transverse load of less than 5000 gm. It has the lowest impact strength and, as expected, the highest water sorption.

Comparison of the fit of denture bases of the four types after processing and after reaching equilibrium in water revealed that the **hydroxyethyl methacrylate types fit the best, followed by the typical acrylic, and then by the rubber-reinforced types.**

Table 13-3. Properties of Modified Acrylic Denture Base Materials

Property	Typical acrylic	Rubber-reinforced acrylic	Hydroxyethyl methacrylate acrylic
Transverse deflection (mm)			
@3500 gm	2.0	2.4	2.5
@5000 gm	4.1	5.0	Fractured
Modulus in bending			
psi	290,000	258,000	239,000
MN/m^2	2000	1780	1650
Impact strength (Charpy)			
N · m	0.26	0.48	0.18
Water sorption (equilibrium)			
mg/cm^2	0.60	0.55	0.90
Ranging of fit (worst = 0; best = 4)	3	2	4
Color stability (24 hours in ultraviolet light)	No change	Slight change	Slight change

On exposure to ultraviolet light, only the typical acrylic shows no discernible color change, whereas the other two types show slight changes that would be clinically insignificant.

Cross-linked heat-cured acrylic is the most widely used denture base material. This material can be described as having low but adequate strength, being fairly flexible, brittle, and soft with a reasonably high-resistance fatigue fracture, low thermal conductivity and heat distortion temperature, fairly high polymerization shrinkage, high water sorption but low water solubility, good resistance to attack by solvents, no adhesion to metal, good color stability and tissue compatibility, moderate wettability by water, and no taste or odor.

Two modifications have special applications. Rubber modified acrylics have improved impact strength but at the expense of increased flexibility. Hydroxyethyl methacrylate modified acrylics have improved wetting by water but at the cost of lower transverse and impact strength.

Manipulation and processing

There is a wide variety of processing technics for acrylic denture bases, and these technics are adequately described in comprehensive textbooks on dental materials and prosthetic dentistry. The most commonly used technic is the dough-molding method, which is described as used for a heat-processing acrylic.

In the dough-molding technic, a powder-liquid system is used, and the materials are mixed in the ratio of about three parts of powder to one part of liquid. The amount of shrinkage and temperature rise during processing are directly related to the amount of monomer used. Both these undesirable effects are minimized by using this 3:1 ratio. The appropriate amount of liquid is poured into a mixing jar, and powder is added until all the liquid is absorbed, as shown in Fig. 13-3, A. The top of the mixing jar is screwed on, and the material is allowed to

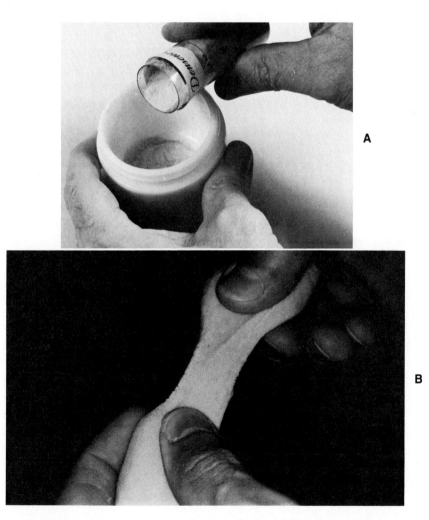

Fig. 13-3. A, Addition of powder to liquid. **B,** Checking for dough consistency.

stand while the solution of the powder and liquid takes place. During the solution process, the material changes from a sandy, to a sticky, to a doughlike consistency. The dough consistency is easily identified because, when this stage is reached, the material separates easily from the side of the mixing jar and breaks cleanly with a snap when pulled apart rapidly, as shown in Fig. 13-3, *B*. When the material reaches this consistency, it is ready to pack into the denture mold contained in a denture flask.

The denture mold is constructed by using a clinically acceptable waxed-up denture on a stone cast, as shown in Fig. 13-4, *A*. The portion of the denture that will be finally constructed in acrylic has been formed with baseplate wax, and the artificial teeth are embedded in the wax in their correct relationship. The waxed-up denture and the stone cast are invested in a split metal denture flask with gypsum products, as illustrated in Fig. 13-4, *B*. After the gypsum has set, the two portions of the flask are separated after the flask has been immersed in boiling water for a few minutes, and the wax is removed by placing the two halves of the flask in boiling water. When the wax has been thoroughly removed and the surface of the gypsum has been cleaned, a liquid alginate separator is applied to all surfaces except those of the teeth, which are embedded in the investment. The two parts of the flask look like the ones shown in Fig. 13-5, *A*.

An excess of the acrylic dough is placed in the part of the flask containing the teeth. A thin plastic sheet is placed over the acrylic, the flask is put together, and pressure is applied with a press to force the dough into all portions of the mold and to eliminate the excess as seen in Fig. 13-5, *B*. The flask is opened, and the excess is trimmed away as shown in Fig. 13-5, *C*. The dough consistency is stiff enough to hold the shape into which it is molded and yet is fluid enough to be forced into all details of the mold. The preceding step is repeated several times (trial packing) until no excess appears; at this point the plastic separating sheet is removed, and the flask is closed and placed in a clamp under pressure.

The denture flask under pressure is placed in a heated polymerization bath, the most common one being a temperature-controlled water bath at 73° C (165° F) for 8 hours or longer (frequently overnight). Processing at 73° C (165° F) provides a sufficiently slow rate of polymerization so that the temperature rise from the reaction does not vaporize the monomer; therefore porosity is avoided. The 8-hour or longer processing time produces nearly complete polymerization with a minimum of unreacted monomer in the denture base. The flask, still under pressure, is then removed from the water bath and allowed to cool to room temperature. The flask is removed from the clamp, and the denture is separated from the investment and is cleaned.

The periphery of the denture is finished with a variety of instruments, and only the non-tissue-bearing surfaces are polished. Polishing is done under wet

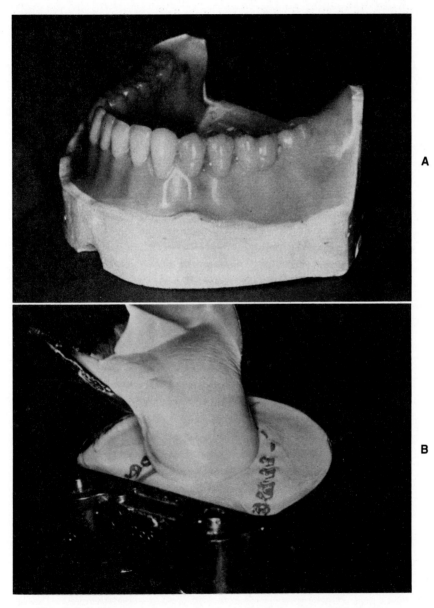

Fig. 13-4. A, Waxed-up denture on a stone cast. **B,** Investing of this denture.

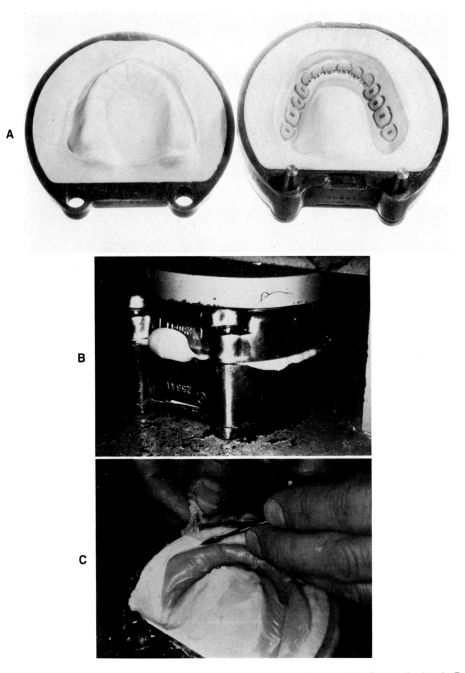

Fig. 13-5. Denture flask. **A,** Two parts of the denture flask just before packing the acrylic dough. **B,** Excess dough is forced out of the flask under pressure. **C,** Excess, or flash, is trimmed away. (**A** from Craig RG, editor: *Restorative dental materials,* ed 8, St. Louis, 1989, Mosby–Year Book; **B** and **C** courtesy Edward R. Dootz, University of Michigan School of Dentistry, Ann Arbor, Mich.)

conditions, since temperatures sufficient to decompose and distort the acrylic plastic can result from dry polishing. The denture is then ready for delivery, adjustment of the occlusion, and any final adjustment by the dentist.

Heat curing is the most popular method of processing denture base acrylics, although the linear dimensional shrinkage is about 0.3% greater than for the chemically cured acrylics. This heat curing system is selected because the accuracy is adequate and the laboratory cost is substantially less. Also, the heat curing procedure results in dentures containing significantly less unreacted methyl methacrylate monomer and thus less chance for tissue irritation on initial insertion.

Care of dentures

Patients should be cautioned to keep the dentures moist when they are not wearing them, since dimensional changes occur on drying. Although the original dimensions will return when water is again absorbed, the dentures will feel tight when first replaced in the mouth. **Patients should be instructed not to use abrasive dentifrices, since the acrylic plastic is soft and can be easily scratched and worn away.** Also the tissue-bearing surface should be brushed carefully with a soft brush, since any material removed alters the fit of the denture. A solution of 1 teaspoon of Clorox and 2 teaspoons of Calgon in one-half glass of water has been recommended for occasional overnight cleaning of acrylic dentures by immersion. It should be emphasized that **this solution is not suitable for dentures containing a base metal or for removable partial dentures in which the metal framework is constructed from a nickel-chromium, cobalt-chromium, or cobalt-chromium-nickel alloy,** since these alloys will turn dark.

Acrylic dentures should not be cleaned in hot water, since processing stresses can be released and can result in permanent deformation and distortion. Adequate denture cleansers are available that can be used with room temperature water. Home ultrasonic (high-frequency vibration) cleansers are available, but studies indicate that they do not clean dentures any better than the other methods described, although they do offer a certain amount of convenience.

PLASTICS AS SOFT LINERS

In general, soft liners have been used for patients with severe undercuts of the ridge or for those patients whose residual ridges are continually sore. They are also useful as a tissue treatment after oral surgery and in obturators for con-

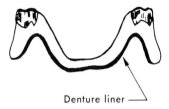

Fig. 13-6. Cross section of a maxillary denture with a soft liner shown in black.

Denture liner

genital or acquired defects of the palate. A cross section through the midline of a maxillary denture with a soft liner is shown in Fig. 13-6. Despite divergent opinions about the use of soft liners, some patients can tolerate dentures significantly better when a soft liner is used.

Soft liners can be classified as long-term (months) or treatment (days) materials. The long-term materials include poly(ethyl methacrylates) or acrylic copolymers plus plasticizers, which may be aromatic esters or these esters and alcohols; these liners may be processed either by heating or at room temperature, depending on their formulation. Long-term materials also include silicone rubber, which is supplied as heat- or room temperature-polymerizing types. The hardness of the long-term acrylic materials increases slowly as the plasticizer is leached out but remains essentially constant with the silicones. The room temperature-polymerizing products can be used as chairside materials, whereas the heat-polymerizing acrylics and all the silicones are processed in the laboratory. The room temperature-polymerizing silicone should not be processed in the mouth because significant quantities of acetic acid are liberated during processing. Silicone liners have presented the problem that they support the growth of yeasts present in the mouth, and with some patients, hard, raised spots result on the surface of the liner. In addition, the silicone liner is difficult to finish at the periphery, and the bond to the hard acrylic base is not always adequate.

Treatment materials consist of a poly(ethyl methacrylate) powder and a liquid containing aromatic esters and ethanol. The materials are used at the chairside, and the liner is replaced frequently or before 3 days have elapsed. The treatment materials flow under static load but are elastic under intermittent loads produced by chewing. As irritated and swollen tissues heal, the liner flows and follows the contour of the tissues. The materials become harder as the plasticizer is leached out by the oral fluids.

Cleaning of soft liners can be accomplished with the method described for acrylic denture bases **and should be done carefully with a soft brush** because of the liners' low hardness and poor abrasion resistance.

Home reliners. Patients should be discouraged from using home or drugstore soft liners or hard reliners, since they can degrade the properties of the acrylic denture base, possibly resulting in improper occlusion that can cause significant damage to the oral structures supporting the denture.

RETENTION OF A COMPLETE DENTURE

The retention of a complete denture is determined by the fit of the tissue-bearing surface; thus any procedure that alters the dimensions of this surface will affect the retention. When the denture is worn, saliva fills the space between the denture and the tissue. The retention of the denture is directly related to the size of its area, the surface tension of the saliva, and the wettability of the denture by saliva. Its retention is inversely related to the thickness of the saliva film. Patients with thin, ropy saliva with low surface tension frequently experience problems with retention, as do those with a poorly fitting denture. Increasing the wetting of the denture by saliva by using hydroxy-containing polymers may increase the retention of a poorly fitting denture but not that of a well-fitting denture.

Surface tension is the attraction of molecules at the surface of the liquid.

Denture adhesives should not be needed with a well-fitting denture. The adhesives are pastes or powders that turn to viscous pastes when mixed with saliva. The viscosity of the paste between the denture and the tissue is much higher than that of the film of saliva. Retention is directly related to viscosity; therefore the retention is increased with a poorly fitting denture. In a well-fitting denture, the use of an adhesive increases the film thickness, and the retention is not improved.

PLASTICS AS PROSTHETIC TEETH

Acrylic and modified acrylic polymers are used in manufacturing plastic teeth. **The principal difference in the composition of plastic teeth and denture base materials is that different pigments are used to produce the various tooth shades.** Plastic teeth are made in layers of different colors, translucencies, and thicknesses, so that the shade is lighter at the incisal or occlusal portion. The gingival, or body, portion of the plastic teeth is prepared from materials that are not cross-linked, or are only slightly cross-linked, since the non-cross-linked polymer bonds better to the denture base material. The coronal portion of the tooth is constructed of cross-linked polymer to provide resistance to crazing. The properties of plastic teeth are the same as those described in Table 13-2 for denture base acrylic materials.

The other material used for denture teeth is porcelain. Both plastic and porcelain materials have certain advantages and disadvantages. **The plastic teeth are tough, but they are also soft and have lower resistance to abrasion, unlike porcelain teeth that are brittle and hard and have high wear resistance.** Plastic teeth chemically bond to the acrylic denture base, and a tensile bond strength of 6000 psi (41 MN/m^2) is not unusual. Porcelain teeth do not bond to acrylic; therefore metal pins or mechanical retention areas must be provided. Examples of porcelain and plastic teeth are shown in Fig. 13-7. The plastic teeth are easy

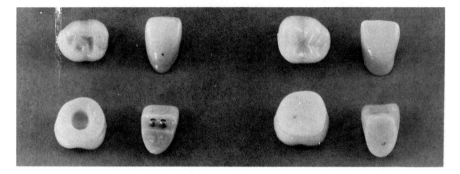

Fig. 13-7. Examples of prosthetic porcelain teeth *(left)* and plastic teeth *(right)*. Note the pins on the anterior porcelain tooth and the diatoric retention hole on the posterior porcelain tooth.

to grind and polish, whereas grinding of porcelain teeth removes the surface glaze, which is impossible to regain. Both plastic and porcelain teeth have a natural lifelike appearance.

The choice between plastic and porcelain teeth depends on the application. In general, **plastic teeth are indicated in low-stress-bearing areas, in patients with poor ridges, when placed opposite natural teeth, and when limited interarch distance exists.** Porcelain teeth are frequently used when patients have good ridge support and adequate interarch distance and when maxillary and mandibular dentures oppose each other. An advantage exists in using opposing plastic and porcelain teeth, since the friction between porcelain and plastic is lower than in any other combination and the clicking sound of porcelain against porcelain is eliminated.

PLASTIC-METAL COMBINATIONS

Plastics have been used in combination with metals in removable prosthodontics, as mentioned in Chapter 11.

In a metal-base complete denture, the metal contacts the tissue-bearing surface, and there is some indication that the rigidity and thermal stimulation as a result of the metal base are advantageous. Acrylic plastics are attached to the metal base by mechanical retention, and the acrylic plastic retains the denture teeth and provides esthetic value.

Partial dentures of the removable type consist of a metal framework that is supported by the remaining teeth and soft tissue. The metals used are rigid (high modulus) alloys such as nickel-chromium, cobalt-chromium, or cobalt-chromium-nickel alloys. The acrylic is mechanically locked to retentive areas in the metal framework (see the meshwork in the posterior area in Fig. 11-6), and

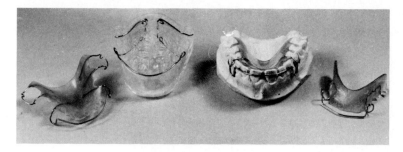

Fig. 13-8. Orthodontic appliances constructed of stainless steel wire and acrylic plastic.

the acrylic also retains the artificial teeth. The processing of either complete or partial dentures containing metals is similar to that described for a complete acrylic denture except that the metal is retained in the investment mold along with the artificial teeth and the acrylic is packed into the space resulting from the loss of the baseplate wax and baseplate.

Acrylic polymers have been used as facings for fixed bridges to improve the esthetic value of the restoration. Porcelain also may be used for this application, but it is more expensive and less easy to repair than acrylic facings, although it is less subject to wear. Individuals involved in athletic activities may be advised to have fixed bridges with acrylic facings because of the probability of fracture. The acrylics used for this application are higher–molecular weight glycol dimethacrylates, which have low vapor pressures and can be polymerized by applying the material to the metal bridge and then heating in an oven at 135° C (275° F) for 8 minutes. Mechanical retention to the gold must be provided for these acrylic facing materials. The advantages of dimethacrylate are obvious in that it can be processed without investing (flasking) and without danger of porosity. The highly cross-linked polymer is easy to finish, and the facing is poorly wetted by chewing gum and lipstick. Clinical experience has established that the dimethacrylate polymer has good stability, is well tolerated by tissues, and can satisfactorily withstand stresses in the mouth.

Acrylics are also used in conjunction with stainless steel wire to construct orthodontic appliances, as shown in Fig. 13-8. It is common practice to form the appliance by using a hand-painting procedure involving the use of a room temperature-processed acrylic. The acrylic liquid is painted on the desired areas, then the acrylic powder is added to the same areas; the procedure is repeated until the proper thickness is attained. The cast containing the framework and the acrylic is placed in a pressure cooker, and 20 psi of air pressure is applied during polymerization. The pressure minimizes the porosity in the acrylic and eliminates investing or flasking.

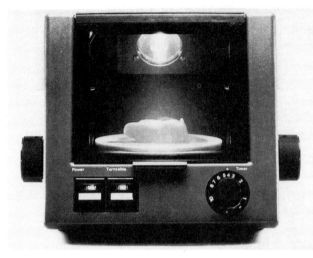

Fig. 13-9. Light-curing oven for polymerizing dimethacrylates.

LIGHT-CURED DIMETHACRYLATES

Dimethacrylates similar to those described in Chapter 4 have been especially **useful in the repair of fractured acrylic dentures.** They have also been used to make orthodontic appliances such as those in Fig. 13-8, to reline dentures, to make impression trays, and even to fabricate dentures.

The dimethacrylate is supplied fully compounded, containing some inorganic filler, blue light absorber, accelerator, and appropriate pigments. It is provided in opaque, tight packages to avoid premature polymerization.

The procedure for repairing a fractured denture involves assembling the broken pieces with sticky wax, pouring a stone model on the inside of the denture, opening up the fracture line with a bur, coating the ground surface with a bonding agent, placing the dimethacrylate repair material into the opened space, carving the surface, painting the dimethacrylate with a liquid to prevent surface inhibition of polymerization, and then placing the model and denture on a turntable in an oven with several high-intensity blue lights as shown in Fig. 13-9. **Polymerization requires 5 to 10 minutes of exposure, and the entire repair can be done in less than 1 hour.** No problems have been observed in repairing a variety of denture acrylics with the dimethacrylate system.

OTHER USES OF PLASTICS IN DENTISTRY

The use of plastics as preventive materials is described in Chapter 3, and their application as tooth restorative materials in Chapter 4; these applications are not discussed further. Several other applications of plastics in dentistry include their use as maxillofacial materials and in the construction of temporary crowns and bridges and individual impression trays.

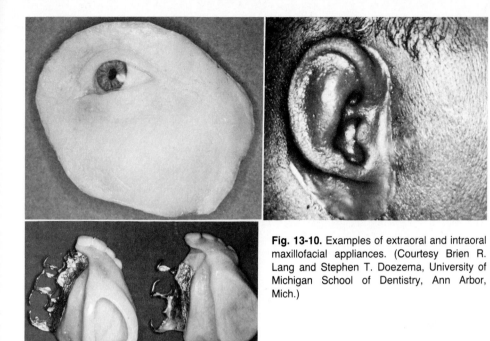

Fig. 13-10. Examples of extraoral and intraoral maxillofacial appliances. (Courtesy Brien R. Lang and Stephen T. Doezema, University of Michigan School of Dentistry, Ann Arbor, Mich.)

Maxillofacial materials. The loss of tissues of the face as a result of accident or disease is generally a problem handled by the prosthodontist. The replacement of a lost ear, nose, eye, or other part requires the construction of a maxillofacial appliance. Since the tissues being replaced are soft, flexible plastics, such as plasticized acrylics and vinyls, as well as elastomers of silicones and urethanes, have been used to construct these appliances. A few of them are illustrated in Fig. 13-10. It is desirable to have some of these prostheses remain soft throughout temperature changes in the environment and with clinical service. They should also resist staining from body oils and should be color stable. The maxillofacial materials should be easily cleaned, and it should be possible to use adhesives to attach the appliance to soft tissue. Since the edges of the appliance are generally thin, the materials should have high resistance to tearing. In addition, the materials should be readily colored to match skin tones and should accept cosmetics. It is not surprising that none of the current materials fulfills all of these requirements; however, the silicone rubbers currently have the best overall properties. Maxillofacial materials are not used in large quantities, but their application is extremely important for patients requiring such service.

Temporary crown and bridge materials. The fabrication of a crown or fixed

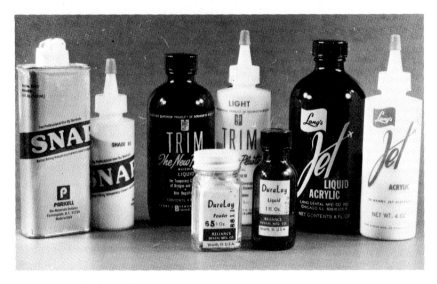

Fig. 13-11. Commercial temporary crown and bridge materials.

bridge is generally a laboratory procedure, and several weeks may lapse between the preparation of the teeth and the cementation of the permanent restoration; thus a temporary restoration must be made. The temporary crown and bridge materials are most commonly acrylic polymers, and some of the available products are shown in Fig. 13-11. The powder and liquid are mixed to a creamy consistency, and the temporary restoration is formed using the mix and a cellulose acetate crown former, a vacuum-formed plastic, or an alginate impression of the area before tooth preparation. A separating medium is used to provide a release from the tooth structure. The creamy mix is flowed into the desired areas of the impression, and when the material reaches a puttylike consistency, the impression is seated in the mouth. The material reaches a rubbery condition in a few minutes, and the temporary restoration is removed and placed in warm water (~57° C) to harden. The temporary restoration is trimmed before cementation with a temporary cement such as zinc oxide–eugenol.

Tray materials. Highly filled powder-liquid acrylics are used for this application, and examples of these tray materials, including the processing equipment, are pictured in Fig. 13-12. The model with or without a wax spacer, or stop, is placed in cold water. The recommended amount of liquid and powder is placed in a disposable cup and thoroughly mixed for 1 minute or until the gloss on the surface disappears and the mix develops a slight firmness. A patty may be prepared with the wooden block and roller or by manipulating the mix between the fingers moistened with water. A U-shaped patty is better for a lower tray. The patty is placed on the palatal area overlapping the ridge of the moist maxillary or

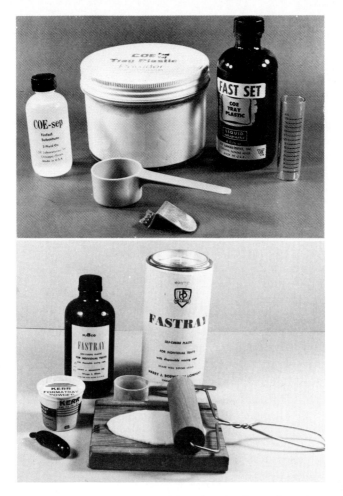

Fig. 13-12. Acrylic tray materials and processing equipment.

mandibular model and is gently adapted over the ridge to the periphery. After a proper thickness is obtained, the excess is trimmed away with a knife. The excess may then be used to form a handle. The acrylic tray material is allowed to polymerize for 6 minutes or so at room temperature, and then the model and tray can be placed in warm water to speed up polymerization. Trimming of the tray is done with acrylic finishing instruments. Retention holes may be drilled into the tray if desired, or the inner surface of the tray may be painted with a rubber adhesive and allowed to dry when a rubber impression material is to be used. If a zinc oxide–eugenol final impression is to be made, no added retention is necessary.

Self-test questions

In the following multiple choice questions, one or more responses may be correct.

1 Methyl methacrylate monomer:
   a. Has a low–molecular weight of about 100
   b. Has a high vapor pressure at room temperature but is nontoxic when inhaled
   c. Is polymerized to a molecular weight of about 50,000 in typical dental processing procedures
   d. When converted to poly(methyl methacrylate) has essentially no vapor pressure
   e. Has a higher density than poly(methyl methacrylate)

2 Which of these statements apply to the polymerization of methyl methacrylate?
   a. Polymerization can be started by decomposing an organic peroxide initiator by heating.
   b. Polymerization can be started by decomposing an organic peroxide at room temperature with an organic amine.
   c. Heat is liberated as a result of polymerization.
   d. Porosity may result during polymerization if the temperature is high.

3 Cross-linked polymers:
   a. Have a network structure
   b. Are formed when monomers with two reactive double bonds are present
   c. Have lower resistance to surface cracking than linear polymers

4 Which of the following statements are true for copolymers or modified acrylic polymers?
   a. Hydroxyethyl methacrylate and methyl methacrylate copolymers are wetted better by saliva than poly(methyl methacrylate).
   b. Rubber-modified acrylic polymers have lower impact strength than poly(methyl methacrylate).
   c. Addition of octyl methacrylate to methyl methacrylate yields a softer polymer than poly(methyl methacrylate).

5 Indicate whether the following components are found in the liquid (l) or the powder (p) of an acrylic denture base material.
   ___ a. Polymer
   ___ b. Monomer
   ___ c. Inhibitor
   ___ d. Methyl methacrylate
   ___ e. Dyed fiber
   ___ f. Titanium dioxide
   ___ g. Amine accelerator
   ___ h. Inorganic pigments
   ___ i. Poly(methyl methacrylate)
   ___ j. Peroxide initiator
   ___ k. Cross-linking agent

6 Indicate the function of the components in acrylic denture base materials listed in the left-hand column by selecting the correct answer listed in the right-hand column.

___ **a.** Methyl methacrylate
___ **b.** Poly(methyl methacrylate)
___ **c.** Titanium dioxide
___ **d.** Organic peroxide
___ **e.** Hydroquinone
___ **f.** Organic amine
___ **g.** Inorganic pigments

1. Accelerator
2. Initiator
3. Inhibitor to provide shelf life
4. Monomer to make a dough and to polymerize
5. Polymer to reduce polymerization shrinkage
6. To add color
7. To control translucency

7 Compared with acrylic denture base polymers:
 a. Rubber-reinforced acrylic polymer has lower transverse deflection.
 b. Hydroxyethyl methacrylate-acrylic polymer has higher water sorption.
 c. Rubber-reinforced acrylic polymer has lower impact strength.

8 Which statements apply to processing of an acrylic denture base material of the dough-molding, heat-polymerizing type?
 a. To control shrinkage a powder-liquid ratio of 1:3 is used.
 b. The dough consistency develops after powder and liquid are mixed because of polymerization of methyl methacrylate.
 c. Polymerization is accomplished by heating at 73° C for 8 hours or longer.

9 Denture patients should be instructed to:
 a. Clean all surfaces of the denture with an abrasive dentifrice to remove any debris.
 b. Avoid placing the denture in hot water.
 c. Keep their dentures in water when not in the mouth.

10 Compared with porcelain teeth, acrylic plastic teeth are:
 a. More brittle
 b. Less abrasion resistant
 c. Able to bond to the denture base
 d. More difficult to polish

11 Acrylic materials used as facings for fixed bridges:
 a. Contain glycol dimethacrylates with low vapor pressure
 b. Can be polymerized at 135° C without flasking or producing porosity
 c. Have poor color stability in the mouth

12 An acrylic tray material:
 a. Is a powder-liquid system highly filled with inorganic powder
 b. Is rolled into a patty on a wooden block with a roller
 c. Is allowed to polymerize in a flask in a water bath at 78° C for 8 hours
 d. Requires an adhesive or mechanical retention for use with a rubber impression material but not with a zinc oxide–eugenol impression material

13 Temporary crown and bridge materials are:
 a. Fabricated in a commercial dental laboratory
 b. Fabricated in the dental office
 c. Applied in the mouth at the creamy consistency stage
 d. Formed using a crown form or an alginate impression

Suggested supplementary readings

Braden M: Selection and properties of some new dental materials, *Dent Update* 1:489. 1974.

Brauer GM: Polymers in dentistry. In Craig RG, editor: *Dental materials review*, Ann Arbor, Mich, 1977, University of Michigan School of Dentistry.

McCabe IF, Wilson HI: Polymers in dentistry, *J Oral Rehabil* 1:335, 1974.

Soni PM, Powers JM, Craig RG: Physical and mechanical properties of acrylic and modified acrylic denture resins, *J Mich Dent Assoc* 59:418, 1977.

chapter fourteen

Dental Porcelain

Porcelain has many applications in restorative dentistry: denture teeth, jacket crowns, porcelain-fused-to-metal bridgework, veneers, and inlays. **Porcelain has excellent esthetics, is mild to tissues, and resists wear extremely well.**

Porcelain is a white translucent ceramic fired at high temperatures.

COMPOSITION

Dental porcelain raw materials contain varying amounts of crystalline ingredients such as silica (SiO_2), feldspar (K_2O-Al_2O_3-6 SiO_2), and alumina (Al_2O_3). These crystalline constituents are held together in glass, which is clear and has a liquidlike structure. The porcelain is manufactured in the factory by heating feldspar and other minerals together with materials called fluxes that form lower-fusing glasses. These fluxes are oxides or carbonates of sodium, potassium, lithium, and boron. The fused mass is called a frit and is quickly cooled or quenched to form the porcelain. The porcelain may then be refired to add metal oxides that give the colors and shades necessary to match natural tooth structure. At least three types of porcelain must be used to fabricate a crown: core or opaque layer, incisal, and gingival. These porcelains are formulated to simulate the different portions of a natural tooth. They are mainly glasses with some crystalline components such as leucite. Colored metal oxides are added in small amounts. The basic pigments used to make up the many shades are yellow, blue, pink, brown, and gray. Generally, these porcelains have coefficients of expansion considerably lower (e.g., $8 \times 10^{-6}/^\circ$ C) than those used for porcelain-fused-to-metal restorations.

Aluminous porcelains contain up to 40% crystalline alumina in the core material. This core material doubles the strength to around 10,000 psi (69 MN/m^2).

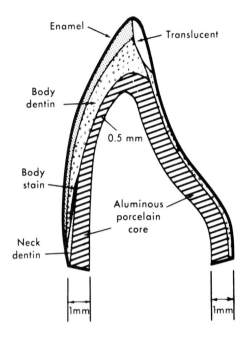

Enamel

Translucent

Body dentin

0.5 mm

Body stain

Aluminous porcelain core

Neck dentin

1mm

1mm

Fig. 14-1. Cross section of an aluminous porcelain crown. (From McLean JW: *J Am Dent Assoc* 75:621, 1967. Copyright by the American Dental Association. Reprinted by permission.)

As seen in Fig. 14-1, this high-alumina porcelain is used to form an inner core on which the rest of the crown is built. However, aluminous porcelain crowns have also been found to occasionally fracture clinically. These failures are thought to be a result of cracks that propagate from inside the crown. To strengthen the crowns further, a platinum foil matrix may be bonded to the inner surface by first plating with tin.

CLASSIFICATION

Porcelains are classified according to their fusing temperatures as follows: high-fusing, 1288° to 1371° C (2350° to 2500° F); medium-fusing, 1093° to 1260° C (2000° to 2300° F); and low-fusing, 871° to 1066° C (1600° to 1950° F). Higher-fusing porcelains contain more crystalline ingredients and usually have a better, or more natural, appearance.

COLOR

One must understand the nature of color and other appearance properties to match tooth shades properly. The three attributes of color are **hue, value,** and **chroma.** Hue is commonly thought of as the color, such as red, green, blue, or orange. The value is the lightness, or the relative amount of light reflected from the color. Chroma refers to the color strength. A brilliant color is high in chroma and light in terms of value. Deep colors are dark and strong in chroma. **It is**

mostly value that makes teeth match as a set. It is this lightness or darkness, rather than differences in hue or chroma, that should be observed. A nonvital tooth is easily perceived, since it may become darker than its neighbors. It is essential that the matching of shades be done under lighting conditions similar to the everyday environment of the patient. **Color and appearance are highly influenced by the nature of the incident light.** Standard light sources are available for matching shades that may be used in every step of the procedure. **Other appearance properties of importance are translucency, surface reflectance, and fluorescence.** Fluorescent materials glow under ultraviolet light. Since natural enamel is fluorescent, oxides are added to dental porcelains to simulate this effect.

Color is a three-dimensional property.

DENTURE TEETH

Porcelain denture teeth are produced in factories by fusing porcelain in metal molds until it is coherent. After removal from the molds, the teeth undergo additional firings in a furnace. Denture teeth are standardized in anatomy and shade. A **shade guide** is a collection of teeth representing all shades available and is used to match the patient's natural teeth. **Initially, both porcelain and plastic teeth have a natural appearance; however, plastic teeth are softer and more subject to wear and abrasion with time.** Recently, posterior denture teeth with ceramic-filled composite occlusal surfaces have been introduced to reduce wear. Plastic denture teeth are also widely used but have different properties from porcelain teeth. **The advantages of plastic teeth are greater resistance to breakage, better bonding to denture base plastics, quiet occlusion, and the ease of making adjustments to them by grinding and polishing.** Plastic teeth are generally used to oppose natural teeth and, in patients with poor ridge conditions, to reduce wear and trauma. Porcelain teeth are more rigid and do not absorb occlusal stresses as well as plastic teeth.

PORCELAIN CROWNS

Porcelain crowns are made by a dental technician from a model of the patient's tooth. The finished crown is cemented over the prepared tooth and simulates the appearance of a natural tooth. Two types of crown construction may be distinguished: the jacket crown and porcelain-fused-to-metal crown. A **jacket crown** may have a ceramic inner core composed of a glass with an oxide added for strength (see Fig. 14-1). Aluminous core materials contain around 40% of crystalline alumina in a glass matrix. The strength of the aluminous core material is about double that of unreinforced porcelain. **The main limitation of jacket crowns is low strength.** They are brittle and cannot withstand pos-

A jacket crown is an all porcelain crown.

terior occlusal stresses without breaking. The clinical failure rate for aluminous core crowns is about 2% for anterior crowns but around 15% for posterior crowns.

Recently, four other jacket crown porcelains have been introduced. The first one is composed of a magnesia core material that is used in place of the aluminous core material. The magnesia core material has a high coefficient of thermal expansion and therefore can be used with the same veneer porcelains that are used with metals.

The second jacket crown development uses an extrusion-molded or injection-molded aluminous core material. Alumina with other ceramics is blended with resins to form a plastic mass when the mixture is heated. Then the plastic mass is injected into a dental stone and plaster mold that was formed by the lost wax process under a pressure of 1500 psi. Next the deflasked core is fired for several hours to a maximum temperature of 1300° C. During the firing the resins are burned off, and a rigid aluminous ceramic core is formed. This method provides a more accurately fitting core than those built up by hand condensation. The outer layers of the crown are built up with a special translucent porcelain by the use of hand condensation. The strength of the extrusion-molded aluminous porcelain crown is comparable to the traditional aluminous core crowns.

The third development is the casting of ceramic crowns by the lost wax process using a phosphate investment mold. The entire crown is cast with a motorized centrifugal casting machine at approximately 1380° C using a fluoride-mica glass. Two cast crowns with sprues attached are shown in Fig. 14-2, *A*. Note they are transparent at this point in their fabrication. The cast glass crown is then heated for several hours to permit crystallization, which forms a strong white ceramic (Fig. 14-2, *B, right*). The final shading is achieved with external staining (Fig. 14-2, *B, left*). The strength of the recrystallized ceramic is also comparable with that of aluminous porcelain. Since the cast crown is converted from a glass to a ceramic by crystallization, it is called a **glass ceramic.**

A fourth development is a translucent porcelain strengthened with the mineral leucite. This porcelain does not need a core porcelain for strength, and it is being used experimentally for small anterior bridges.

The porcelain-fused-to-metal crown consists of an outer layer of porcelain bonded to an inner alloy casting (Fig. 14-3). **Because of the higher strengths of alloys, porcelain-fused-to-metal bridges are routinely used in dental practice.** On the other hand, all porcelain bridges do not have sufficient strength to resist breakage.

Fabrication involving hand condensation

Porcelain powder is mixed with water or another special liquid to form a paste that is used to fabricate the anatomy of a crown using a small brush and carving

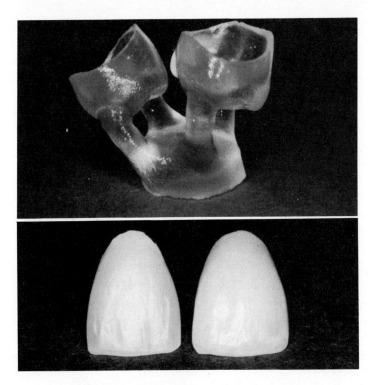

Fig. 14-2. A, Glass ceramic castings of crowns. **B,** *right,* Ceramed crown. **B,** *left,* Ceramed and stained crown.

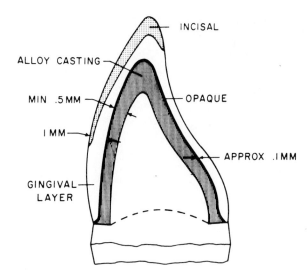

INCISAL

ALLOY CASTING

MIN .5 MM

I MM

OPAQUE

APPROX .1 MM

GINGIVAL
LAYER

Fig. 14-3. Cross section of a ceramic-metal crown with full coverage. (From O'Brien WJ, Ryge G, editors: *Outline of dental materials,* Philadelphia, 1978, WB Saunders.)

instruments (Fig. 14-4). In the case of a jacket crown, the aluminous porcelain is first applied to a **platinum foil matrix** formed on a die made from an impression of the patient's prepared tooth. In the case of a porcelain-fused-to-metal crown, the opaque porcelain is the first layer applied to the surface of the casting. The purpose of the opaque layer is to hide the color of the metal oxides on the casting. After application of a core or opaque layer, excess moisture is removed by the use of vibration and a paper tissue in a procedure called hand condensation.

The platinum foil matrix is a thin sheet of pure platinum that is swaged over a die to form a support for firing the porcelain.

After condensation, the platinum matrix with the applied core material or the casting with an opaque layer is dried in front of the porcelain furnace for a few minutes and then placed inside. The temperature of the furnace is raised to the firing temperature of the porcelain. This temperature is 1066° C in the case of the aluminous core material and 982° C for most opaque porcelains. Densification of the porcelain during firing occurs by the process of **sintering,** which involves partial fusion and bonding of adjacent surfaces of particles rather than

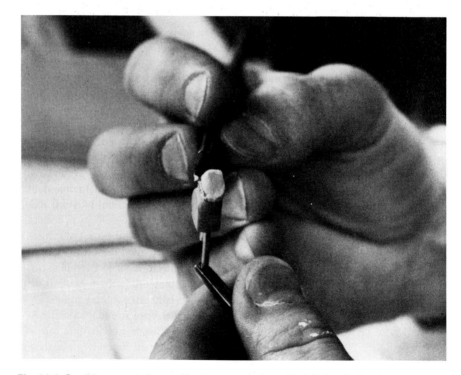

Fig. 14-4. Small increment of ceramic-water paste being added during the buildup of porcelain.

complete melting. The sintered core or opaque layers are then covered with the more translucent body and incisal porcelains. The same procedures of condensation and sintering are repeated. As a result of sintering, the porcelain shrinks. This shrinkage is anticipated and is provided for by building up a larger size crown before the firing. Usually the porcelain on a crown or bridge is completed after three firings. In the final firing, the porcelain is brought to a glaze that is formed by the flow of fused porcelain over the surface. This glaze gives the porcelain surface the gloss necessary to simulate a natural tooth surface. Glazing may also be accomplished by firing a layer of a low-fusing glass or by overglazing on the surface of the crown. The color or shade of the porcelain may also be modified in this step by using colored glazes. However, this practice is questionable, since low-fusing glazes are soluble and gradually wear off over a period of years in the mouth.

PORCELAIN-METAL BONDING

Porcelain-fused-to-metal crowns are fabricated by firing a porcelain directly to a crown made from a specially formulated alloy (Fig. 14-5). The surface of the metal alloy oxidizes as shown in Fig. 14-6. The first layer of the porcelain, called the opaque, bonds to this oxide layer. **Good wetting by the glass phase of the**

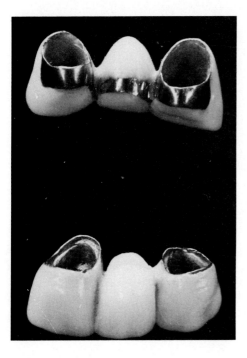

Fig. 14-5. Views of a cast metal bridge with Ceramco porcelain fused to the surface. (Courtesy J. Aderer, Long Island City, NY.)

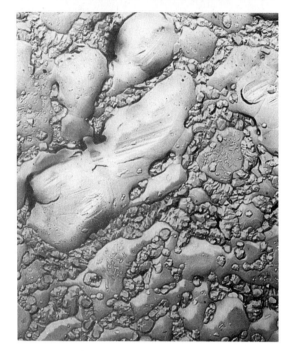

Fig. 14-6. Surface oxide formed on a Ceramco alloy. (×8000.) (From Kelly M, Asgar K, O'Brien WJ: *J Biomed Mater Res* 3:403, 1969.)

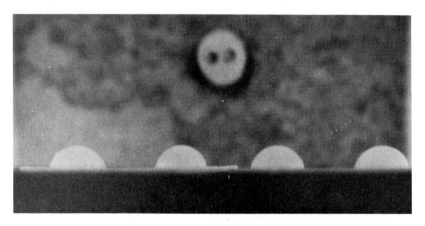

Fig. 14-7. Drops of fused porcelain on a Ceramco alloy showing wetting. (From O'Brien WJ, Ryge G: *J Prosthet Dent* 15:1094, 1965.)

porcelain is essential to the bonding. Drops of porcelain wetting gold alloys are shown in Fig. 14-7. **It is essential that the coefficients of thermal expansion of the metal and porcelain be matched to prevent cracking during cooling.** The coefficient of thermal expansion of the currently available porcelains is 13 to 14 × 10^{-6}/° C. The term porcelain enamel is often used for ceramics that are fired directly on metals.

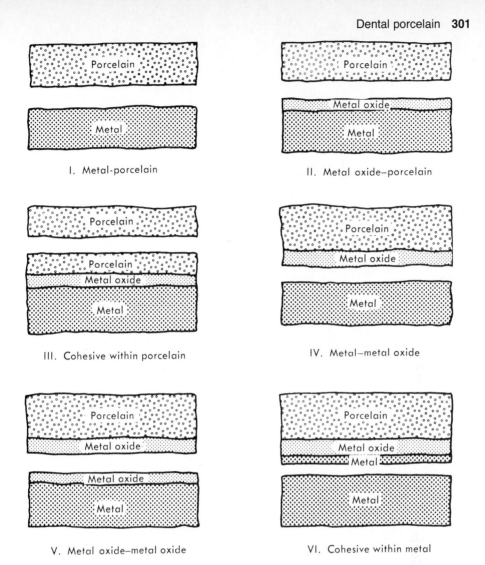

Fig. 14-8. Classification of porcelain-enamel failures according to interfaces formed. (From O'Brien WJ. In Craig RG, editor: *Dental materials review,* Ann Arbor, Mich, 1977, University of Michigan.)

A proper bond between the porcelain and the alloy is one that is stronger than the porcelain itself. Therefore the porcelain rather than the bond will fail cohesively. Six types of bond failures are possible near the porcelain-metal interface as shown in Fig. 14-8. Type III represents a cohesive failure indicative of a proper bond. Fig. 14-9 shows an example of a Type I failure. These porcelain-metal failures are usually the result of coating the casting with a layer of pure gold to improve the appearance of the crown. **This action results in a weak bond, since the oxides that are associated with good bonding do not form;**

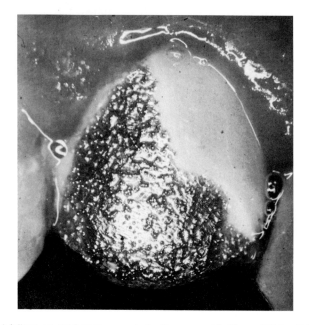

Fig. 14-9. Type I failure on gold casting coated with pure gold. (From O'Brien WJ. In Yamada H, editor: *Dental porcelain: the state of the art—1977,* Los Angeles, 1977, University of Southern California.)

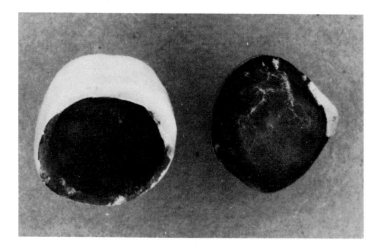

Fig. 14-10. Example of Type V failure through oxide layer of nickel-chromium alloy. (From O'Brien WJ. In Yamada H, editor: *Dental porcelain: the state of the art—1977,* Los Angeles, 1977, University of Southern California.)

with gold alloys, these are tin, indium, and iron oxides. Fig. 14-10 illustrates a Type V failure in which the porcelain has separated because of a weak boundary oxide on a nickel-chromium alloy. These alloys must be oxidized carefully according to the manufacturer's instructions for a thin adherent oxide layer to form. Observations of clinical failures often show the presence of mixed types of failure.

The bond strength increases with the **cohesive site density** as shown in Fig. 14-11. Fig. 14-12 shows areas on the surface of a nickel-chromium casting surface with cohesive sites. A sufficient number of these sites must be present for the bond strength to approach the cohesive strength of the porcelain. It is difficult to tell if bonding is chemical or mechanical, since the oxides are so complex in composition and structure. Several bond tests have been employed, and the results obtained are difficult to relate to each other. However, they all indicate a proper bond if there is cohesive attachment of the porcelain on the alloy surface after the test has been completed. A tensile bond test will indicate

The cohesive site density is the number of good attachment sites per unit area.

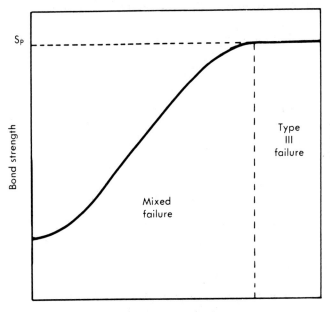

Fig. 14-11. Relation between density of cohesive attachment sites and observed bond strengths. (From O'Brien WJ. In Yamada H, editor: *Dental porcelain: the state of the art—1977,* Los Angeles, 1977, University of Southern California.)

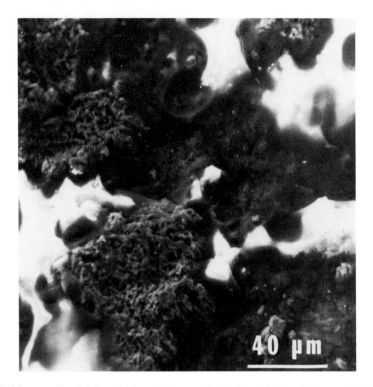

Fig. 14-12. Microscopic cohesive attachment sites on the fracture interface between nickel-chromium alloy and porcelain. (From O'Brien WJ. In Yamada H, editor: *Dental porcelain: the state of the art—1977,* Los Angeles, 1977, University of Southern California.)

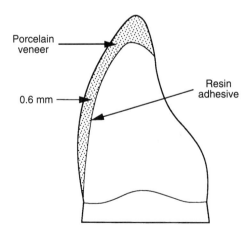

Porcelain veneer

0.6 mm

Resin adhesive

Fig. 14-13. Porcelain veneer bonded to facial surface of tooth.

a bond strength of 5000 psi (35 MN/m^2) with Type III failure, since this is the strength of the porcelain. However, a pull-through shear test will give maximum values of around 17,000 psi (117 MN/m^2), since the strength of the porcelain is near this value in shear.

VENEERS

Porcelain veneers are cosmetic facings that are bonded to the facial surfaces of anterior teeth to improve appearance, as shown in Fig. 14-13. They are bonded to the enamel by means of the acid etch technic and the use of resin cements. They can be fabricated by firing on platinum foil or on refractory dies similar in composition to phosphate-bonded casting investments. The porcelains used most are made from feldspar and are low fusing. **The main advantage of porcelain veneers is greater resistance to wear and staining as is the case with porcelain denture teeth.**

INLAYS

Inlays made from porcelain have the advantage of a natural appearance. Porcelain inlays are usually fabricated by firing porcelain on a refractory die of the prepared tooth. They can also be fabricated by casting a glass ceramic and by computer assisted design and computer assisted machining (CAD-CAM). The advantage of the CAD-CAM system is production of the inlay in one visit. However, commercial CAD-CAM systems are too expensive for the average practice, and the average accuracy of the procedure on a production basis has not yet been established.

The uses and types of dental porcelain have been growing in the past decade. Porcelains are used mainly for porcelain-fused-to-metal crowns and bridgework. These porcelains have high expansion coefficients and are low-fusing. The growing emphasis in esthetics has resulted in using more all ceramic crowns, inlays, and veneers. Although the traditional condensation and oven firing method is still the main one, casting glass is being used and computer assisted matching (CAD-CAM) is being developed.

Self-test questions

In the following multiple choice questions, one or more responses may be correct.
 1 The raw materials used to make dental porcelain include:
   a. Zinc oxide
   b. Alumina
   c. Silica

d. Feldspar

e. Oxides or carbonates of sodium, potassium, lithium, and boron

f. Fluxes

2 Factors that can influence the color and appearance of a porcelain restoration include:

a. Nature of the incident light

b. Translucency of the porcelain

c. Surface reflectance of the porcelain

d. Fluorescence of the porcelain

3 Which of the following statements apply to porcelain used for jacket crowns?

a. They are mainly glasses with some crystalline components and small amounts of colored metal oxides.

b. Their esthetics are inferior to porcelain-fused-to-metal restorations.

c. Their use is restricted to the anterior portion of the mouth where esthetics are important and stresses are lower.

4 In the fracture of a porcelain-fused-to-metal restoration, which of these statements apply?

a. Failure at the porcelain-gold interface usually results from too thick a gold coating on the casting, which prevents oxides of tin, indium, and iron in the gold alloy from bonding with the porcelain.

b. Failure in the oxide layer attached to a nickel-chromium alloy results from a weak boundary layer of oxide.

c. Failure in the porcelain indicates that the porcelain-metal bond was stronger than the tensile or shear strength of the porcelain.

5 Match the dental porcelains according to the fusion temperatures listed:

___ **a.** 1288° to 1371° C   1. High-fusing

___ **b.** 1093° to 1260° C   2. Medium-fusing

                          3. Low-fusing

6 Which of the following statements is true in comparing porcelain and plastic denture teeth?

a. Porcelain teeth wear less than acrylic teeth.

b. Acrylic teeth absorb more and transmit lower biting forces.

c. Porcelain and acrylic teeth are both easily adjusted by grinding and polishing.

7 The coefficient of thermal expansion values of porcelains used for porcelain-fused-to-metal restorations are approximately:

a. $10 \times 10^{-6}/°$ C

b. $8 \times 10^{-6}/°$ C

c. $14 \times 10^{-6}/°$ C

8 During the sintering of porcelain:

a. The porcelain completely liquefies.

b. Shrinkage occurs.

c. Adjacent particles fuse at points of contact.

9 The coefficient of thermal expansion values for aluminous porcelains are:

a. $10 \times 10^{-6}/°$ C

   b. $8 \times 10^{-6}/^\circ$ C

   c. $14 \times 10^{-6}/^\circ$ C

10 The following are true regarding the strength of porcelain:

   a. Porcelain is strong in compression but weak in tension and bending.

   b. Alumina additions strengthen porcelain.

   c. Surface scratches strengthen porcelain.

11 Factors that promote strong porcelain-to-metal bonds are:

   a. An oxide layer on the alloy surface

   b. A gold coating on the alloy surface

   c. Matched coefficient of thermal expansion values

Suggested supplementary readings

McLean JW: *The science and art of dental ceramics,* New Orleans, 1976, Louisiana State University School of Dentistry.

O'Brien WJ: Cohesive plateau theory of porcelain-alloy bonding. In Yamada H, editor: *Dental porcelain: the state of the art—1977,* Los Angeles, 1977, University of Southern California.

O'Brien WJ: Dental porcelains. In Craig RG, editor: *Dental materials review,* Ann Arbor, Mich, 1977, University of Michigan.

O'Brien WJ: Evolution of dental casting. In Valega TM, editor: *Alternatives to gold alloys in dentistry.* HEW Pub. No. (NIH)77-1227, Washington. DC, 1977, U.S. Government Printing Office.

Answers to self-test questions

Chapter 1

1 b
2 a, c
3 a, c
4 b
5 a, d
6 a, b, c
7 b, c, d
8 c
9 a, b, c, d
10 b, c

Chapter 2

1 b, d
2 b
3 a
4 c
5 a, b, c
6 b, c
7 a, c, d
8 a, b, c, d
9 a
10 a, b
11 a, c, d
12 c
13 b
14 d
15 a, b, c
16 b
17 c
18 a, c
19 a, c, d, e
20 a

Chapter 3

1 a
2 c, d
3 a, b, c
4 b, d
5 a, b, c, d
6 a, c, d
7 a, b, c, d
8 a, b, c, d
9 a, b, d
10 b, d
11 a, c, d
12 b
13 a, c, d
14 a, b, c
15 a, b, d

Chapter 4

1 d
2 a, b, c, d
3 d
4 a, c
5 b
6 d
7 a
8 none
9 a, c
10 a, c
11 d
12 a, b, c, d
13 c, d

Chapter 5

1 a, b
2 c, d
3 d
4 a. Ag-Sn, Ag-Hg, Sn-Hg
   b. Ag-Sn-Cu, Ag-Hg, Cu-Sn
5 a, c
6 a. Sn-Hg
   b. Sn-Hg
   c. Sn-Hg
7 a. Spherical high-copper
   b. Spherical high-copper
   c. Comminuted
8 a, c
9 a, d
10 a
11 a, b
12 a, b, c, d
13 b, c, d

Chapter 6

1 a, b, c
2 c, d
3 b, d, e, f—finishing
   a, c, g, h—polishing
4 c
5 c, d
6 b
7 a
8 c
9 a, b, c, d
10 a, b, c, d
11 a, b, e, f, g
12 a, c, d

Chapter 7

1 a, b, c
2 a, b, c
3 a, c, d
4 a, b
5 a, b, c, d
6 b, c, d
7 a, b, c
8 b, c
9 a
10 a, b, d
11 c, d
12 a, b
13 a, b, d
14 a
15 c
16 b, c, d

Chapter 8

1 a, c, e
2 a, b, d, e, f—flexible
c, g, h—rigid
3 a, b, c, d, e
4 a, b, c, d, e, g
5 a. 5
b. 1
c. 4, 6
d. 2
e. 3, 4
f. 6
6 a, c, d
7 b, c, d
8 a, c, d
9 a, b, c, d
10 a, c, d, e
11 b, c, d, e
12 a, b
13 a. 1
b. 3
c. 4
d. 2
e. 1

14 c
15 a, c, d
16 a. 3; 6
b. 2; 6
c. 1; 6
d. 2; 5
e. 1; 5
f. 3; 5
g. 1, 2, 4; 7
h. 4; 5
17 b, c, d, e
18 b
19 b, c
20 a, b
21 b, d
22 d
23 c, d
24 b, c

Chapter 9

1 a. 1, 2, 3
b. 1
c. 1
d. 1, 2, 3, 4
e. 1
f. 1, 4
g. 1, 2
2 d
3 a, c, d
4 a, d
5 b, c, d
6 b
7 a, b, c, d
8 a, d
9 a, d
10 a, b
11 b, e, f, g, h—retarders
a, c, d—accelerators
12 b, c, d, e
13 c, d, e
14 c, d

Chapter 10

1 a, c
2 d
3 a, c, d
4 c
5 a, b
6 d
7 a, b, c, d, e
8 a, d

Chapter 11

1 a, b, c
2 a, b, c
3 b
4 d
5 a, b, e
6 a, c, f
7 b, d
8 b
9 b, d
10 a, c
11 a. 2, 4
b. 1, 7, 8
c. 1, 8, 9
d. 6, 7
e. 1, 3, 4, 5, 9
f. 1, 3, 4, 5, 9
g. 3
12 a
13 a, b, c
14 b, d
15 a, b, c
16 a, c, d
17 a, b
18 a. 1, 4
b. 1, 2, 3
c. 5
d. 1
e. 6
f. 1, 2
g. 2
19 b, c
20 a, b, c

Chapter 12

1 b, d
2 a, c, d
3 a, b, c
4 b, c
5 a, b, c
6 c
7 a, b, d
8 a, b, d
9 a, b
10 a, b, c

Chapter 13

1 a, c, d
2 a, b, c, d
3 a, b
4 a, c
5 a. *p*
  b. *l*
  c. *l*
  d. *l*
  e. *p*
  f. *p*
  g. *l*
  h. *p*
  i. *p*
  j. *p*
  k. *l*

6 a. 4
  b. 5
  c. 7
  d. 2
  e. 3
  f. 1
  g. 6
7 b
8 c
9 b, c
10 b, c
11 a, b
12 a, b, d
13 b, d

Chapter 14

1 b, c, d, e, f
2 a, b, c, d
3 a, c
4 a, b, c
5 a. 1
  b. 2
6 a, b
7 c
8 b, c
9 b
10 a, b
11 a, c

Appendix

Conversion factors

1 inch (in)	= 2.54 centimeters (cm)	= 25.4 millimeters (mm)
1 micrometer (μm)	= 0.001 millimeter (mm)	= 1 micron (μ)
1 meter (m)	= 100 centimeters (cm)	= 1000 millimeters (mm)

1 pound (lb)   = 453.6 grams (gm)
1 gram (gm)   = 10^6 micrograms (μg) = 10^9 nanograms (ng)
1 milligram (mg) = 0.001 gram (gm)
1 kilogram (kg) = 9.8 newtons (N)   = 1000 grams (gm)
1 grain (gr)   = 0.065 gram (gm)
1 quart (qt)   = 0.946 liter (L)
1 liter (L)   = 1000 milliliters (ml) = 1000 cubic centimeters (cc)

1 square inch (in^2)   = 6.45 square centimeters (cm^2)
1 cubic inch (in^3)   = 16.39 cubic centimeters (cm^3)
1 kilogram/square centimeter (kg/cm^2) = 14.2 pounds/square inch (psi)
1 pound/square inch (psi)   = 0.07 kilogram/square centimeter (kg/cm^2)
1 meganewton/square meter (MN/m^2) = 145 pounds/square inch (psi)
1 meganewton/square meter (MN/m^2) = 1 megapascal (MPa)

Temperature in degrees Fahrenheit (° F) = (9/5 temperature in centigrade [° C]) + 32°
Temperature in degrees centigrade (° C) = 5/9 (temperature in Fahrenheit [° F] − 32°)

1×10^{-6} (or 10^{-6}) = 0.000001
1×10^0 = 1
1×10^6 (or 10^6)   = 1,000,000
1×10^9 (or 10^9)   = 1,000,000,000

index

Page numbers in italics indicate an illustration; *t* indicates a table.